Metformin

Edited by Anca Mihaela Pantea Stoian
and Manfredi Rizzo

Published in London, United Kingdom

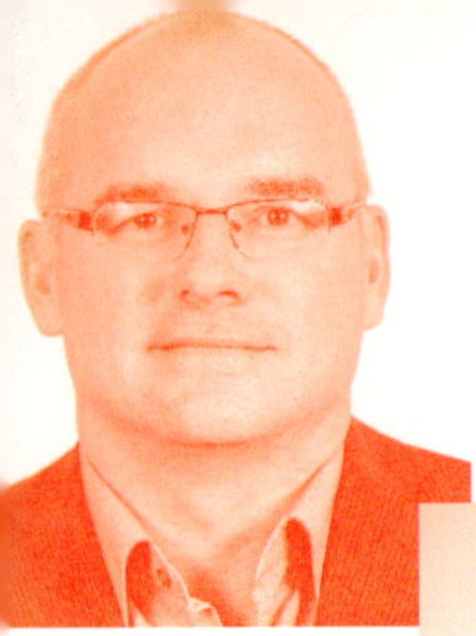
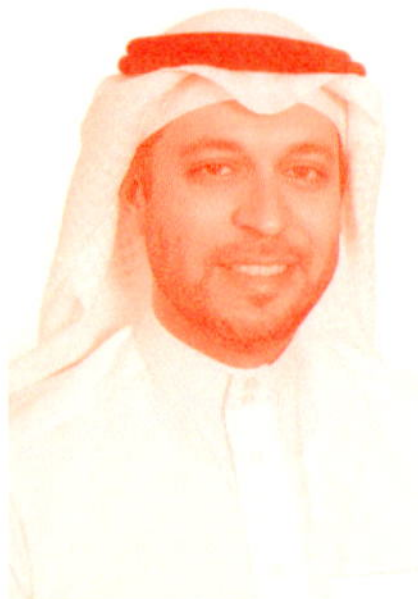
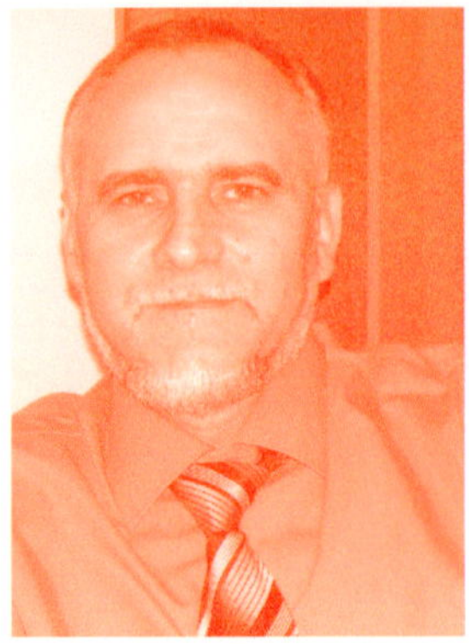
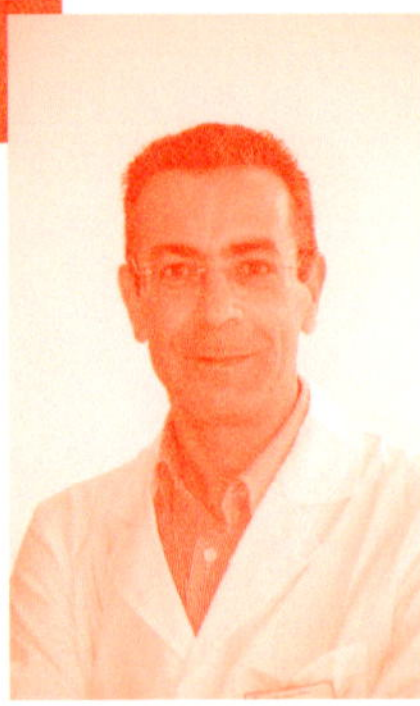
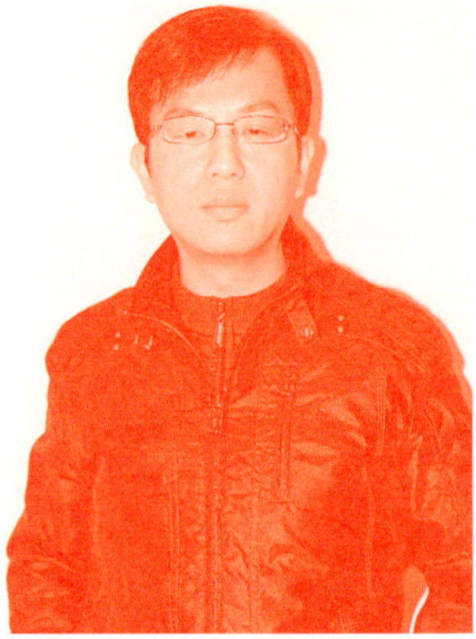
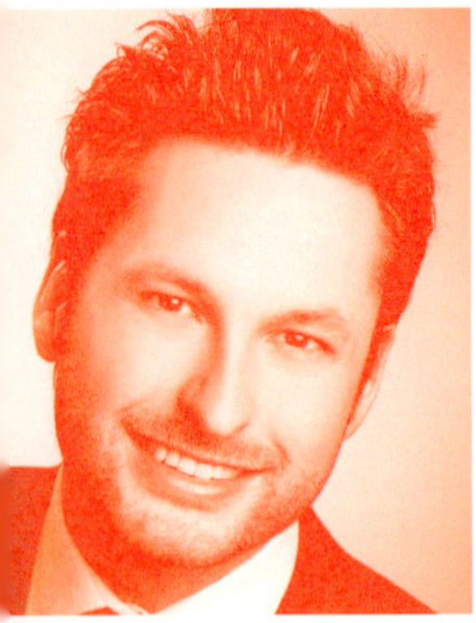
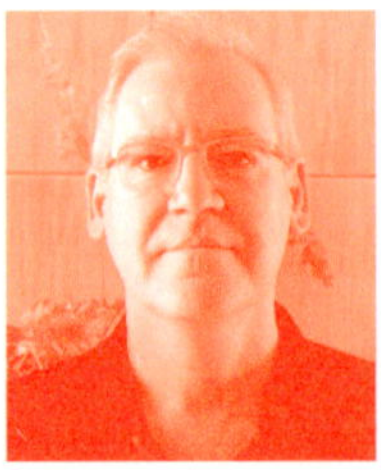

IntechOpen

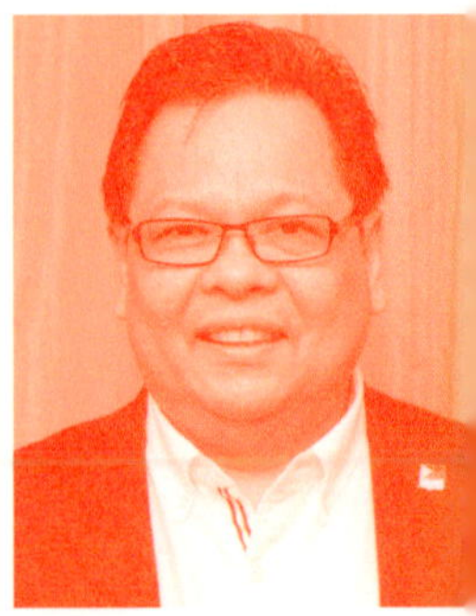
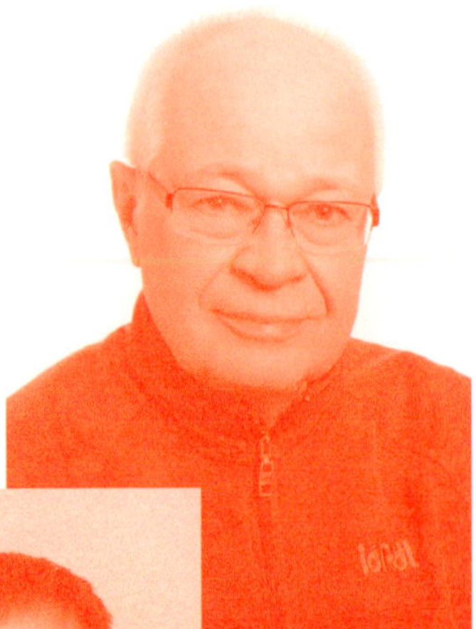
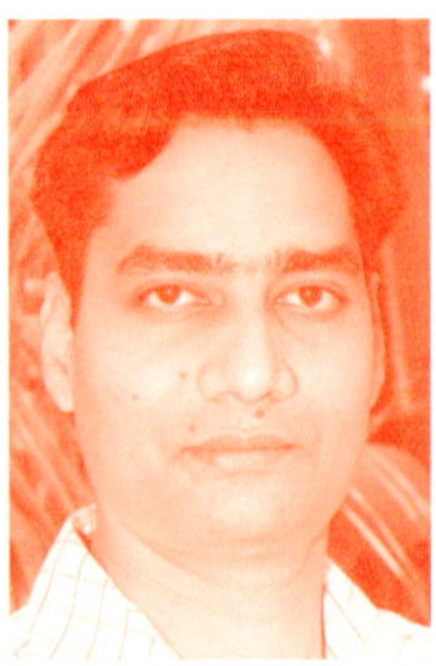
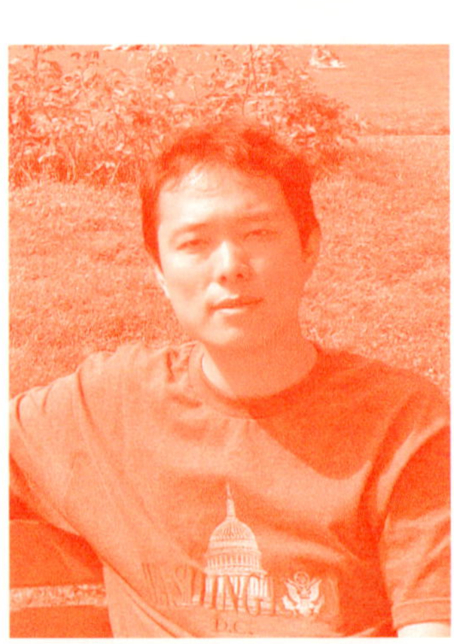
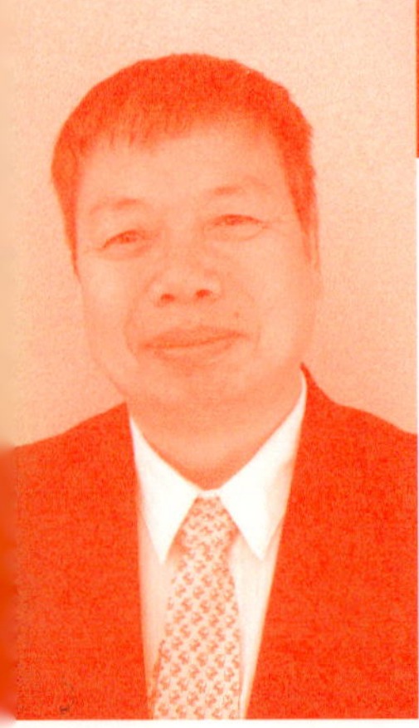
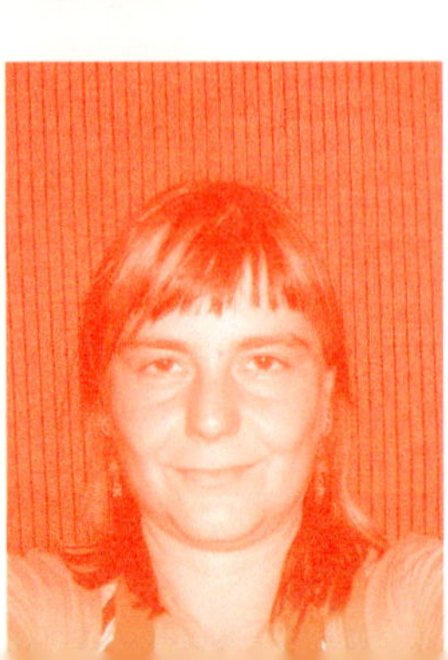

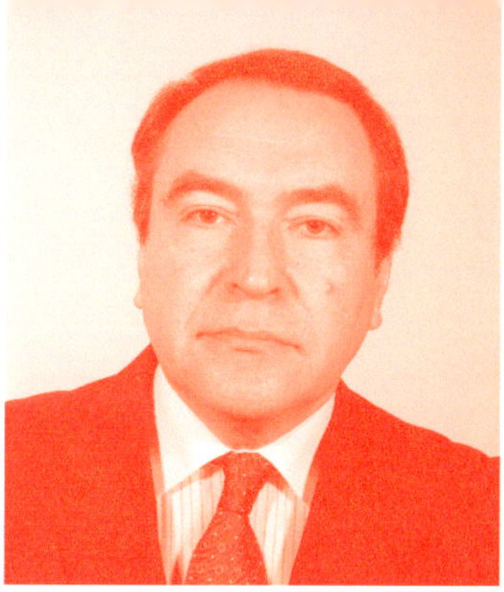
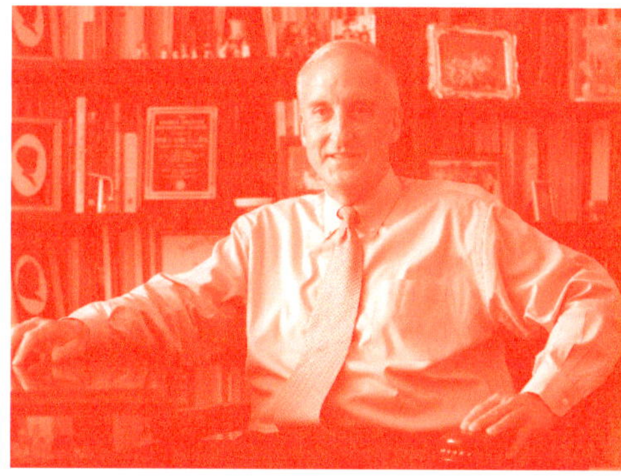
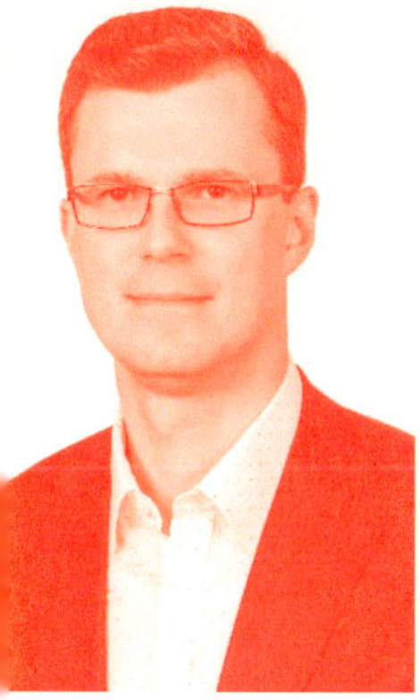
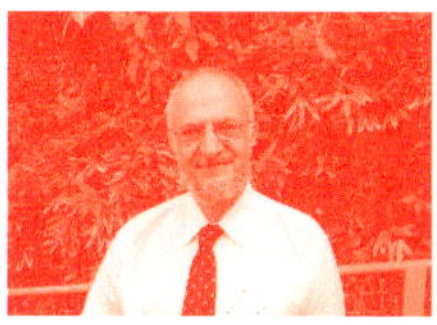
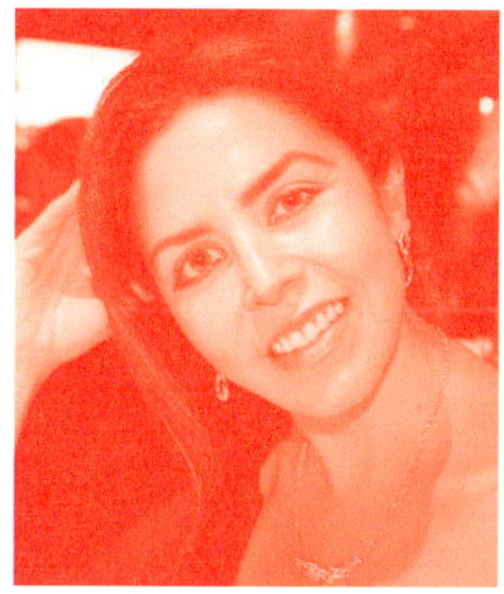

Supporting open minds since 2005

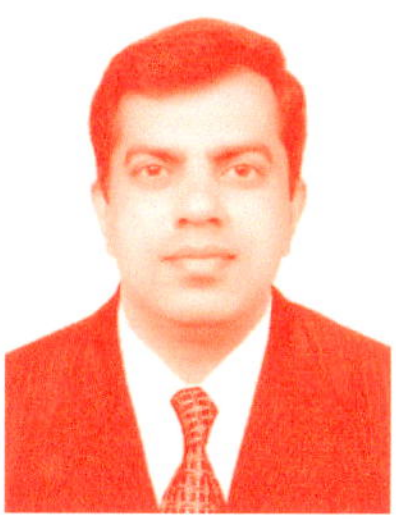
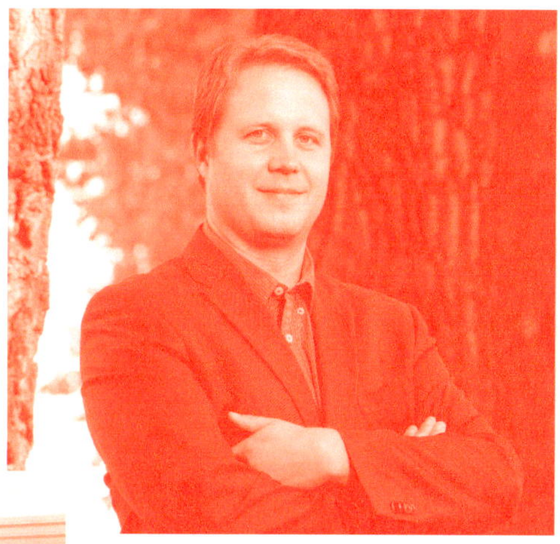
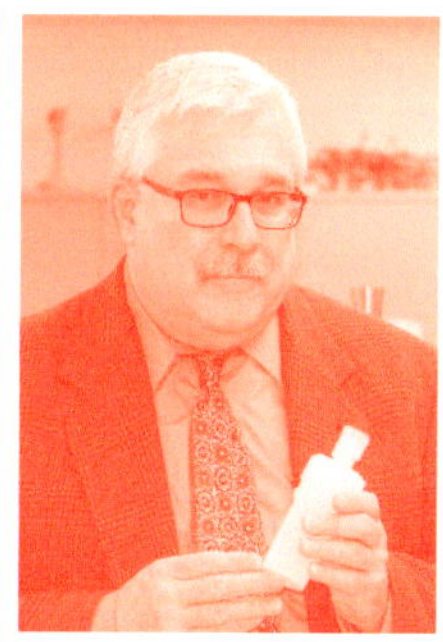
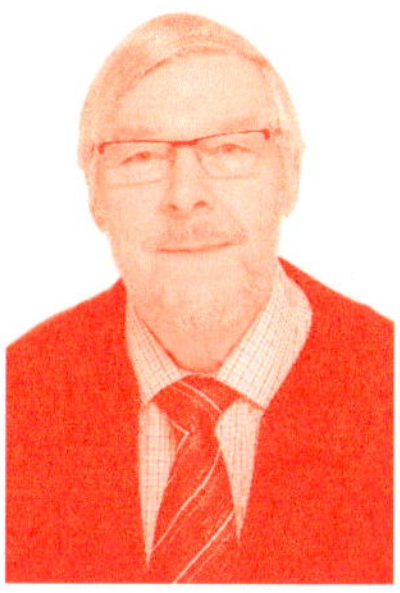
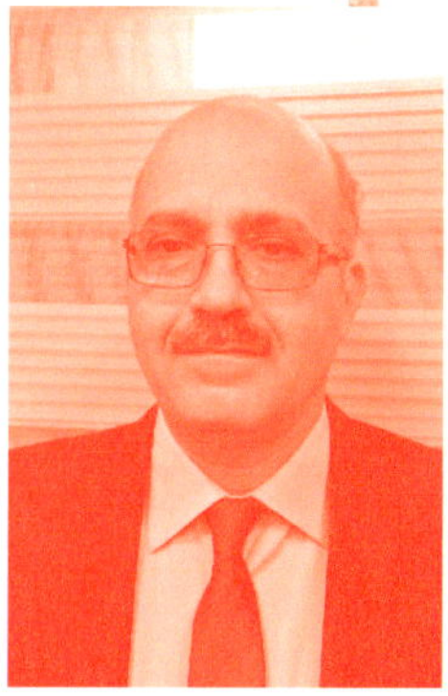
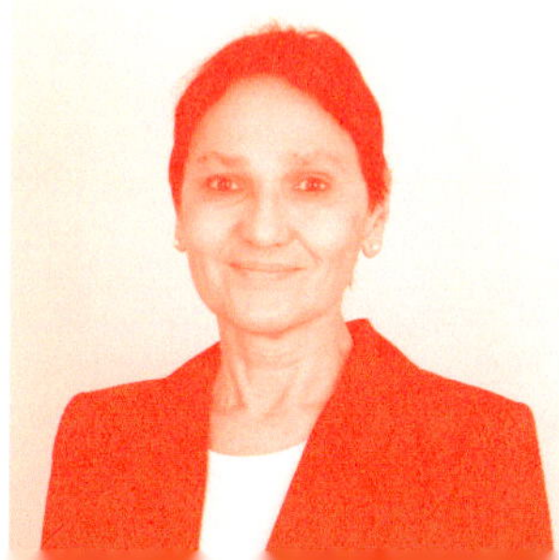
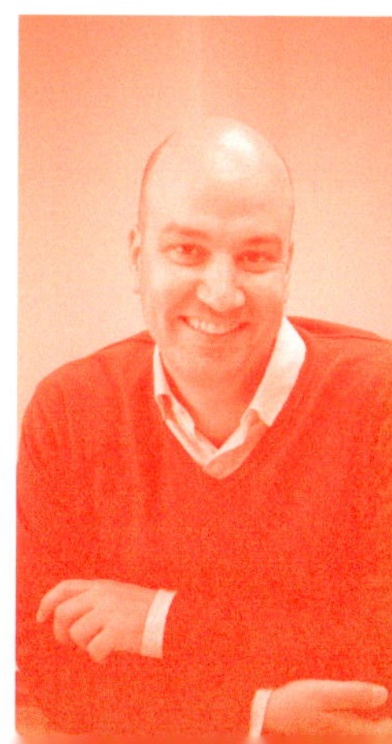

Metformin
http://dx.doi.org/10.5772/intechopen.77824
Edited by Anca Mihaela Pantea Stoian and Manfredi Rizzo

Contributors
Roxana Adriana Stoica, Simona Diana Stefan, Anca Pantea Stoian, Manfredi Rizzo, Andra-Iulia F. Suceveanu, Adrian-Paul Suceveanu, Cristian Serafinceanu, Elham Pourmatroud, Sergiu Ioan Micu, Madalina Elena Manea, Claudia Voinea, Laura Mazilu, Doina Catrinoiu, Irinel Parepa, Carmen Romero, Maritza P Garrido, Margarita Vega, Andreea Arsene, Adriana Florinela Catoi, Andreea Corina, Dan Cristian Vodnar, Felix Voinea, Andreea Gheorghe, Dana Stanculeanu, Malgorzata Tyszka-Czochara, Marcin Majka, Yun Yan, Karen Kover, Wayne V. Moore, Mariia Nagalievska, Halyna Hachkova, Nataliia Sybirna, Zhijun Luo, Xiaochen Wang, Yile Jiao, Jasna Kusturica, Aida Kulo Ćesić, Maida Rakanović-Todić, Lejla Burnazović-Ristić, Sanita Maleškić Kapo, Reema Wahdan-Alaswad, Ann D. Thor

First published in London, United Kingdom, 2020 by IntechOpen
IntechOpen is the global imprint of INTECHOPEN LIMITED, registered in England and Wales, registration number: 11086078, 7th floor, 10 Lower Thames Street, London, EC3R 6AF, United Kingdom
Printed in Croatia

British Library Cataloguing-in-Publication Data
A catalogue record for this book is available from the British Library

Additional hard and PDF copies can be obtained from orders@intechopen.com

Metformin
Edited by Anca Mihaela Pantea Stoian and Manfredi Rizzo
p. cm.
Print ISBN 978-1-83880-427-5
Online ISBN 978-1-83880-428-2
eBook (PDF) ISBN 978-1-83880-760-3

For EU product safety concerns:
IN TECH d.o.o., Prolaz Marije Krucifikse Kozulić 3, 51000 Rijeka, Croatia, info@intechopen.com or visit our website at intechopen.com.

Meet the editors

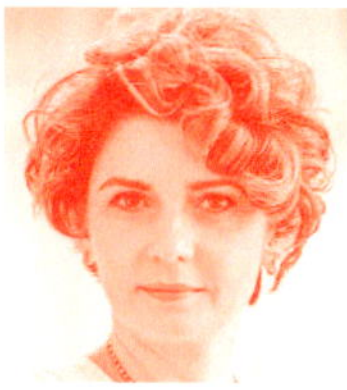

Dr Pantea Stoian is a diabetes, nutrition and metabolic diseases specialist, a senior specialist in health food hygiene, a resident in nephrology, and is competent in medical aesthetics and general ultrasonography. She has held an Associate Professor in the Diabetes, Nutrition, and Metabolic Diseases Department since 2019 at "Carol Davila" University of Medicine, Bucharest, Romania. Her field of activity is closely related to the micro- and macro-vascular complications in diabetes as well as their new therapies. Its main directions of activity are nutritional intervention in chronic pathology, as well as cardio-renal-metabolic risk assessment, and diabetes in cancer. In diabetes, she is currently engaged in new therapy and technology tools that screen and prevent diabetes and educate patients. She is a member of the European Association for the Study of Diabetes, Cardiometabolic Academy, Romanian Society of Diabetes, Nutrition and Metabolic Diseases, Romanian Diabetes Federation and Association for Renal Metabolic and Nutrition Studies. She has authored or co-authored 110 papers in national and international peer-reviewed journals.

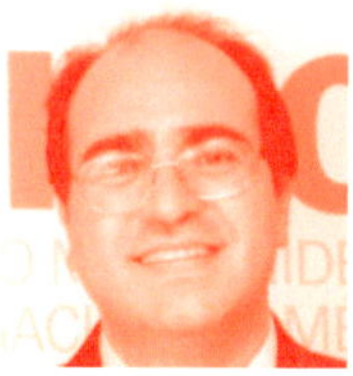

Prof. Manfredi Rizzo, MD, PhD. Prof. Rizzo studied medicine and received training in Internal Medicine in Italy. He spent several years in the United States, working at the University of California. There he was able to gain clinical and research experience on patients with different metabolic disorders, including dyslipidemia, diabetes, obesity, and metabolic syndrome. He is also the Head of the Cardiometabolic Research Laboratory of the Department of Internal Medicine at the University of Palermo. Prof. Rizzo maintains a faculty position in the USA, where he is Adjunct Associate Professor of Internal Medicine at the School of Medicine, University of South Carolina, with a research position in the Division of Endocrinology, Diabetes, and Metabolism. Currently, Prof. Rizzo is on sabbatical leave since he joined Novo Nordisk in 2019 as a Director of the Clinical, Medical & Regulatory Department, Novo Nordisk Europe East and South. Prof. Rizzo sits on the editorial board of 10 international journals. The research work of Prof. Rizzo combines translational and primary research, with 250+ scientific publications in international journals. Finally, Prof. Rizzo has been the Coordinator, Vice-Chairman or Co-Chairman of international expert panel documents in the field of dyslipidemia, diabetes, and metabolic syndrome. He is currently a National Board Member of the Italian Society of Nutraceuticals (SINUT) and Executive Board Member of the Mediterranean Group for the Study of Diabetes (MGSD).

Contents

Preface XI

Section 1
Metformin and Diabetes Mellitus 1

Chapter 1 3
Metformin Indications, Dosage, Adverse Reactions, and Contraindications
by Roxana Adriana Stoica, Diana Simona Ștefan, Manfredi Rizzo, Andra Iulia Suceveanu, Adrian Paul Suceveanu, Cristian Serafinceanu and Anca Pantea-Stoian

Chapter 2 21
New Insight into Metformin Mechanism of Action and Clinical Application
by Yun Yan, Karen L. Kover and Wayne V. Moore

Chapter 3 45
Metformin and Its Benefits in Improving Gut Microbiota Disturbances in Diabetes Patients
by Andra Iulia-Suceveanu, Sergiu Ioan Micu, Claudia Voinea, Madalina Elena Manea, Doina Catrinoiu, Laura Mazilu, Anca Pantea Stoian, Irinel Parepa, Roxana Adriana Stoica and Adrian-Paul Suceveanu

Chapter 4 61
Potential Protective Effects of Metformin on Ocular Complications in Patients with Type 2 Diabetes
by Jasna Kusturica, Aida Kulo, Maida Rakanović-Todić, Lejla Burnazović-Ristić and Sanita Maleškić

Chapter 5 75
Galega officinalis L. and Immunological Status in Diabetes Mellitus
by Mariia Nagalievska, Halyna Hachkova and Nataliia Sybirna

Section 2
Metformin and Reproductive System 97

Chapter 6 99
Metformin in Health Issues and Reproductive System
by Elham Pourmatroud

Section 3
Metformin and Cancer 111

Chapter 7 113
Metformin and Its Implication in Cancer Therapy
by Laura Mazilu, Dana Stanculeanu, Andreea Gheorghe, Adrian-Paul Suceveanu, Irinel Parepa, Felix Voinea, Doina Catrinoiu and Andra-Iulia Suceveanu

Chapter 8 127
Preventive and (Neo)Adjuvant Therapeutic Effects of Metformin on Cancer
by Yile Jiao, Xiaochen Wang and Zhijun Luo

Chapter 9 149
Metformin in Cervical Cancer: Metabolic Reprogramming
by Malgorzata Tyszka-Czochara and Marcin Majka

Chapter 10 163
Antitumoral Effects of Metformin in Ovarian Cancer
by Maritza P. Garrido, Margarita Vega and Carmen Romero

Chapter 11 181
Metformin Activity against Breast Cancer: Mechanistic Differences by Molecular Subtype and Metabolic Conditions
by Reema S. Wahdan-Alaswad and Ann D. Thor

Section 4
Metformin and Ageing 209

Chapter 12 211
Metformin Modulates the Mechanisms of Ageing
by Adriana Florinela Cătoi, Andra Diana Andreicuț, Dan Cristian Vodnar, Katalin Szabo, Andreea Corina, Andreea Arsene, Simona Diana Stefan, Roxana Adriana Stoica and Manfredi Rizzo

Preface

Metformin has been in clinical practice since 1957, having a sinuous route to date. There have been many books, articles, and studies related to metformin, thus discovering many therapeutic values. The book brings to light both the standard therapeutic recommendations, namely, the first-intention therapy in patients with type 2 diabetes and current trends in use. Metformin can now be regarded as a panacea, the valences of its therapeutics being increasingly appreciated, both in the background treatmen t of diabetes, prediabetes, but also in reproductive pathology, cancer, cardiovascular disease, and antiaging. In this respect, the mechanisms of action and the pharmacodynamics of metformin seem to be incompletely known; several current studies have revealed new action valences. The function of these pharmacogenetic mechanisms, as well as the mode of action of metformin, needs to be known because they also predict the recommendations of future therapeutics.

Its significant role in the treatment of type 2 diabetes is recognized by all international guidelines in the field, placing it in the first line of treatment along with lifestyle optimization. New evidence also appears in the use of metformin in patients with type 1 diabetes, especially in those who develop insulin resistance. Some chapters explain adverse effects, indications, and contraindications of metformin and also its implication in gut microbiota. Immunological status in diabetes and the role of metformin was described very extensively by Prof. Mariia Nagalievska et al. in their chapter, and Prof. Yun Yan et al. elaborated several new insights in metformin action.

The international specialty literature brings new evidence in initiating metformin therapy in prediabetes, but also the prevention of cancer or reproductive system diseases, and cardiovascular or gastrointestinal disorders. In this way, several chapters have been dedicated to the reproductive system and to the role of metformin in cancer therapy, especially in cervical cancer, ovarian cancer, and breast cancer.

An important role of metformin is immune system modulation as well as antiaging therapy. A chapter was dedicated to the mechanism of ageing and the part of metformin in preventing ageing.

I hope this book is a key for every reader to open new insights to metformin.

Anca Mihaela Pantea Stoian
Diabetes, Nutrition and Metabolic Diseases Department,
Carol Davila University of Medicine,
Bucharest, Romania

Manfredi Rizzo
Division of Endocrinology, Diabetes and Metabolism, Department of Medicine,
University of South Carolina,
Columbia, SC, USA

Department of Health Promotion, Mother and Child Care,
Internal Medicine and Medical Specialties,
University of Palermo,
Italy

Section 1

Metformin and Diabetes Mellitus

Chapter 1

Metformin Indications, Dosage, Adverse Reactions, and Contraindications

Roxana Adriana Stoica, Diana Simona Ștefan, Manfredi Rizzo, Andra Iulia Suceveanu, Adrian Paul Suceveanu, Cristian Serafinceanu and Anca Pantea-Stoian

Abstract

Metformin or dimethyl biguanide is the oral antidiabetic drug with the most extensive experience of prescribing in the clinical practice of type 2 diabetes mellitus. In this chapter, we reviewed the indications, contraindications, and adverse drug reactions (ADR) of metformin. The most significant adverse drug reactions of metformin are lactic acidosis, allergies, hypoglycemia, vitamin B12 deficiency, altered taste, and gastrointestinal intolerance. Metformin is contra-indicated in severe chronic diseases (hepatic, renal, and cardiac failure) or acute complications of diabetes (ketoacidosis and hyperosmolar state). Metformin is considered by all international guidelines the first-line treatment in type 2 diabetes mellitus (T2DM) together with medical, nutritional therapy. It is one of the most prescribed molecules worldwide. Furthermore, metformin can also be prescribed for other diseases like polycystic ovary syndrome or prediabetes (impaired glucose tolerance/fasting hyperglycemia). Recent studies have shown positive results concerning the use of metformin for cardiovascular or neuro-protective effects; also, several scientific papers are suggesting an antitumor or antiaging effect of metformin. Having such an excellent efficiency in practice, thus predicting its sustainability on the pharmaceutical market, research is directed toward characterizing metformin action on bacteria genera in the gut. Modifying the microbiota composition by pre- and probiotics could improve metformin action.

Keywords: metformin, indication, adverse reaction, gastric intolerance, lactic acidosis, diabetes

1. Introduction

Metformin or dimethyl biguanide has its origin in traditional herbal medicine (*Galega officinalis* or goat's rue) that is rich in guanidine. Guanidine was proven to have the capacity to lower blood glucose and was used as an antidiabetic treatment from the 1920s to 1930s. Its administration was interrupted prematurely due to toxicity. The medicine was valued again between the 1940s and 1950s when Jean Sterne observed the low blood glucose values of patients that were treated with metformin for influenza. Since then, the drug class of biguanides has received much consideration, especially buformin and phenformin in the 1970s and metformin after the 1990s [1].

The 60-year history of biguanides' use is filled with victories and defeats, being the oral antidiabetic drug with the most extensive experience of prescribing in the clinical practice.

We will review in the following pages the indications, contraindications, and adverse drug reactions (ADR) of metformin and the single biguanide approved globally for use nowadays.

An ADR according to the World Health Organization is "a response to a drug which is noxious and unintended, and which occurs at doses normally used in man for the prophylaxis, diagnosis, or therapy of a disease, or the modification of physiological function." A side effect is "an unintended effect occurring at normal dose related to the pharmacological properties" [2].

A contraindication represents "something (such as a symptom or condition) that makes a particular treatment or procedure inadvisable" [3].

2. Indications

2.1 Type 2 diabetes mellitus (T2DM)

All international guidelines consider metformin and lifestyle intervention as the first-line treatment in adults with T2DM in order to improve glycemic control [4]. It can be used either as monotherapy or combination therapy with glucagon-like peptide-1 receptor agonist (GLP-1 RA), sodium-glucose co-transporter inhibitor (SGLT2i), dipeptidyl peptidase-4 inhibitor (DPP4-I), thiazolidinedione (TZD), sulfonylurea (SU), and insulin. Metformin therapy should be continued as long as it is well tolerated and not contraindicated. All other agents, including insulin, should be added to metformin treatment [4].

2.2 Prediabetes

Metformin can be used in order to prevent or delay the onset of T2DM [5]. Although other pharmacological agents have been used in clinical trials (acarbose [6–8], orlistat [9], and rosiglitazone [10]), it appears that metformin has the most reliable evidence base [11–16]. The vast majority of international guidelines recommend metformin use in prediabetes. It can be used together with a combination of a lifestyle intervention for patients with prediabetes: impaired glucose tolerance (2-h post-load glucose 140–199 mg/dL), fasting hyperglycemia (100–125 mg/dl), or A1C 5.7–6.4% [17–23]. Metformin appears to have a more significant advantage when used in patients who are <60 years old and have a BMI >35 kg/m^2 or women with prior gestational diabetes mellitus [16].

2.3 Type 1 diabetes mellitus (T1DM)

Metformin is sometimes used in T1DM to limit insulin dose requirement [24, 25]. The American Diabetes Association states that adding metformin leads to the reduction in body weight and can improve lipid levels, but not HbA1c [4, 26]. The REMOVAL study suggests that metformin might also reduce atherosclerosis progression, thus suggesting to improve CVD risk management in type 1 diabetes [27, 28].

2.4 Gestational diabetes mellitus (GDM)

Lifestyle modification is the first-line therapy for GDM. If glycemic targets are not achieved, then insulin treatment is required for lowering blood glucose; metformin can also be considered if the patient cannot take or declines insulin [29]. Some controlled randomized trials are proving limited efficacy of metformin during pregnancy [30, 31]. Metformin therapy is associated with a lower risk of neonatal hypoglycemia and less maternal weight gain than insulin in systematic reviews [32–34]; metformin may slightly increase the risk of prematurity, and it crosses the placenta [35]. Thus, the ADA considers that metformin should not be used as first-line agents [36].

2.5 Polycystic ovary syndrome (PCOS)

PCOS patients suffer from insulin resistance and hyperinsulinemia [37]. Metformin has been used for PCOS treatment [38] for treating the metabolic abnormalities of PCOS. A recent meta-analysis [39] demonstrated that metformin could decrease testosterone and insulin level in women with PCOS.

2.6 Antitumor or antiaging effect of metformin

Several studies showed an increased life-span when using metformin (4–6% in different mouse breeds or a mean life-span increased by 14% and maximum life-span increased by 1 month of treatment with metformin is started early in life) [40, 41]. In the United Kingdom Prospective Diabetes Study (UKPDS), the use of metformin decreased the risk of cardiovascular disease, cancer incidence, and overall mortality, compared with other antidiabetic drugs [42].

Epidemiological studies reported a positive result of metformin concerning ovarian [43, 44], breast, prostate, or colorectal tumors [45–48] enhancing the antitumor effect of metformin. Furthermore, studies are demonstrating a reduced incidence of several gastroenterological cancers and a reduction in cancer mortality when using metformin [49, 50].

2.7 Cardiovascular or neuroprotective effects

UKPDS was the first study that demonstrated the cardiovascular benefit of metformin; the risk of all-cause mortality and acute myocardial infarction was significantly reduced in overweight patients with T2DM [42]. The 10-year post-interventional follow-up of the UKPDS survivor cohort revealed that metformin treatment had a long-term benefit on cardiovascular risk [51].

The cardiovascular protective effects of metformin could be explained by the reduced level of LDL cholesterol [52], the limitation of weight gain, [53] and the improvement of oxidative stress, inflammatory response, and the endothelial cell function [54].

It has been reported that patients treated with metformin have lower risk of dementia than those with other diabetes medications [55]. Metformin has a better protective effect on the domain of verbal learning, working memory, and executive function than other diabetic treatments [56].

2.8 Antipsychotic-induced weight gain

Results of meta-analyses of RCTs (primarily in patients with schizophrenia and schizoaffective disorder) support the use of metformin for weight loss, preventing weight gain associated with second-generation antipsychotics in adult patients [57].

Metformin can be recommended as a second-line option after nonpharmacologic strategies for managing weight gain in patients with mood disorders and is recognized as often being used as a secondary prevention strategy for antipsychotic-related weight gain [58].

3. Dosage

The dose for glucose-lowering efficacy is usually in the range of 500–2000 mg/day. There is no standard dosage regimen for the management of hyperglycemia in patients with type 2 diabetes. On the other side, clinically significant responses are not seen at doses below 1500–2000 mg per day.

The dosage of metformin must be individualized for every patient considering effectiveness and tolerance while not exceeding the maximum recommended daily doses (2550 mg in adults and 2000 mg in pediatric patients >10 years of age) (**Table 1**).

Patients that are receiving immediate-release metformin treatment may be switched to extended form once daily with the same total daily dose (up to 2000 mg daily).

In the case of renal impairment, the dosage of metformin must be adjusted (**Table 2**).

		Initial dose	Titration dose	Maximum dose
Adults	Immediate-release metformin	500 mg/daily or 850 mg/daily	500 mg/weekly or 850 mg/2 weeks	2550 mg/daily
	Extended-release metformin	500 mg/daily or 1000 mg/daily	500 mg/weekly	2000 mg/daily
Geriatric use	With caution; to start at the low end of the dosing range, assess renal function more frequently			
Pediatric use >10 years old	Immediate release	500 mg/daily	500 mg/weekly	2000 mg/daily
	Extended release		Not yet established	

Table 1.
Dosage of metformin.

Renal impairment	eGFR		
	<30	30–45	>45
Initiation	Contraindicated	Not recommended	No dose adjustment needed
If eGFR falls during treatment	Stop	Assess the benefit-risk of continuing therapy	No dose adjustment needed

Table 2.
Dosage of metformin for renal impairment.

4. Adverse drug reactions of metformin

4.1 Lactic acidosis (very rare)

Phenformin and buformin were two potent biguanides that were used in the 1970s for type 2 diabetes treatment. The Swedish Adverse Drug Reaction Committee analyzed the reports from 1965 to 1977 that involved biguanides (0.6% of the total). The fact that attracted attention was that in 6% of the cases in which the patient died (the majority with lactic acidosis), phenformin was administered [59]. After this committee report analysis, the class was used with precaution, and metformin was favored over phenformin because there was an early study that showed that type 2 diabetic patients admitted in the hospital had a higher mean lactate level when they were treated with other medicine instead of the first-mentioned earlier [59, 60].

A Cochrane meta-analysis that was published in 2006 that analyzed data from 206 trials and cohort studies did not find any case of lactic acidosis in metformin-treated patients or the control group. Also, the lactate level was not significantly raised in the metformin group, although there was a small difference between patients treated with this biguanide and phenformin [61].

A case-control study with 10.652 Danish type 2 diabetic patients showed that the lactic acidosis incidence in patients treated with metformin was 391/100.000 person-years, but the use of the drug itself did not elevate the risk; associated diseases had greater importance [62].

4.2 Allergic reactions (infrequent)

Systemic allergic reactions to metformin are infrequent [63, 64]. It can be used in patients with asthma that have hypersensitivity, without increasing the risk of related outcomes, meaning hospitalizations, asthma-related emergency room visits, or exacerbations [65].

Cutaneous allergic reactions have been described scarcely ever, but clinicians should be aware of their existence [66].

4.3 Hypoglycemia (very rare)

In monotherapy as a first-line agent, metformin was proven to be safe and beneficial in a recent meta-analysis. The hypoglycemic risk was lower than for monotherapy with sulfonylurea [67].

Rare cases in elderly patients, with comorbidities and polypharmacy (angiotensin-converting enzyme inhibitors or nonsteroidal anti-inflammatory drugs) or combined with malnutrition, have been described [68].

4.4 Vitamin B12 deficiency (rare)

The American Diabetes Association Guidelines recommend that potential vitamin B12 deficiency should be taken into consideration and screened in type 2 diabetes patients long-treated with high-dose metformin (more than 2 g/day) [59]. A meta-analysis of 29 studies showed that the metformin-treated group had a significantly lower level of this vitamin [69]. The implied mechanisms are:

- The drug acts as a competitor for vitamin B12 absorption.
- It affects the intrinsic factor action.
- It generates bacterial overgrowth because it alters bowel movement [70].

4.5 Altered taste (frequent)

Taste disturbance is an adverse effect that can be caused by the accumulation and secretion of metformin in saliva. Lee N et al. demonstrated that the salivary glands express the organic cation transporter-3 (OCT3) in high amounts that is responsible for metformin carriage and could be involved in the mechanism of this side effect. In animal studies, the OCT3(−/−) mice, the uptake of metformin in the saliva was downregulated [71].

4.6 Gastrointestinal intolerance (widespread)

Gastrointestinal side effects include diarrhea, nausea, meteorism, and constipation and affect approximately 20% of the patients [71, 72].

The hydrochloride salt of metformin is usually administered orally and is absorbed mostly by the small intestine. The concentration inside the enterocyte can reach up to 300 times the level in the circulation and depends on drug transport by organic cation transporter 1 (OCT1) [67]. Also, metformin increases glucose use in the anaerobic cycle and lactate production inside the enterocyte. Local higher production of lactate could be associated with adverse reactions [73].

Scarpello et al. demonstrated that metformin slows the absorption of bile acids, consequently leading to osmotic diarrhea [74]. On the contrary, the serum measures of lactate, serotonin, or bile acids were similar in normal and intolerant volunteers after a 500-mg dose of metformin, making the authors conclude that the intolerance is probably related to local factors within the lumen or enterocyte [73].

Some authors suggested that a reduced function of OCT1 could have an effect on the tolerability of metformin in the digestive system. The population with a reduced-function OCT1 alleles also had a higher increase of metformin intolerance. If this population was additionally treated with an OCT1 inhibitor, the risk increased even more [75]. Thus, patients that are under treatment with other medications that interact with OCT1 could have a higher risk for gastrointestinal ADR [75].

There are several formulations like the immediate-release (IR) tablets that result in high local concentration, extended-release tablets (XR) that have a prolonged discharge of the active molecule due to a dual polymer matrix, and delayed-release tablets (DR). The XR and the DR forms help in uniformly spreading out molecules along the intestinal membrane and prevent intolerance [75].

4.7 Hypothyroidism (controversial)

Metformin acts by activating adenosine monophosphate-activated protein kinase (AMPK), an enzyme that also activates thyroid iodine in vitro models. Thus, it was assumed that metformin could alter thyroid function [76]. In healthy volunteers, only the level of T3 was decreased by metformin administration, but not the iodine uptake, TSH, or fT4 [76].

Following this idea, observational studies proved that metformin treatment could reduce thyroid-stimulating hormone (TSH) level, but randomized control trials performed afterward failed to certify this hypothesis [77].

5. Contraindications

The indications and efficiency of metformin in type 2 diabetes are clearly stated in current guidelines [4] and continue to extend to other branches of medicine. For example, the UKPDS study revealed that metformin is associated with a lower risk of mortality [37], and some researchers tried to use metformin as an antiaging drug. Besides its broad indications, metformin remains contraindicated in many conditions associated with hypoxemia because it can lead to lactic acidosis [78].

5.1 Ketoacidosis

In type 2 diabetes patients with severe hyperglycemia and ketoacidosis or type 1 diabetes, insulin treatment should be initiated [4]. When the glycemic values are balanced, and if the patient does not have other contraindications, metformin treatment can be started in type 2 diabetes [4].

In type 1 diabetes, metformin is solely administered as an adjuvant because it can reduce the insulin requirements [25]. A randomized controlled trial found that metformin increases the risk for gastrointestinal adverse events in overweight type 1 diabetes patients, with no benefit for glycemic control, so a clinician should reach a decision depending on patient particularities and response [79].

5.2 Cardiac failure

After the warning regarding lactic acidosis, cardiac failure was put on the list with contraindications. Afterward, observational studies [80] and systematic reviews [81, 82] showed that metformin could be used in stable heart failure. If patients develop congestive heart failure or concomitantly have other contraindications or acute diseases, metformin should be stopped. The studies realized and included in the meta-analysis are very heterogeneous, most of them comparing different medications, but with no specifications regarding the mean dose of metformin or other classes. Overall, the mortality rate was 22% lower in patients with heart failure and type 2 diabetes treated with metformin [82].

5.3 Chronic kidney disease (CKD)

Metformin is restricted in patients with eGFR less than 30 ml/min/1.73 m2 (stage IV CKD), and dose must be adjusted beginning with an eGFR below 45 ml/min/1.73 m2 (stage IIIb) [4]. In a cohort study of a national registry, metformin was associated with a lower rate of mortality and serious adverse events at an eGFR between 45 and 60 ml/min/1.73 m2 and had neutral effects on the same variables at eGFR between 30 and 45 ml/min/1.73 m2. Although its effect is less evident in stage IV chronic kidney disease, the benefit of biguanide treatment outweighs the ADR risk in a 4-year follow-up [82, 83].

5.4 Hepatic failure and cirrhosis

Impaired hepatic function is another warning from the FDA [64]. This term includes a broad spectrum of liver pathology, and metformin treatment should be tailored. In a retrospective study that included patients with cirrhosis, metformin had a protective effect for encephalopathy development [84]. Likewise, in another retrospective study, biguanide treatment was continued after cirrhosis diagnosis and was associated with improved survival [85]. In patients with cirrhosis secondary to hepatitis C virus infection, the risk of hepatocellular carcinoma was reduced during a 5-year follow-up [86].

5.5 Respiratory insufficiency

Because the risk of lactic acidosis is higher in patients with altered blood gas exchange like in chronic obstructive pulmonary disease (COPD), asthma, restrictive pulmonary pathologies, the FDA and EMA recommend precaution [63, 64].
A randomized clinical trial used metformin in a rapidly escalated dose after a COPD exacerbation and showed no amelioration in glycemic profile. This could be since

mean in-hospital glycemia was assessed and it usually takes 1–2 weeks for metformin to reach its maximum hypoglycemic potential; there were no cases of lactic acidosis, and mean serum lactate was similar in the intervention and placebo group [87].

6. Special populations

6.1 Children

Metformin is indicated now in children above 10 years [63, 64], although there were studies that included obese participants above 7 years without side effects [88].

6.2 Pregnancy

There are limited data that could not identify a drug-associated risk of miscarriage or congenital disabilities. Metformin use was not associated with any of these maternal or fetal outcomes in post-marketing studies with small sample size or in meta-analyses of the randomized clinical trials that included pregnant women. The risk of stillbirth, congenital disabilities, and macrosomia can be increased if the patients do not have reasonable control under this oral treatment. Thus, the risk is falsely attributed to metformin [89].

6.3 Lactation

Metformin is present in the human milk in insignificant concentration. The potential adverse effect on the child or milk production has not been described [89].

6.4 Elderly

There is a study which compared pharmacokinetics and pharmacodynamics of metformin in the older population (65–85 years) versus young controls. Results showed that the glucose-lowering effect was similar in both groups, although the maximum concentration and exposure were two times higher in the advanced age population. Usually, it is not recommended in patients above 85 years old because they have a reduced eGFR [90].

7. Overdosage

A retrospective cohort study performed in the emergency department analyzed 56 of self-reported metformin overdose from a total of 2872 cases (1.9%). The incidence of hyperlactatemia was 56.4%, and that of metformin-associated lactic acidosis (MALA) was 17.9%. When the patient is co-ingested with acetaminophen, the risk of MALA was higher. No case resulted in death [91].

Treatment in metformin overdose includes supportive care, gastrointestinal decontamination (gastric lavage), alkalinization, and even emergency hemodialysis in severe cases [92].

8. Future directions: metformin and metagenome

There were some studies on human microbiota, which suggested that metformin induces dysbiosis and promotes nutritional imbalances for specific bacterial types in healthy volunteers [93, 94]. *Escherichia* sp. has a selective advantage over other organisms [95].

Twelve bacterial species that were present at baseline predicted the appearance of gastrointestinal adverse events (self-reported) [94]. Characterizing these bacteria genera and modifying the microbiota composition by pre- and probiotics could improve metformin action. Also, these bacteria could be set as new targets for diabetes treatment.

9. Conclusions

Besides its controversial history, metformin remains the most used medicine in type 2 diabetes treatment. Progressive dose increases should be encouraged in order to prevent gastrointestinal adverse effects. Lactic acidosis is obsolete if the patient does not have other severe comorbidities. The indications of metformin currently extend to other areas like oncology, endocrinology, and gastroenterology and should offer the scientific world more information about its adverse effects.

Conflict of interest

Anca Pantea Stoian, MD, PhD; Cristian Serafinceanu MD, PhD; and Manfredi Rizzo, MD, PhD, were advisory boards for AstraZeneca, Eli Lilly, Merck, Novo Nordisk, Sanofi. Anca Pantea Stoian, MD, PhD, is the Vicepresident of Romanian National Committee of Diabetes, Nutrition and Metabolic Diseases, and speaker for Astra Zeneca, Eli-Lilly, Coca-Cola, NovoNordisk, Sanofi. Manfredi Rizzo, MD, PhD, is the Director, Clinical Medical & Regulatory Affairs, Novo Nordisk Europe East and South. Simona Diana Stefan, MD, received speaker fees from Merck, Novo Nordisk, Sanofi. Andra Iulia Suceveanu, MD, PhD; Adrian Paul Suceveanu, MD, PhD; and Roxana Adriana Stoica, MD, declare no conflict of interest.

Author details

Roxana Adriana Stoica[1†], Diana Simona Ștefan[1,2†*], Manfredi Rizzo[3,4†], Andra Iulia Suceveanu[5†], Adrian Paul Suceveanu[5†], Cristian Serafinceanu[1,2†] and Anca Pantea-Stoian[1†]

1 University of Medicine and Pharmacy "Carol Davila" Bucharest, Romania

2 National Institute of Diabetes, Nutrition and Metabolic Diseases "Prof. Paulescu N.C." Bucharest, Romania

3 Biomedical Department of Internal Medicine and Medical Specialties School of Medicine, University of Palermo, Palermo, Italy

4 Division of Endocrinology, Diabetes and Metabolism University of South Carolina School of Medicine Columbia, South Carolina, USA

5 University of Medicine "Ovidius" Constanta, Romania

*Address all correspondence to: simona_ds2002@yahoo.com

† All authors are with an equal scientific contribution.

References

[1] Bailey CJ. Metformin: Historical overview. Diabetologia. 2017;**60**(9):1566-1576. DOI: 10.1007/s00125-017-4318-z

[2] Available at: https://www.who.int/medicines/areas/quality_safety/safety_efficacy/trainingcourses/definitions.pd [Accessed at 29.06.2019]

[3] Available at: https://www.merriam-webster.com/dictionary/contraindication [Accessed at 29.06.2019]

[4] American Diabetes Association et al. Diabetes Care. 2019;**42**(Suppl. 1):S90-S102. DOI: 10.2337/dc19-S009

[5] Cefalu WT, Riddle M. More evidence for a prevention-related indication for metformin: Let the arguments resume! Diabetes Care. 2019;**42**:499-501. DOI: 10.2337/dci18-0062

[6] Wenying Y, Lixiang L, Jinwu Q, Guangwei L, Zhiqing Y, Xiaoren P. The preventive effect of acarbose and metformin on the IGT population from becoming diabetes mellitus: A 3-year multicentral prospective study. Chinese Journal of Endocrinology and Metabolism. 2001;**17**:131-134. http://en.cnki.com.cn/Article_en/CJFDTotal-ZHNF200103001.htm

[7] Chiasson JL, Josse RG, Gomis R, Hanefeld M, Karasik A, Laakso M. Acarbose for prevention of type 2 diabetes mellitus: The STOP-NIDDM randomised trial. Lancet. 2002;**359**:2072-2077. DOI: 10.1016/S0140-6736(02)08905-5

[8] Chiasson JL, Josse RG, Gomis R, Hanefeld M, Karasik A, Laakso M. Acarbose treatment and the risk of cardiovascular disease and hypertension in patients with impaired glucose tolerance: The STOP-NIDDM trial. Journal of the American Medical Association. 2003;**290**:486-494. DOI: 10.1001/jama.290.4.486

[9] Torgerson JS, Hauptman J, Boldrin MN, Sjöstrom L. XENical in the prevention of diabetes in obese subjects (XENDOS) study. Diabetes Care. 2004;**27**:155-161. DOI: 10.2337/diacare.27.1.155

[10] Gerstein HC, Yusuf S, Bosch J, Pogue J, Sheridan P, Dinccag N, et al. Effect of rosiglitazone on the frequency of diabetes in patients with impaired glucose tolerance or impaired fasting glucose: A randomised controlled trial. Lancet. 2006;**368**:1096-1105. DOI: 10.1016/S0140-6736(06)69420-8

[11] Diabetes Prevention Program Research Group. Reduction in the incidence of type 2 diabetes with lifestyle intervention or metformin. The New England Journal of Medicine. 2002;**346**:393-403. PMID: 11832527

[12] Knowler WC, Fowler SE, Hamman RF, Christophi CA, Hoffman HJ, Brenneman AT, et al. 10-year follow-up of diabetes incidence and weight loss in the diabetes prevention program outcomes study. Lancet. 2009;**374**:1677-1686. DOI: 10.1016/S0140-6736(09)61457-4

[13] Zinman B, Harris SB, Neuman J, Gerstein HC, Retnakaran RR, Raboud J, et al. Low-dose combination therapy with rosiglitazone and metformin to prevent type 2 diabetes mellitus (CANOE trial): A double-blind randomised controlled study. Lancet. 2010;**376**:103-111. DOI: 10.1016/S0140-6736(10)60746-5

[14] Ramachandran A, Snehalatha C, Mary S, Mukesh B, Bhaskar AD, Vijay V. The Indian diabetes prevention programme shows that lifestyle modification and metformin prevent type 2 diabetes in Asian Indian subjects

with impaired glucose tolerance (IDPP1). Diabetologia. 2006;**49**:289-297. DOI: 10.1007/s00125-005-0097-z

[15] Andreadis EA, Katsanou PM, Georgiopoulos DX, Tsourous GI, Yfanti GK, Gouveri ET, et al. The effect of metformin on the incidence of type 2 diabetes mellitus and cardiovascular disease risk factors in overweight and obese subjects–the Carmos study. Experimental and Clinical Endocrinology & Diabetes. 2009;**117**:175-180. DOI: 10.1055/s-0028-1087177

[16] Metformin for prediabetes. JAMA. 2017;**317**(11):1171. DOI: 10.1001/jama.2016.17844

[17] American Diabetes Association. Standards of medical care in diabetes—2019. Diabetes Care. 2019;**42**(Suppl 1):S29-S33

[18] Rydén L, Grant PJ, Anker SD, Berne C, Cosentino F, Danchin N, et al. ESC guidelines on diabetes, pre-diabetes, and cardiovascular diseases developed in collaboration with the EASD: The task force on diabetes, pre-diabetes, and cardiovascular diseases of the European Society of Cardiology (ESC) and developed in collaboration with the European Association for the Study of diabetes (EASD). European Heart Journal. 2013;**34**:3035-3087

[19] Paulweber B, Valensi P, Lindström J, Lalic NM, Greaves CJ, McKee M, et al. A European evidence-based guideline for the prevention of type 2 diabetes. Hormone and Metabolic Research. 2010;**42**(Suppl 1):S3-S36. DOI: 10.1055/s-0029-1240928

[20] Twigg SM, Kamp MC, Davis TM, Neylon EK, Flack JR, Australian Diabetes Educators Association. Prediabetes: A position statement from the Australian Diabetes Society and Australian diabetes educators association. The Medical Journal of Australia. 2007;**186**:461-465. PMID:17484708

[21] Eastern Mediterranean Regional Office (WHO). Guidelines for the Prevention, Management and Care of Diabetes Mellitus. EMRO Technical Publications Series 32. [Internet] Available at: www.emro.who.int/dsaf/dsa664.pdf

[22] Committee Canadian Diabetes Association Clinical Practice Guidelines Expert. Reducing the risk of developing diabetes. Canadian Journal of Diabetes. 2013;**37**:S16-S19. DOI: 10.1016/j.jcjd.2013.01.013

[23] Hostalek U, Gwilt M, Hildemann S. Therapeutic use of metformin in prediabetes and diabetes prevention. Drugs. 2015;**75**(10):1071-1094. DOI: 10.1007/s40265-015-0416-8

[24] What role for metformin in type 1 diabetes? Drug and Therapeutics Bulletin. 2018;**56**(7):78-80. DOI: 10.1136/dtb.2018.7.0645

[25] Vella S, Buetow L, Royle P, et al. The use of metformin in type 1 diabetes: A systematic review of efficacy. Diabetologia. 2010;**53**:809-820. DOI: 10.1007/s00125-009-1636-9

[26] Meng H, Zhang A, Liang Y, Hao J, Zhang X, Lu J. Effect of metformin on glycaemic control in patients with type 1 diabetes: A meta-analysis of randomized controlled trials. Diabetes/Metabolism Research and Reviews. 2018;**34**:e2983r. DOI: 10.1002/dmrr.2983

[27] Petrie JR, Chaturvedi N, Ford I, REMOVAL Study Group, et al. Cardiovascular and metabolic effects of metformin in patients with type 1 diabetes (REMOVAL): A double-blind, randomised, placebo-controlled trial. The Lancet Diabetes and Endocrinology. 2017;**5**:597-609. DOI: 10.1016/S2213-8587(17)30194-8

[28] Petrie JR, Chaturvedi N, Ford I, et al. Metformin in adults with type 1 diabetes: Design and methods of reducing with metformin vascular adverse lesions (REMOVAL): An international multicentre trial. Diabetes, Obesity & Metabolism. 2017;**19**:509-516. DOI: 10.1111/dom.12840

[29] Committee on Practice Bulletins – Obstetrics. ACOG practice bulletin No. 190: Gestational diabetes mellitus. Obstetrics and Gynecology. 2018;**131**(2):e49-e63. DOI: 10.1097/AOG.0000000000002501

[30] Rowan JA, Hague WM, Gao W, Battin MR, Moore MP, Trial Investigators MG. Metformin versus insulin for the treatment of gestational diabetes. The New England Journal of Medicine. 2008;**358**:2003-2015. DOI: 10.1056/NEJMoa0707193

[31] Gui J, Liu Q, Feng L. Metformin vs insulin in the management of gestational diabetes: A meta-analysis. PLoS One. 2013;**8**:e64585. DOI: 10.1371/journal.pone.0064585

[32] Balsells M, Garćıa-Patterson A, Sola I, RoqúéM, Gich I, Corcoy R. Glibenclamide, metformin, and insulin for the treatment of gestational diabetes: A systematic review and meta-analysis. BMJ. 2015;**350**:h102. DOI: 10.1136/bmj.h102

[33] Jiang Y-F, Chen X-Y, Ding T, Wang X-F, Zhu Z-N, Su S-W. Comparative efficacy and safety of OADs in management of GDM: Network meta-analysis of randomized controlled trials. The Journal of Clinical Endocrinology and Metabolism. 2015;**100**:2071-2080. DOI: 10.1210/jc.2014-4403

[34] Camelo Castillo W, Boggess K, Sturmer T, Brookhart MA, Benjamin DK Jr, Jonsson Funk M. Association of adverse pregnancy outcomes with glyburide vs insulin in women with gestational diabetes. JAMA Pediatrics. 2015;**169**:452-458. DOI: 10.1001/jamapediatrics.2015.74

[35] Vanky E, Zahlsen K, Spigset O, Carlsen SM. Placental passage of metformin in women with polycystic ovary syndrome. Fertility and Sterility. 2005;**83**:1575-1578. DOI: 10.1016/j.fertnstert.2004.11.051

[36] American Diabetes Association. Management of Diabetes in pregnancy: Standards of medical Care in Diabetes. Diabetes Care. 2019;**42**(Suppl. 1):S165-S172

[37] Carmina E, Lobo RA. Use of fasting blood to assess the prevalence of insulin resistance in women with polycystic ovary syndrome. Fertility and Sterility. 2004;**82**(3):661-665. DOI: 10.1016/j.fertnstert.2004.01.041

[38] Velazquez EM, Mendoza S, Hamer T, Sosa F, Glueck CJ. Metformin therapy in polycystic ovary syndrome reduces hyperinsulinemia, insulin resistance, hyperandrogenemia, and systolic blood pressure, while facilitating normal menses and pregnancy. Metabolism. 1994;**43**(5):647-654. PMID:8177055

[39] Morley LC, Tang T, Yasmin E, Norman RJ, Balen AH. Insulin-sensitising drugs (metformin, rosiglitazone, pioglitazone, D-chiro-inositol) for women with polycystic ovary syndrome, oligo amenorrhoea and subfertility. Cochrane Database of Systematic Reviews. 2017;**11**(11):CD003053. DOI: 10.1002/15151858.CD003053.pub6

[40] Martin-Montalvo A, Mercken EM, Mitchell SJ, et al. Metformin improves healthspan and lifespan in mice. Nature Communications. 2013;**4**:2192. DOI: 10.1038/ncomms3192

[41] Anisimov VN, Berstein LM, Popovich IG, et al. If started early in life, metformin treatment increases

life span and postpones tumors in female SHR mice. Aging (Albany NY). 2011;**3**(2):148-157. DOI: 10.18632/aging.100273

[42] UK Prospective Diabetes Study (UKPDS) Group. Effect of intensive blood-glucose control with metformin on complications in overweight patients with type 2 diabetes (UKPDS 34). Lancet. 1998;**352**(9131):854-865. PMID:9742977

[43] Bodmer M, Becker C, Meier C, Jick SS, Meier CR. Use of metformin and the risk of ovarian cancer: A case-control analysis. Gynecologic Oncology. 2011;**123**(2):200-204. DOI: 10.1016/j.ygyno.2011.06.038

[44] Tseng CH. Metformin reduces ovarian cancer risk in Taiwanese women with type 2 diabetes mellitus. Diabetes/Metabolism Research and Reviews. 2015;**31**(6):619-626. DOI: 10.1002/dmrr.2649

[45] Jiralerspong S, Palla SL, Giordano SH, et al. Metformin and pathologic complete responses to neoadjuvant chemotherapy in diabetic patients with breast cancer. Journal of Clinical Oncology. 2009;**27**(20):3297-3302. DOI: 10.1200/JCO.2009.19.6410

[46] Campagnoli C, Pasanisi P, Abbà C, et al. Effect of different doses of metformin on serum testosterone and insulin in non-diabetic women with breast cancer: A randomized study. Clinical Breast Cancer. 2012;**12**(3):175-182. DOI: 10.1016/j.clbc.2012.03.004

[47] Tseng CH. Metformin significantly reduces incident prostate cancer risk in Taiwanese men with type 2 diabetes mellitus. European Journal of Cancer. 2014;**50**(16):2831-2837. DOI: 10.1016/j.ejca.2014.08.007

[48] Sehdev A, Shih YC, Vekhter B, Bissonnette MB, Olopade OI, Polite BN. Metformin for primary colorectal cancer prevention in patients with diabetes: A case-control study in a US population. Cancer. 2015;**121**(7):1071-1078. DOI: 10.1002/cncr.29165

[49] Monami M, Colombi C, Balzi D, et al. Metformin and cancer occurrence in insulin-treated type 2 diabetic patients. Diabetes Care. 2011;**34**(1):129-131. DOI: 10.2337/dc10-1287

[50] Landman GW, Kleefstra N, van Hateren KJ, Groenier KH, Gans RO, Bilo HJ. Metformin associated with lower cancer mortality in type 2 diabetes: ZODIAC-16. Diabetes Care. 2010;**33**(2):322-326. DOI: 10.2337/dc09-1380

[51] Holman RR, Paul SK, Bethel MA, Matthews DR, Neil HA. 10-year follow-up of intensive glucose control in type 2 diabetes. The New England Journal of Medicine. 2008;**359**(15):1577-1589. DOI: 10.1056/NEJMoa0806470

[52] Xu T, Brandmaier S, Messias AC, et al. Effects of metformin on metabolite profiles and LDL cholesterol in patients with type 2 diabetes. Diabetes Care. 2015;**38**(10):1858-1867. DOI: 10.2337/dc15-0658

[53] Malin SK, Nightingale J, Choi SE, Chipkin SR, Braun B. Metformin modifies the exercise training effects on risk factors for cardiovascular disease in impaired glucose tolerant adults. Obesity (Silver Spring). 2013;**21**(1):93-100. DOI: 10.1002/oby.20235

[54] Isoda K, Young JL, Zirlik A, et al. Metformin inhibits proinflammatory responses and nuclear factor-kappaB in human vascular wall cells. Arteriosclerosis, Thrombosis, and Vascular Biology. 2006;**26**(3):611-617. DOI: 10.1161/01.ATV.0000201938.78044.75

[55] Cheng C, Lin CH, Tsai YW, Tsai CJ, Chou PH, Lan TH. Type 2 diabetes and

antidiabetic medications in relation to dementia diagnosis. The Journals of Gerontology. Series A, Biological Sciences and Medical Sciences. 2014;**69**(10):1299-1305. DOI: 10.1093/gerona/glu073

[56] Herath PM, Cherbuin N, Eramudugolla R, Anstey KJ. The effect of diabetes medication on cognitive function: Evidence from the PATH through life study. BioMed Research International. 2016;**2016**:7208429. DOI: 10.1155/2016/7208429

[57] Mizuno Y et al. Pharmacological strategies to counteract antipsychotic-induced weight gain and metabolic adverse effects in schizophrenia: A systematic review and meta-analysis. Schizophrenia Bulletin. 2014;**40**(6): 1385-1340. DOI: 10.1093/schbul/sbu030

[58] McIntyre RS et al. The Canadian network for mood and anxiety treatments (CANMAT) task force recommendations for the management of patients with mood disorders and comorbid metabolic disorders. Annals of Clinical Psychiatry. 2012 Feb;**24**(1):69-81

[59] Bergman U, Boman G, Wiholm BE. Epidemiology of adverse drug reactions to phenformin and metformin. British Medical Journal. 1978;**2**(6135):464-466. DOI: 10.1136/bmj.2.6135.464

[60] Daubresse JC, Luyckx A, Lefèbvre P. Lactic acidosis. [Article in French]. Revue Médicale de Liège. 1975;**30**(14):453-460. PMID: 1135540

[61] Salpeter S, Greyber E, Pasternak G, Salpeter E. Risk of fatal and nonfatal lactic acidosis with metformin use in type 2 diabetes mellitus. Cochrane Database of Systematic Reviews. 2006;(1):CD002967. DOI: 10.1002/14651858.CD002967.pub2

[62] Aharaz A, Pottegård A, Henriksen DP, Hallas J, Beck-Nielsen H, Lassen AT. Risk of lactic acidosis in type 2 diabetes patients using metformin: A case control study. PLoS One. 2018;**13**(5):e0196122. DOI: 10.1371/journal.pone.0196122

[63] Available at: [Internet] https://www.ema.europa.eu/en/medicines/human/referrals/metformin-metformin-containing-:medicines [Accessed: 29.06.2019]

[64] Available at: [Internet]: https://www.fda.gov/drugs/postmarket-drug-safety-information-patients-and-providers/metformin-information, [Accessed : 29.06.2019]

[65] Li CY, Erickson SR, Wu CH. Metformin use and asthma outcomes among patients with concurrent asthma and diabetes. Respirology. 2016;(7):1210-1218. DOI: 10.1111/resp.12818

[66] Steber CJ, Perkins SL, Harris KB. Metformin-induced fixed-drug eruption confirmed by multiple exposures. American Journal of Case Reports. 2016;**17**:231-234. DOI: 10.12659/ajcr.896424

[67] Maruthur NM, Tseng E, Hutfless S, et al. Diabetes medications as monotherapy or metformin-based combination therapy for type 2 diabetes: A systematic review and meta-analysis. Annals of Internal Medicine. 2016;**164**(11):740-751. DOI: 10.7326/M15-2650

[68] Zitzmann S, Reimann IR, Schmechel H. Severe hypoglycemia in an elderly patient treated with metformin. International Journal of Clinical Pharmacology and Therapeutics. 2002;**40**(3):108-110. DOI: 10.5414/cpp40108

[69] Niafar M, Hai F, Porhomayon J, Nader ND. The role of metformin on vitamin B12 deficiency: A meta-analysis review. Internal and Emergency

Medicine. 2015;**10**(1):93-102. DOI: 10.1007/s11739-014-1157-5

[70] Andrès E, Noel E, Goichot B. Metformin-associated vitamin B12 deficiency. Archives of Internal Medicine. 2002;**162**(19):2251-2252. PMID: 12390080

[71] Lee N, Duan H, Hebert MF, Liang CJ, Rice KM, Wang J. Taste of a pill: Organic cation transporter-3 (OCT3) mediates metformin accumulation and secretion in salivary glands. The Journal of Biological Chemistry. 2014;**289**(39):27055-27064. DOI: 10.1074/jbc.M114.570564

[72] McCreight LJ, Bailey CJ, Pearson ER. Metformin and the gastrointestinal tract. Diabetologia. 2016;**59**:426-435. DOI: 10.1007/s00125-015-3844-9

[73] McCreight LJ, Stage TB, Connelly P, et al. Pharmacokinetics of metformin in patients with gastrointestinal intolerance. Diabetes, Obesity & Metabolism. 2018;**20**(7):1593-1601. DOI: 10.1111/dom.13264

[74] Scarpello JH, Hodgson E, Howlett HC. Effect of metformin on bile salt circulation and intestinal motility in type 2 diabetes mellitus. Diabetic Medicine. 1998;**15**:651-656. DOI: 10.1002/(SICI)1096-9136(199808)15:8<651::AID-DIA628>3.0.CO;2-A

[75] Dujic T, Zhou K, Donnelly LA, Tavendale R, Palmer CN, Pearson ER. Association of organic cation transporter 1 with intolerance to metformin in type 2 diabetes: A GoDARTS study. Diabetes. 2015;**64**:1786-1793. DOI: 10.2337/db14-1388

[76] Sloot YJE, Janssen MJR, van Herwaarden AE, et al. The influence of energy depletion by metformin or hypocaloric diet on thyroid iodine uptake in healthy volunteers: A randomized Trial. Scientific Reports. 2019;**9**(1):5396. DOI: 10.1038/s41598-019-41997-2

[77] Palui R, Sahoo J, Kamalanathan S, et al. Effect of metformin on thyroid function tests in patients with subclinical hypothyroidism: An open-label randomised controlled trial. Journal of Endocrinological Investigation. 2019. DOI: 10.1007/s40618-019-01059-w [Epub ahead of print]

[78] Lazarus B, Shin JI, Grams ME. Lactic acidosis, metformin use, and dose-response association-reply. JAMA Internal Medicine. 2018;**178**(10):1427-1428. DOI: 10.1001/jamainternmed.2018.4430

[79] Libmam IM, Miller KM, DiMeglio LA, T1D Exchange Clinic Network Metformin RCT Study Group, et al. Effect of metformin added to insulin on glycemic control among overweight/obese adolescents with type 1 diabetes: A randomized clinical trial. JAMA. 2015;**314**:2241-2250. DOI: 10.1001/jama.2015.16174

[80] Roberts F, Ryan GJ. The safety of metformin in heart failure. The Annals of Pharmacotherapy. 2007;**41**(4):642-646. DOI: 10.1345/aph.1H523

[81] Eurich DT, Weir DL, Majumdar SR. Comparative safety and effectiveness of metformin in patients with diabetes mellitus and heart failure: Systematic review of observational studies involving 34,000 patients. Circulation. Heart Failure. 2013;**6**:395-402. DOI: 10.1161/CIRCHEARTFAILURE.112.000162

[82] Crowley MJ, Diamantidis CJ, JR MD, Cameron CB, Stanifer JW, Mock CK, et al. Clinical outcomes of metformin use in populations with chronic kidney disease, congestive heart failure, or chronic liver disease: A systematic review. Annals of Internal Medicine. 2017;**166**(3):191-200. DOI: 10.7326/M16-1901

[83] Ekström N, Schiöler L, Svensson AM, Eeg-Olofsson K, Jonasson JM, Zethelius B, et al. Effectiveness and safety of metformin in 51 675 patients with type 2 diabetes and different levels of renal function: A cohort study from the Swedish National Diabetes Register. BMJ Open. 2012;**2**:4. DOI: 10.1136/ bmj open-2012-001076

[84] Ampuero J, Ranchal I, Nunez D, Diaz-Herrero Mdel M, Maraver M, del Campo JA, et al. Metformin inhibits glutaminase activity and protects against hepatic encephalopathy. PLoS One. 2012;**7**:e49279. DOI: 10.1371/ journal.pone.0049279

[85] Zhang X, Harmsen WS, Mettler TA, Kim WR, Roberts RO, Therneau TM, et al. Continuation of metformin use after a diagnosis of cirrhosis significantly improves survival of patients with diabetes. Hepatology. 2014;**60**:2008-2016. DOI: 10.1002/ hep.27199

[86] Nkontchou G, Cosson E, Aout M, Mahmoudi A, Bourcier V, Charif I, et al. Impact of metformin on the prognosis of cirrhosis induced by viral hepatitis C in diabetic patients. The Journal of Clinical Endocrinology and Metabolism. 2011;**96**:2601-2608. DOI: 10.1210/ jc.2010-2415

[87] Hitchings AW, Lai D, Jones PW, Baker EH, Metformin in COPD Trial Team. Metformin in severe exacerbations of chronic obstructive pulmonary disease: A randomised controlled trial. Thorax. 2016 Jul;**71**(7):587-593. DOI: 10.1136/ thoraxjnl-2015-208035

[88] Pastor-Villaescusa B, Cañete MD, Caballero-Villarraso J, et al. Metformin for obesity in Prepubertal and pubertal children: A randomized controlled Trial. Pediatrics. 2017;**140**(1):e20164285. DOI: 10.1542/peds.2016-4285

[89] Priya G, Kalra S. Metformin in the management of diabetes during pregnancy and lactation. Drugs Context. 2018;**7**:212523. DOI: 10.7573/ dic.212523

[90] Jang K, Chung H, Yoon JS, Moon SJ, Yoon SH, Yu KS, et al. Pharmacokinetics, safety, and tolerability of metformin in healthy elderly subjects. Journal of Clinical Pharmacology. 2016;**6**(9):1104-1110. DOI: 10.1002/jcph.699

[91] Taub ES, Hoffman RS, Manini AF. Incidence and risk factors for hyperlactatemia in ED patients with acute metformin overdose. The American Journal of Emergency Medicine. 2019;(19):30184-30186. DOI: 10.1016/j.ajem.2019.03.033

[92] Wang GS, Hoyte C. Review of Biguanide (metformin) toxicity. Journal of Intensive Care Medicine. 2018;**21**:885066618793385. DOI: 10.1177/0885066618793385

[93] Elbere I, Kalnina I, Silamikelis I, et al. Association of metformin administration with gut microbiome dysbiosis in healthy volunteers. PLoS One. 2018;**13**(9):e0204317. DOI: 10.1371/ journal.pone.0204317

[94] Bryrup T, Thomsen CW, Kern T, et al. Metformin-induced changes of the gut microbiota in healthy young men: Results of a non-blinded, one-armed intervention study. Diabetologia. 2019;**62**(6):1024-1035. DOI: 10.1007/ s00125-019-4848-7

[95] Rosario D, Benfeitas R, Bidkhori G, et al. Understanding the representative gut microbiota dysbiosis in metformin-treated type 2 diabetes patients using genome-scale metabolic modeling. Frontiers in Physiology. 2018;**9**:775. DOI: 10.3389/fphys.2018.00775

Chapter 2

New Insight into Metformin Mechanism of Action and Clinical Application

Yun Yan, Karen L. Kover and Wayne V. Moore

Abstract

Metformin is the first-line medication for Type 2 diabetes (T2D) treatment, and it is the only US FDA approved oral antidiabetic medication for pediatric patients with T2D 10 years and older. Metformin is also used to treat polycystic ovary syndrome (PCOS), another condition with underlying insulin resistance. The clinical applications of metformin are continuing to expand into other fields including cancer, aging, cardiovascular diseases, and neurodegenerative diseases. Metformin modulates multiple biological pathways. Its novel properties and effects continue to evolve; however, its molecular mechanism of action remains incompletely understood. In this chapter, we focus on the recent translational research and clinical data on the molecular action of metformin and the evidence linking the effects of metformin on insulin resistance, prediabetes, diabetes, aging, cancer, PCOS, cardiovascular diseases, and neurodegenerative diseases.

Keywords: metformin, insulin, insulin resistance, diabetes, aging, PCOS, cancer, cardiovascular, neurodegenerative

1. Introduction

Synthesis of metformin was reported in 1922 and its effect of lowering glucose was reported soon after. Metformin was first reported to be used for the treatment of diabetes by French physician Jean Steme in 1957. The effect of metformin on improvement of morbidity and mortality in type 2 diabetes (T2D) was confirmed in the United Kingdom Prospective Diabetes Study (UKPDS), a large clinical trial performed in 1980–1990s [1]. It was approved for T2D treatment in adults by US FDA in 1994 and for pediatric patients 10 years and older in 2000. Metformin is prescribed world-wide as the first-line oral drug for adults and children with T2D. Its physiological effects related to T2D include increase in insulin sensitivity, reduction of gluconeogenesis in the liver, enhanced glucose uptake by muscle, and reduced intestinal glucose absorption. Several molecular mechanisms of action have been proposed but more remain to be discovered. In this chapter, we will review molecular mechanisms of action of metformin and its prospect for clinical application.

2. Mechanisms of action

The potential mechanisms of metformin action involve several pathways. The AMPK-pathway plays an important role in metformin actions [2, 3]. Metformin inhibits the mitochondrial respiratory chain (complex I), which increases the AMP to ATP ratio, leading to the phosphorylation of AMP-activated protein kinase (AMPK) at Thr-172. We have demonstrated that metformin treatment increases protein level of phosphorylated AMPK in high-glucose-treated endothelial cells [4]. The phosphorylated AMPK subsequently phosphorylates multiple downstream effectors to regulate cellular metabolism and energy homeostasis [5]. These downstream effectors include thioredoxin interacting protein (TXNIP) and TBC1D1, a RAB-GTPase activating protein and a member of the tre-2/BUB2/cdc1 domain family. Phosphorylated TXNIP and TBC1D1 increase the plasma membrane localization of glucose transporter 1 (GLUT1) and GLUT4, respectively [6, 7], and regulate glycogen synthases (GYS1 and GYS2) to prevent the storage of glycogen [8]. Some actions of metformin have been found to be AMPK-independent [9].

In diabetic mice, metformin has an effect on gut microbiota by inducing a profound shift in the gut microbial community profile, resulting in an increase in the Akkermansia spp. population [10] and cAMP-induced agmatine production [11], which may decrease absorption of glucose from the gastrointestinal tract and increase lipid metabolism respectively. In addition, metformin decreases insulin-induced suppression of fatty acid oxidation and lowers lipid content of hepatic cells [12].

3. Insulin resistance

Insulin resistance (IR) is a condition in which the cellular response to insulin is decreased resulting in elevated insulin levels (hyperinsulinism). When the beta cells are not able to overcome the resistance by producing more insulin, hyperglycemia develops. Insulin resistance is more prevalent in certain racial populations suggesting a genetic basis for the resistance. The major "environmental" risk factors for insulin resistance are obesity and sedentary lifestyle. Exercise and weight loss are established approaches to improve insulin sensitivity and decrease insulin resistance [13]. Insulin resistance may also be the basis for polycystic ovary syndrome (PCOS) in women. Some studies have suggested that metabolic syndrome (insulin resistance, type 2 diabetes, obesity, hyperlipidemia, and hypertension) and PCOS (insulin resistance, hyperandrogenism, amenorrhea, non-obese) are the ends of a spectrum of insulin resistance. The loss of microvascular insulin response and reduction of muscle glucose uptake are early events in the pathogenesis of insulin resistance [14, 15].

Metformin can increase insulin receptor tyrosine kinase activity, enhance glycogen synthesis, and increase the recruitment and activity of GLUT4 glucose transporters. In high-fat-diet-fed insulin resistant rats, metformin improved the insulin sensitivity of vascular and skeletal muscle and restored glucose uptake in insulin resistant skeletal muscle [16]. In adipose tissue, metformin promoted the re-esterification of free fatty acids and inhibited lipolysis, which indirectly improved insulin sensitivity through reduced lipotoxicity [17].

Insulin resistance is a risk factor for the development of T2D [18] and occurs earlier than hyperglycemia. Blood-based biomarker that identify insulin resistance earlier than current glycemia-based approaches, including fasting glucose and HbA1C [19] might identify individual's at risk for developing diabetes, and provide a novel tool to monitor metformin treatment in the high risk population. Several blood-based biomarkers of insulin resistance have been identified [19]. Branched-chain amino acids [20] and asymmetric dimethylarginine (ADMA) [21] show an association with insulin resistance. Metformin decreases the level of circulating branched-chain amino acids and reduces insulin resistance in a high-fat diet mouse model [22]. Metformin treatment lowers plasma ADMA which is associated with improved glycemic control in patients with T2D [23].

Recent studies indicate that phosphatidylinositol-3-kinase/protein kinase B protein (PI3K/PKB, also known as Akt) signaling pathway is associated with insulin resistance, and plays a critical role in insulin stimulation of glucose transport into cells [24–30]. The key molecules involved in this pathway are PI3K, Akt, 3-phosphoinositide-dependent protein kinase 1 (PDK1), and phosphoinositide 3.4.5 trisphosphate (PIP3).

Akt has three isoforms Akt1, Akt2 and Akt3 (also referred to as protein kinase B (PKB) α, −β and −γ, respectively). Their domain structures are similar, including a pleckstrin homology (PH) kinase domain at the amino-terminal and a hydrophobic motif (HM) domain at the carboxyl-terminal [31]. Three isoforms share many substrates, but each isoform also has specific substrate. Akt2 is specific for the insulin signaling pathway and plays a critical role in glucose homeostasis. Akt2 deficient mice have insulin resistance, hyperglycemia, and loss of pancreatic β cells while Akt1 deficient mice do not exhibit diabetes phenotypes [32, 33].

PIP3 binds to PDK1 and Akt protein and recruits Akt protein to the plasma membrane. PDK1 phosphorylates Akt at Thr308/309 of Akt1/Akt2, respectively of the kinase domain leading to partial Akt activation. PI3K might directly phosphorylate Akt1 at Thr308 [34]. Full Akt activation is associated with a second PI3K phosphorylation of Akt at Ser473/474 of Akt1/Akt2, respectively in the carboxyl-terminal hydrophobic motif [34]. Subsequently, the phosphorylated Akt2 recruits insulin-regulated GLUT1 and GLUT4 glucose transporters from the cytoplasm onto the cell membrane surface and thereby increases glucose uptake [35].

GLUT1 is an insulin independent transporter whereas GLUT4 is an insulin dependent transporter. Insulin increases GLUT4 in the cell membrane and promotes the glucose transport into muscle and fatty cells (**Figure 1**). Any defect in Akt pathway along with the downstream molecules could result in insulin resistance [29]. Clinical data indicate that acute myocardial insulin resistance that occurs after cardiac surgery with cardiopulmonary bypass is attributed to Akt inactivation.

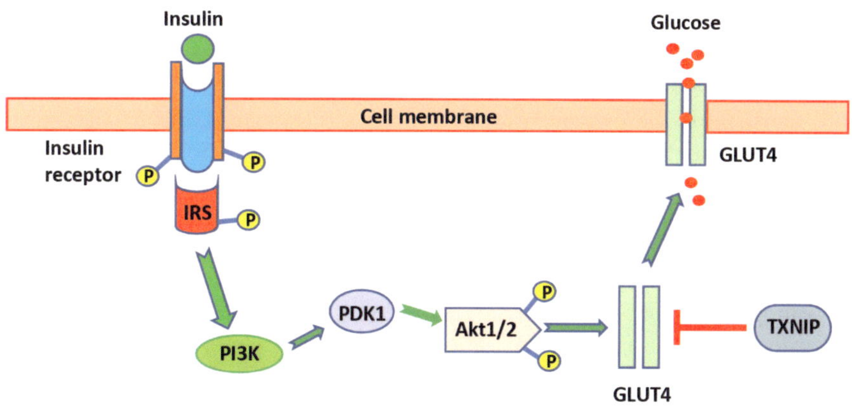

Figure 1.
Insulin binds to insulin receptor and induces its dimerization and auto phosphorylation of tyrosine residues in two transmembrane β subunits, which further lead to the phosphorylation of tyrosine residues on the IRS protein. These molecules can further activate PI3K, resulting in activation of PDK1/2. AKT is recruited and gets phosphorylated by PDK1/2. Once activated, AKT promotes GLUT4 translocation to plasma membrane and facilitates glucose into cell. TXNIP inhibits glucose transporter by promoting GLUT4 endocytosis.

Inactivated Akt impairs the membrane transposition of GLUT4, which results in insulin resistance accompanied with hyperinsulinemia, hyperglycemia and cardiac dysfunction [36]. It has been reported that metformin attenuates insulin resistance by restoring PI3K/Akt/GLUT4 signaling in the hepatocytes of T2D rats [37]. Metformin combined with phloretin, a dihydrochalcone found in fruits, promoted glucose consumption and suppressed gluconeogenesis in skeletal muscle via PI3K/Akt/GlUT4 signaling pathway in T2D rat models [38].

TXNIP is being considered as a novel mediator of insulin resistance [39, 40]. TXNIP induced by high-glucose concentration is a key intracellular regulator of glucose and lipid metabolism [6]. We have demonstrated that metformin improves endothelial cell function via down-regulation of high-glucose-induced TXNIP transcription [4].

Over expression of TXNIP induces apoptosis of pancreatic β cells and endothelial cells, decreases muscle and adipose insulin sensitivity, promotes GLUT4 endocytosis and reduces glucose uptake in myocytes and adipocytes [4, 41–43]. Reduction of TXNIP expression by RNA interference gene-silencing significantly improves insulin induced glucose uptake in cultured human skeletal muscle cells [41]. TXNIP knockout mice had improved insulin sensitivity and increased glucose uptake in both adipose and skeletal muscle [39]. In PCOS, metformin improved insulin resistance in a PCOS rat model via an AMPK alpha-SIRT1 pathway [44].

4. Prediabetes

New criteria defining prediabetes includes the presence of one or more of the following, impaired fasting glucose (IFG), impaired glucose tolerance (IGT) and HbA1C of 5.7–6.4% [45]. The progression from prediabetes to diabetes is related to insulin resistance and β-cell dysfunction. Prediabetes is a serious health condition which increases the risk of developing T2D, heart disease and stroke. In the US, approximately 84 million American adults (more than 1 out of 3) have prediabetes but 90% patients with prediabetes are not aware of their condition [46]. Metformin improves insulin sensitivity and provides an attractive pharmacological intervention for prediabetes [47, 48]. Results from several clinical trials in the prediabetes population, including children, adolescents and adults, have indicated that metformin can delay or halt the progression from prediabetes to diabetes [49–51]. Metformin is generally well tolerated and has no significant safety issues with long-term use for diabetes prevention [48]. In the long-term "Diabetes Prevention Program Outcomes Study (DPPOS)", either lifestyle intervention or metformin significantly reduced diabetes development over 15 years. Lifestyle intervention has been shown similar or greater effectiveness than metformin in clinical trials [52] and remains the cornerstone of care for patients with prediabetes. However, lifestyle interventions are difficult for patients to maintain and often fail to control weight over the long term. Metformin therapy was shown to be just as effective as lifestyle intervention in individual with prediabetes <60 years of age, BMI ≥ 35 $kg/m^{2,}$ and in women with a history of gestational diabetes mellitus [51, 53]. A study showed that metformin was underused in patients with prediabetes and only 3.7% of adult patients with prediabetes were prescribed metformin [54]. Currently metformin is not approved by FDA for prediabetes. Overweight patients with comorbidities may be at increased risk of diabetes. New guidelines recommended that metformin therapy for T2D prevention should be considered in those with prediabetes, especially those with BMI ≥ 35 kg/m^2, those aged <60 years, and women with prior gestational diabetes mellitus [55]. The combinations of metformin with lifestyle or other treatments have shown more beneficial effects in diabetes prevention [48, 49].

5. Diabetes

Metformin is approved for use in patients with T2D. It is still under debated whether metformin can be an adjunct therapy for T1D though many overweight T1D patients have been prescribed metformin due to its beneficial effects on improving insulin resistance.

5.1 Adult T2D

Metformin is considered first-line therapy to treat T2D due to its blood glucose-lowering effects, safety and relatively low cost. Metformin lowers blood glucose level by decreasing glucose production in liver, reducing intestinal glucose absorption, increasing insulin sensitivity and promoting muscle glucose uptake in muscle. Metformin treatment can be combined with lifestyle modification and other anti-diabetic drugs, such as dipeptidyl peptidase-4 (DPP-4) inhibitors, glucagon-like peptide-1 (GLP-1) receptor agonists or sodium-glucose cotransporter-2 (SGLT2) [56, 57]. Combined therapy is individualized depending on effectiveness, safety, tolerability, and the characteristics of each patient [58].

Metformin is safe and tolerable with the exception of the risk of lactic acidosis in patients with risk factors for lactic acidosis [59], including impairment of renal, cardiac, and hepatic function [60–62]. Another concern is metformin-induced vitamin B12 deficiency; patients who receive long-term metformin treatment (>6 months) at large doses have developed B12 deficiency [63, 64], so that annual screening of vitamin B12 level is recommended [65].

5.2 Adult T1D

Insulin resistance in T1D patients may contribute to poor glycemic control and is associated with increased insulin dose requirement [66]. Metformin treatment has been shown to increase insulin sensitivity, improve glycemic control, and reduce cardiovascular risk in patients with T1D [67]. The studies reported that metformin used as an adjunct therapy in T1D reduced insulin dose and body weight with no improvement in HbA1c and glycemic control [68, 69]. Another short term adjunct therapy with metformin demonstrated improved glycemic control, insulin sensitivity, and quality of life without weight gain, while long-term (2 years) metformin treatment was associated with decreased BMI [70]. A 1 year retrospective investigation reported an association between metformin as adjunct therapy and decreased glucose levels, decreased prevalence metabolic syndrome traits, and decreased insulin dose [71].

5.3 Pediatric T2D

Metformin was shown to be safe and effective for treatment of pediatric patients with T2D age 10 to 16 years old [72]. Treatment Options for Type 2 Diabetes in Adolescents and Youth (TODAY) recruited 699 youth and adolescents over a 4-year period. In this cohort study, metformin was used alone or in combination with life style modification or other antidiabetics drugs [73]. Metformin treatment was associated with decreased HbA1c and improved glycemic control in more than half of the participants. Metformin plus rosiglitazone was significantly better than metformin monotherapy [74].

5.4 Pediatric T1D

Using metformin to improve glycemic control and insulin sensitivity in youth and adolescents with T1D has been reported in several clinical trials. Studies that report a positive association of metformin have reported: 1. Decreased insulin dose, BMI and waist circumference in adolescents with T1D [75]. 2. Lower daily insulin dose improved whole-body and peripheral insulin resistance in adolescents with T1D who were overweight/obese [76]. 3. Lower insulin dose and improved vascular smooth muscle function and HbA1c children with T1D [77]. 4. Decreased cardiovascular disease risk factors in youth with T1D [78]. 5. Improvement in HbA1c level in adolescents with T1D [79, 80]. In contrast, some trials did not observe improvement in HbA1c [76, 81], or glycemic control. As expected, there was an increased gastrointestinal adverse event in overweight adolescents with T1D [81].

6. Aging

Metformin has attracted interest for its potential effects on aging [82]. Metformin treatment has a positive association with reduction in the incidence of mortality from age-related diseases including diabetes, cancer, cardiovascular diseases, and neurodegenerative diseases. Metformin is reported to increase lifespan in several animal models. Cohort clinical trials, Metformin in Longevity Study (MILES) and Targeting Aging with Metformin (TAME), have been initiated to investigate metformin's anti-aging effects in human.

In several animal models, including nematodes and rodents, metformin has been shown to delay aging. Metformin treated female outbred mice (100 mg/kg in drinking water) showed an increased mean lifespan 37.8% [83]. The effects of metformin treatment were shown to be age dependent in mice. When treatment was started at the early stage of life, middle-age and late stages of life, the mean lifespan was increased by 21%, 7% and 13% respectively compared to the controls [84]. In a mouse breast cancer model, metformin delayed the onset of mammary adenocarcinoma and increased lifespan by a mean of 8% compared to the control group [85]. Metformin prolonged the survival time of male mice with Huntington's disease by 21.1%, but had no effects in female [86]. A recent study found that metformin reduced oxidative stress and inflammation, extended both lifespan and healthspan by 4–6% in different strains of mice, and attenuated the deleterious effects of aging in male mice [87].

Gut microbiota has been shown to affect health status and longevity and play a role in resistance to infection, inflammation, autoimmunity, and cancer, and the regulation of the brain-gut axis [88, 89]. Metformin acts directly on gut bacteria to decrease absorption of glucose, improve lipid metabolism and elevate agmatine production to extend host lifespan [10, 90].

The reported effects of metformin on microbiota and animals have promoted interest in evaluating its effects on human longevity. In 2014, Metformin in Longevity Study (MILES, NCT02432287) clinical trial was initiated to examine the effects of metformin treatment on the biology of aging in humans, and to determine if treatment with metformin (1700 mg/day) could restore more youthful gene expression in elderly people with impaired glucose tolerance. Results from MILES showed that 6-weeks of metformin treatment in older adults (~70-year-old participants) improved age-associated gene expression, and significantly influenced metabolic and non-metabolic pathways in skeletal muscle and subcutaneous adipose tissue [91]. Currently, MILES has progressed to a phase 4 trial. Targeting Aging with Metformin (TAME) is managed by America Federation for Aging Research (AFAR) to investigate metformin's ability to delay the onset of comorbidities related to aging. The plan is to recruit 3000 older adults (aged 65–79 years old) without diabetes who will be randomly assigned to 1500 mg metformin daily or placebo for 6 years, with a mean follow-up time of more than 3–5 years (https://www.afar.org/research/TAME). These ongoing trials are expected to further evaluate and update the roles of metformin in antiaging.

7. PCOS

Polycystic ovary syndrome (PCOS) is a common endocrine disorder affecting about 5–15% of reproductive age women [92, 93]. PCOS is associated with insulin resistance and hyperinsulinemia, even in lean women. The condition puts women at risk for infertility, obesity, diabetes, as well as cardiovascular disease [94]. Metformin has been used to treat PCOS for 25 years and is currently recommended in combination with other therapy.

Clinically, metformin was first reported as a treatment for PCOS in 1994 [95]. A 6-month trial of metformin or placebo in women with PCOS found that metformin improved menstruation and insulin sensitivity, and reduced hyperinsulinemia and hyperandrogenemia [96]. In addition, metformin has been found to inhibit androgen production by repressing the steroidogenic enzymatic activities of 17α-hydroxylase/17,20 lyase (CYP17A1) and 3β-hydroxysteroid dehydrogenase type 2 (HSD3B2) in the theca cells taken from the ovaries of women with PCOS [97].

Women treated with metformin had increased rates of ovulation and pregnancy [93], reduced rates of early pregnancy loss, preterm delivery, preeclampsia, and fetal growth restriction [98, 99], and improved live birth rates [93]. There were no serious adverse effects in pregnant women with PCOS treated with metformin or their offspring [98–100]. These results indicate that the roles of metformin are not only in glucose metabolism, but also in regulating ovarian hormonal activities and functions in women with PCOS.

There is not enough evidence to recommend metformin as first-line therapy for women with PCOS but adding metformin to other PCOS treatment seems an optimal option. Gastrointestinal side effects were more common in metformin combined with clomiphene citrate than clomiphene citrate alone, but the combined therapy may have beneficial effects in the rates of ovulation and pregnancy [93, 101]. Combination of metformin with clomiphene citrate can be considered as the first line therapy in anovulatory PCOS women without other infertility factors [102]. Metformin was less effective than clomiphene citrate in obese women with PCOS [93, 102]. Combined therapy of metformin and spironolactone showed greater improvement in menstrual cycles and hyperinsulinemia. Adding metformin to ethinyl estradiol-cyproterone acetate treatment in non-obese women with PCOS resulted in significant decreases in androgen levels and increases sex hormone-binding globulin level, which confirmed that metformin also, has some beneficial effects in non-obese women with PCOS [103]. In a DHEA-induced PCOS rat animal model, metformin treatment restored ovarian angiogenesis and follicular development [104].

8. Cardiovascular diseases

Cardiovascular diseases (CVD) are the leading cause of death and disability in the world. Metformin might have sustained beneficial role on reducing CVD risk and mortality [105, 106]. The cardioprotective effects include reduction of weight gain and hyperinsulinemia, improvement of endothelial function and fibrinolysis, and reduction of low-grade inflammation, oxidative stress, and glycation.

Recent clinical studies have shown that metformin has protective effects on vascular endothelial function and angiogenesis in patients with T2D [107]. Several clinical trials have reported that metformin treatment reduced CVD risk in T2D [1, 108]. Recently the efficacy of metformin in modifying CVD outcomes has been challenged [109–111] but updated evidence support that metformin is cardiovascular protective [112]. A meta-analysis that included 40 clinical trials comprising 1,066,408 patients has shown that metformin reduced cardiovascular mortality, all-cause mortality and cardiovascular events in coronary artery disease [105].

Diabetes increases CVD risk and mortality. More than 75% of male and more than 57% female T2D patients died from cardiovascular disease. The mortality of CVD with T2D patients is twice those without T2D [113]. Patients with chronic cardiovascular disease (CVD) comorbidity are likely to benefit from metformin treatment [1, 105, 108]. Metformin is recommended to be used alone or in combination with other drugs as the first line therapy in T2D patients with high risk of CVD, including atherosclerotic cardiovascular disease [114, 115].

Several clinical trials for metformin on participants with or without T1D diabetes have been completed [106]. Trials Metformin in Insulin Resistant Left Ventricular Dysfunction (TAYSIDE, NCT00473876) and Reducing with Metformin Vascular Adverse Lesions of Type 1 Diabetes (REMOVAL, NCT01483560) have promising data. TAYSIDE found that metformin had a beneficial effect in participants with nondiabetic chronic heart failure and insulin resistance, significantly improved the secondary endpoint of the slope of the ratio of minute ventilation to carbon dioxide production, fasting insulin resistance and weight loss [116]. REMOVAL showed that metformin reduced the prespecified tertiary end point of carotid artery intima-media thickness in T1D suggesting a cardiovascular protective effect [117]. In an 8-week period of metformin treatment for nondiabetic participants with cardiac syndrome X, metformin improved endothelium-dependent microvascular response, maximal ST-segment depression, Duke score, and chest pain incidence, which suggested that metformin may improve vascular function and decrease myocardial ischemia [118]. However, several studies reported that metformin was not found to be effective in their participants [106].

Investigation of Metformin in Pre-diabetes on Atherosclerotic Cardiovascular OuTcomes (VA-IMPACT, NCT02915198) and Glucose Lowering in Non-diabetic Hyperglycemia Trial (GLINT, ISRCTN34875079) are current ongoing studies to further evaluate the effects of metformin on CVD [119]. The trials will evaluate the incidence of cardiovascular death and non-fatal myocardial infarction events. Their data will provide more insight on the association of metformin treatment on CVD.

The role of metformin in inhibiting mitochondrial enzymes and activating AMPK pathway are the most likely cellular mechanisms in cardiovascular protection. We have demonstrated that AMPK activated by metformin improved cellular function, decreased apoptosis, and reduced inflammation in vascular endothelial cells [4, 42]. TXNIP is a key regulator of cellular redox state induced by high glucose and promotes high-glucose-induced macrovascular endothelial dysfunction. We have also reported that metformin down-regulated high-glucose-induced TXNIP expression by inactivating ChREBP and Forkhead box O1 (FOXO1) through AMPK pathway (**Figure 2**) [4].

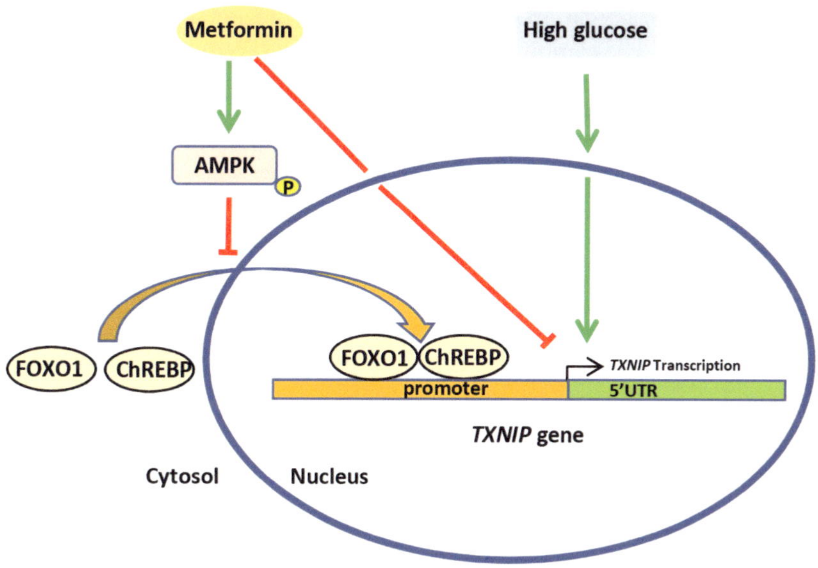

Figure 2.
Metformin inhibits the nuclear entry of ChREBP and FOXO1 from cytosol and their binding capacity to the TXNIP promoter, thus potently and effectively suppresses TXNIP transcription induced by high glucose at last. The inhibitory effect of metformin on nuclear translocation is AMPK-phosphorylation-dependent.

9. Cancer

Preexisting diabetes is a risk factor for cancers, including liver, pancreas, endometrium, colon, breast, and bladder cancers [120]. Epidemiological studies show that the incidence of cancer is decreased in patients with T2D treated with metformin [121]. Metformin has shown to inhibit cancer cell growth in clinical trials including cancer patients without diabetes [122–124]. Based on http://ClinicalTrials.gov in January 2020, there are more than 300 clinical trials investigating metformin in cancer treatment, more than 100 of them have been completed. The results were published or posted on http://ClinicalTrials.gov. These trials included patients with or without diabetes with different cancers using metformin treatment or combination of metformin with other anticancer drugs. Accumulating evidence from clinical trials and a national cohort study suggest that metformin treatment may improve therapeutic response and have potential beneficial effects on cancer prevention and therapy [125–127].

The effect of metformin on inhibiting cell proliferation can be classified as AMPK independent and AMPK dependent [128]. Metformin inhibits the electron transport chain, resulting in an elevated $NADH/NAD^+$ ratio and decrease of ATP production in mitochondrial complex I ATP as well as activation of AMPK [129, 130]. AMPK activated by metformin subsequently regulates cell growth and survival by targeting metabolic enzymes and transporters [131, 132]. AMPK downregulates mTOR activity that plays a central role in the regulation of cell proliferation, growth, differentiation, migration, and survival [133–135].

Tumor protein 53 (p53) plays a central role in the cellular responses to repair of DNA damage, cell survival and apoptosis. p53 mutations occur in almost every type of human cancer cells and more than 50% of human cancers have a somatic p53 mutation [136]. AMPK activation induced phosphorylation at Ser15 of p53, leading to cell-cycle arrest [137].

Metformin was reported to inhibit melanoma cell invasion and metastasis via an AMPK/p53 dependent manner [138]. In a pre-clinical lymphoma model, metformin treatment resulted in activation of p53, leading to cell apoptosis [139]. In the prostate cancer cells, the combination of metformin and 2-deoxyglucose resulted in p53-dependent cell apoptosis [140]. Metformin has been found to inhibit human cervical cancer cell proliferation and induce apoptosis via modulating p53 and cyclin D1 expression [141].

The effect of metformin on anti-cancer also has a p53-independent mechanism. Metformin has been shown to induce G2M arrest in p53-deficient colorectal cancer cells and tumors. When combined with ionizing radiation metformin therapy enhanced antitumor effects in radioresistant p53-deficient colorectal cancer cells [142]. Treatment with metformin increased apoptosis in p53-deficient human colon cancer cell and reduced tumor growth in xenografts of p53-deficient human colon cancer cells [143].

The p53 homologs, P63 and p73 have overlapping function in tumorigenesis and development [144]. P63 and P73 mutations are rare in human tumors, but they can be overexpressed. P63 plays a critical role in development of squamous epithelium and is overexpressed in squamous cell carcinoma [145]. Metformin inhibited p63 protein expression in squamous carcinoma cell, resulting in decreased cell viability and xenographic tumor growth [146]. P73 overexpression induces apoptosis and cell cycle arrest of tumor cells [147]. AMPK activated by metformin phosphorylated Ser426 of p73 leading to p73 accumulation and cell apoptosis in human colon cancer cells [148].

Metformin may prevent tumorigenesis by inhibiting the insulin like growth factor (IGF)-1 signaling pathway and increasing insulin sensitivity. The proliferation marker Ki-67 was significantly decreased in patients with endometrial cancer cell after metformin treatment [149]. Metformin enhances cytotoxic T lymphocyte (CTL) antitumor activity via activating AMPK to phosphorylate Ser195 of PDL-1 in a murine model of breast cancer which is consistent with the finding that tumor tissues from metformin-treated breast cancer patients exhibited reduced PDL-1 level with AMPK activation [150].

These findings suggest that metformin could be a useful adjuvant agent and has therapeutic benefits in several tumor types, including colorectal, prostate and breast cancers. However, there is limited evidence in other tumor types, and further clinical investigations are needed to evaluate metformin effects in cancer therapy.

10. Neurodegenerative diseases

Metformin is described to have a beneficial effect in neurodegenerative diseases (ND), including dementia, Alzheimer's disease, Parkinson's disease, Huntington's disease and mild cognitive impairment [151, 152].

Population-based studies support an association between the elevated risk of ND in patients with T2D [153–155]. A large population cohort study used Taiwan's National Health Insurance Database to investigate the relationship between dementia, T2D, and metformin treatment. They found that the prevalence of dementia was increased in patients with T2D and that metformin therapy was associated with a 24% decrease in the incidence of dementia in patients with T2D. The combination treatment of metformin with sulfonylureas was associated with a 35% decrease in the risk of dementia in T2D patients over 8 years of observation [156]. In a recent study, long-term (>2 years) metformin therapy was associated with lower incidence of dementia among elderly adults with T2D. Longer term treatment (>4 years) was associated with reduced risk of Alzheimer's and Parkinson's diseases, and none with mild cognitive impairment [157]. A large T2D population cohort study found that sulfonylureas therapy increased the risk of Parkinson's disease, but adding metformin as a co-therapy significantly reduced the risk of Parkinson's disease in T2D

[158]. Long-term (>6 years) metformin treatment significantly reduced the risk of cognitive impairment among older adults with T2D [159].

In contrast, other studies have shown that the metformin therapy of T2D is associated with: 1. a slightly higher risk of Alzheimer's disease [160], 2. increased risk for cognitive impairment [161], and 3. no beneficial effects on preventing development of Alzheimer's disease after adjusting for underlying risk factors and the duration of diabetes since diagnosis [162]. In addition, metformin treatment aggravated neurodegenerative process in ApoE knockout mice [163].

The current evidence suggests that the neuroprotective effects of metformin occur via activation of AMPK/mTOR pathway and inhibition of tau phosphorylation [164, 165]. In addition, it is known that metformin enhances angiogenesis and neurogenesis, induces autophagy, reduces oxidative stress, and improves neurological deficits [166–170].

Despite the different findings from these studies, a recent meta-analysis suggests that metformin may prevent development of dementia in patients with diabetes indicating that metformin should be continued in patients with T2D patients at risk of the dementia or Alzheimer's disease. Use of metformin to prevent neurodegenerative diseases in people without diabetes is not supported by current evidence [152].

11. Conclusions

Metformin is currently approved and widely prescribed for patients with T2D and PCOS. The clinical trial data and clinical experience over several decades have demonstrated its safety and efficacy. The interest in metformin therapy has dramatically increased as the population-based cohort studies indicate that metformin can decrease the risk of cancer, cardiovascular and cerebral disease. Current studies indicate that metformin has potential for treatment of T1D, cancer, aging, cardiovascular and neurodegenerative diseases. Translational and clinical trials need to be continued and expanded to determine if there are indications for metformin therapy in diseases other than T2D.

Conflict of interest

The authors declare no conflict of interest.

Author details

Yun Yan*, Karen L. Kover and Wayne V. Moore
Department of Pediatrics, Division of Endocrinology, Children's Mercy Kansas City, School of Medicine, University of Missouri Kansas City, Kansas City, USA

*Address all correspondence to: yyan@cmh.edu

References

[1] UKPDS G. Effect of intensive blood-glucose control with metformin on complications in overweight patients with type 2 diabetes (UKPDS 34). UK prospective Diabetes study (UKPDS) group. Lancet. 1998;**352**:854-865. DOI: 10.1016/S0140-6736(98)07037-8

[2] Zhou G, Myers R, Li Y, Chen Y, Shen X, Fenyk-Melody J, et al. Role of AMP-activated protein kinase in mechanism of metformin action. The Journal of Clinical Investigation. 2001;**108**:1167-1174. DOI: 10.1172/JCI13505

[3] Coughlan KA, Valentine RJ, Ruderman NB, Saha AK. AMPK activation: A therapeutic target for type 2 diabetes? Diabetes, Metabolic Syndrome and Obesity: Targets and Therapy. 2014;7:241-253. DOI: 10.2147/DMSO.S43731

[4] Li X, Kover KL, Heruth DP, Watkins DJ, Moore WV, Jackson K, et al. New insight into metformin action: Regulation of ChREBP and FOXO1 activities in endothelial cells. Molecular Endocrinology. 2015;**29**:1184-1194. DOI: 10.1210/ME.2015-1090

[5] Mihaylova MM, Shaw RJ. The AMPK signalling pathway coordinates cell growth, autophagy and metabolism. Nature Cell Biology. 2011;**13**:1016-1023. DOI: 10.1038/ncb2329

[6] Wu N, Zheng B, Shaywitz A, Dagon Y, Tower C, Bellinger G, et al. AMPK-dependent degradation of TXNIP upon energy stress leads to enhanced glucose uptake via GLUT1. Molecular Cell. 2013;**49**:1167-1175. DOI: 10.1016/j.molcel.2013.01.035

[7] Chavez JA, Roach WG, Keller SR, Lane WS, Lienhard GE. Inhibition of GLUT4 translocation by Tbc1d1, a Rab GTPase-activating protein abundant in skeletal muscle, is partially relieved by AMP-activated protein kinase activation. The Journal of Biological Chemistry. 2008;**283**:9187-9195. DOI: 10.1074/jbc.M708934200

[8] Bultot L, Guigas B, Von Wilamowitz-Moellendorff A, Maisin L, Vertommen D, Hussain N, et al. AMP-activated protein kinase phosphorylates and inactivates liver glycogen synthase. The Biochemical Journal. 2012;**443**:193-203. DOI: 10.1042/BJ20112026

[9] Miller RA, Birnbaum MJ. An energetic tale of AMPK-independent effects of metformin. The Journal of Clinical Investigation. 2010;**120**:2267-2270. DOI: 10.1172/JCI43661

[10] Shin NR, Lee JC, Lee HY, Kim MS, Whon TW, Lee MS, et al. An increase in the Akkermansia spp. population induced by metformin treatment improves glucose homeostasis in diet-induced obese mice. Gut. 2014;**63**:727-735. DOI: 10.1136/gutjnl-2012-303839

[11] MacNeil LT, Schertzer JD, Steinberg GR. Bacteria transmit metformin-associated lifespan extension. Nature Reviews. Endocrinology. 2019;**16**:9-10. DOI: 10.1038/s41574-019-0278-3

[12] Collier CA, Bruce CR, Smith AC, Lopaschuk G, Dyck DJ. Metformin counters the insulin-induced suppression of fatty acid oxidation and stimulation of triacylglycerol storage in rodent skeletal muscle. American Journal of Physiology. Endocrinology and Metabolism. 2006;**291**:E182-E189. DOI: 10.1152/ajpendo.00272.2005

[13] Grapov D, Fiehn O, Campbell C, Chandler CJ, Burnett DJ, Souza EC, et al. Exercise plasma metabolomics and xenometabolomics in obese, sedentary, insulin-resistant women: Impact of a fitness and weight loss intervention. American Journal of Physiology.

Endocrinology and Metabolism. 2019;**317**:E999-E1014. DOI: 10.1152/ajpendo.00091.2019

[14] Zhao L, Fu Z, Wu J, Aylor KW, Barrett EJ, Cao W, et al. Inflammation-induced microvascular insulin resistance is an early event in diet-induced obesity. Clinical Science (London, England). 2015;**129**:1025-1036. DOI: 10.1042/CS20150143

[15] Sjoberg KA, Rattigan S, Jeppesen JF, Lundsgaard AM, Holst JJ, Kiens B. Differential effects of glucagon-like peptide-1 on microvascular recruitment and glucose metabolism in short- and long-term insulin resistance. The Journal of Physiology. 2015;**593**:2185-2198. DOI: 10.1113/JP270129

[16] Bradley EA, Premilovac D, Betik AC, Hu D, Attrill E, Richards S, et al. Metformin improves vascular and metabolic insulin action in insulin resistant muscle. The Journal of Endocrinology. 2019;**243**:85-96. DOI: 10.1530/JOE-19-0067

[17] Giannarelli R, Aragona M, Coppelli A, Del Prato S. Reducing insulin resistance with metformin: The evidence today. Diabetes & Metabolism. 2003;**29**:6S28-6S35. DOI: 10.1016/s1262-3636(03)72785-2

[18] Adeva-Andany MM, Martinez-Rodriguez J, Gonzalez-Lucan M, Fernandez-Fernandez C, Castro-Quintela E. Insulin resistance is a cardiovascular risk factor in humans. Diabetes and Metabolic Syndrome: Clinical Research and Reviews. 2019;**13**:1449-1455. DOI: 10.1016/j.dsx.2019.02.023

[19] Varvel SA, Voros S, Thiselton DL, Pottala JV, Dall T, Warnick GR, et al. Comprehensive biomarker testing of glycemia, insulin resistance, and beta cell function has greater sensitivity to detect diabetes risk than fasting glucose and HbA1c and is associated with improved glycemic control in clinical practice. Journal of Cardiovascular Translational Research. 2014;**7**:597-606. DOI: 10.1007/s12265-014-9577-1

[20] Newgard CB, An J, Bain JR, Muehlbauer MJ, Stevens RD, Lien LF, et al. A branched-chain amino acid-related metabolic signature that differentiates obese and lean humans and contributes to insulin resistance. Cell Metabolism. 2009;**9**:311-326. DOI: 10.1016/j.cmet.2009.02.002

[21] Lee W, Lee HJ, Jang HB, Kim HJ, Ban HJ, Kim KY, et al. Asymmetric dimethylarginine (ADMA) is identified as a potential biomarker of insulin resistance in skeletal muscle. Scientific Reports. 2018;**8**:2133. DOI: 10.1038/s41598-018-20549-0

[22] Zemdegs J, Martin H, Pintana H, Bullich S, Manta S, Marques MA, et al. Metformin promotes anxiolytic and antidepressant-like responses in insulin-resistant mice by decreasing circulating branched-chain amino acids. The Journal of Neuroscience. 2019;**39**:5935-5948. DOI: 10.1523/JNEUROSCI.2904-18.2019

[23] Asagami T, Abbasi F, Stuelinger M, Lamendola C, McLaughlin T, Cooke JP, et al. Metformin treatment lowers asymmetric dimethylarginine concentrations in patients with type 2 diabetes. Metabolism. 2002;**51**:843-846. DOI: 10.1053/meta.2002.33349

[24] Granado M, Amor S, Martin-Carro B, Guerra-Menendez L, Tejera-Munoz A, Gonzalez-Hedstrom D, et al. Caloric restriction attenuates aging-induced cardiac insulin resistance in male Wistar rats through activation of PI3K/Akt pathway. Nutrition, Metabolism, and Cardiovascular Diseases. 2019;**29**:97-105. DOI: 10.1016/j.numecd.2018.09.005

[25] Fang P, Yu M, Zhang L, Wan D, Shi M, Zhu Y, et al. Baicalin against obesity and insulin resistance through

activation of AKT/AS160/GLUT4 pathway. Molecular and Cellular Endocrinology. 2017;**448**:77-86. DOI: 10.1016/j.mce.2017.03.027

[26] Ke B, Ke X, Wan X, Yang Y, Huang Y, Qin J, et al. Astragalus polysaccharides attenuates TNF-alpha-induced insulin resistance via suppression of miR-721 and activation of PPAR-gamma and PI3K/AKT in 3T3-L1 adipocytes. American Journal of Translational Research. 2017;**9**:2195-2206

[27] Ooi J, Adamu HA, Imam MU, Ithnin H, Ismail M. Polyphenol-rich ethyl acetate fraction isolated from *Molineria latifolia* ameliorates insulin resistance in experimental diabetic rats via IRS1/AKT activation. Biomedicine & Pharmacotherapy. 2018;**98**:125-133. DOI: 10.1016/j.biopha.2017.12.002

[28] Yang S, Chen Z, Cao M, Li R, Wang Z, Zhang M. Pioglitazone ameliorates Abeta42 deposition in rats with diet-induced insulin resistance associated with AKT/GSK3beta activation. Molecular Medicine Reports. 2017;**15**:2588-2594. DOI: 10.3892/mmr.2017.6342

[29] Zhang Z, Liu H, Liu J. Akt activation: A potential strategy to ameliorate insulin resistance. Diabetes Research and Clinical Practice. 2017;**156**:107092. DOI: 10.1016/j.diabres.2017.10.004

[30] Hajduch E, Litherland GJ, Hundal HS. Protein kinase B (PKB/Akt)—A key regulator of glucose transport? FEBS Letters. 2001;**492**:199-203. DOI: 10.1016/s0014-5793(01)02242-6

[31] Chan TO, Rittenhouse SE, Tsichlis PN. AKT/PKB and other D3 phosphoinositide-regulated kinases: Kinase activation by phosphoinositide-dependent phosphorylation. Annual Review of Biochemistry. 1999;**68**:965-1014. DOI: 10.1146/annurev.biochem.68.1.965

[32] Garofalo RS, Orena SJ, Rafidi K, Torchia AJ, Stock JL, Hildebrandt AL, et al. Severe diabetes, age-dependent loss of adipose tissue, and mild growth deficiency in mice lacking Akt2/PKB beta. The Journal of Clinical Investigation. 2003;**112**:197-208. DOI: 10.1172/JCI16885

[33] Thomas H, Reynold EM, Cinquino N, Gaugler M. Effects of aging on insulin action and AkT signaling is isoform specific AKT knockout mice. The FASEB Journal. 2011;**25**:supplement-Ib-1

[34] Tsuchiya A, Kanno T, Nishizaki T. PI3 kinase directly phosphorylates Akt1/2 at Ser473/474 in the insulin signal transduction pathway. The Journal of Endocrinology. 2014;**220**:49-59. DOI: 10.1530/JOE-13-0172

[35] Beg M, Abdullah N, Thowfeik FS, Altorki NK, McGraw TE. Distinct Akt phosphorylation states are required for insulin regulated Glut4 and Glut1-mediated glucose uptake. eLife. 2017;**6**:1-22. DOI: 10.7554/eLife.26896

[36] Wang Z, Wang Y, Han Y, Yin Q, Hu S, Zhao T, et al. Akt is a critical node of acute myocardial insulin resistance and cardiac dysfunction after cardiopulmonary bypass. Life Sciences. 2019;**234**:116734. DOI: 10.1016/j.lfs.2019.116734

[37] Garabadu D, Krishnamurthy S. Metformin attenuates hepatic insulin resistance in type-2 diabetic rats through PI3K/Akt/GLUT-4 signalling independent to bicuculline-sensitive GABAA receptor stimulation. Pharmaceutical Biology. 2017;**55**:722-728. DOI: 10.1080/13880209.2016.1268635

[38] Shen X, Wang L, Zhou N, Gai S, Liu X, Zhang S. Beneficial effects of combination therapy of phloretin and metformin in streptozotocin-induced

diabetic rats and improved insulin sensitivity in vitro. Food & Function. 2020;**11**:392-403. DOI: 10.1039/c9fo01326a

[39] Chutkow WA, Birkenfeld AL, Brown JD, Lee HY, Frederick DW, Yoshioka J, et al. Deletion of the alpha-arrestin protein Txnip in mice promotes adiposity and adipogenesis while preserving insulin sensitivity. Diabetes. 2010;**59**:1424-1434. DOI: 10.2337/db09-1212

[40] Nasoohi S, Parveen K, Ishrat T. Metabolic syndrome, brain insulin resistance, and Alzheimer's disease: Thioredoxin interacting protein (TXNIP) and Inflammasome as Core amplifiers. Journal of Alzheimer's Disease. 2018;**66**:857-885. DOI: 10.3233/JAD-180735

[41] Parikh H, Carlsson E, Chutkow WA, Johansson LE, Storgaard H, Poulsen P, et al. TXNIP regulates peripheral glucose metabolism in humans. PLoS Medicine. 2007;**4**:e158. DOI: 10.1371/journal.pmed.0040158

[42] Li X, Kover KL, Heruth DP, Watkins DJ, Guo Y, Moore WV, et al. Thioredoxin-interacting protein promotes high-glucose-induced macrovascular endothelial dysfunction. Biochemical and Biophysical Research Communications. 2017;**493**:291-297. DOI: 10.1016/j.bbrc.2017.09.028

[43] Waldhart AN, Dykstra H, Peck AS, Boguslawski EA, Madaj ZB, Wen J, et al. Phosphorylation of TXNIP by AKT mediates acute influx of glucose in response to insulin. Cell Reports. 2017;**19**:2005-2013. DOI: 10.1016/j.celrep.2017.05.041

[44] Tao X, Cai L, Chen L, Ge S, Deng X. Effects of metformin and Exenatide on insulin resistance and AMPKalpha-SIRT1 molecular pathway in PCOS rats. Journal of Ovarian Research. 2019;**12**:86. DOI: 10.1186/s13048-019-0555-8

[45] American Diabetes A. 2. Classification and diagnosis of Diabetes: Standards of medical Care in Diabetes-2019. Diabetes Care. 2019;**42**:S13-S28. DOI: 10.2337/dc19-S002

[46] CDCP. Center for Disease Control and Prevention, Prediabetes: Your Chance to Prevent Type 2 Diabetes. 2020. Available from : http://cdc.gov/diabetes

[47] Metformin for Prediabetes. JAMA. 2017;**317**:1171. DOI: 10.1001/jama.2016.17844

[48] Hostalek U, Gwilt M, Hildemann S. Therapeutic use of metformin in prediabetes and diabetes prevention. Drugs. 2015;**75**:1071-1094. DOI: 10.1007/s40265-015-0416-8

[49] Naidoo P, Wing J, Rambiritch V. Effect of sitagliptin and metformin on prediabetes progression to type 2 Diabetes - a randomized, double-blind, double-arm, multicenter clinical trial: Protocol for the Sitagliptin and metformin in PreDiabetes (SiMePreD) study. JMIR Research Protocols. 2016;**5**:e145. DOI: 10.2196/resprot.5073

[50] Khokhar A, Umpaichitra V, Chin VL, Perez-Colon S. Metformin use in children and adolescents with Prediabetes. Pediatric Clinics of North America. 2017;**64**:1341-1353. DOI: 10.1016/j.pcl.2017.08.010

[51] Knowler WC, Barrett-Connor E, Fowler SE, Hamman RF, Lachin JM, Walker EA, et al. Reduction in the incidence of type 2 diabetes with lifestyle intervention or metformin. The New England Journal of Medicine. 2002;**346**:393-403. DOI: 10.1056/NEJMoa012512

[52] Diabetes Prevention Program Research G. Long-term effects of

lifestyle intervention or metformin on diabetes development and microvascular complications over 15-year follow-up: The Diabetes prevention program outcomes study. The Lancet Diabetes and Endocrinology. 2015;**3**:866-875. DOI: 10.1016/S2213-8587(15)00291-0

[53] Ratner RE, Christophi CA, Metzger BE, Dabelea D, Bennett PH, Pi-Sunyer X, et al. Prevention of diabetes in women with a history of gestational diabetes: Effects of metformin and lifestyle interventions. The Journal of Clinical Endocrinology and Metabolism. 2008;**93**:4774-4779. DOI: 10.1210/jc.2008-0772

[54] Moin T, Li J, Duru OK, Ettner S, Turk N, Keckhafer A, et al. Metformin prescription for insured adults with prediabetes from 2010 to 2012: A retrospective cohort study. Annals of Internal Medicine. 2015;**162**:542-548. DOI: 10.7326/M14-1773

[55] American Diabetes A. 3. Prevention or delay of type 2 Diabetes: Standards of medical Care in Diabetes-2019. Diabetes Care. 2019;**42**:S29-S33. DOI: 10.2337/dc19-S003

[56] Diabetes Canada Clinical Practice Guidelines Expert C, Houlden RL. Introduction. Canadian Journal of Diabetes. 2018;**42**(Suppl 1): S1-S5. DOI: 10.1016/j.jcjd.2017.10.001

[57] Cahn A, Cernea S, Raz I. An update on DPP-4 inhibitors in the management of type 2 diabetes. Expert Opinion on Emerging Drugs. 2016;**21**:409-419. DOI: 10.1080/14728214.2016.1257608

[58] Marin-Penalver JJ, Martin-Timon I, Sevillano-Collantes C, Del Canizo-Gomez FJ. Update on the treatment of type 2 diabetes mellitus. World Journal of Diabetes. 2016;**7**: 354-395. DOI: 10.4239/wjd.v7.i17.354

[59] Flory JH, Hennessy S, Bailey CJ, Inzucchi SE. Reports of lactic acidosis attributed to metformin, 2015-2018. Diabetes Care. 2019;**43**:244-246. DOI: 10.2337/dc19-0923

[60] Deden LN, Aarts EO, Aelfers SCW, van Borren M, Janssen IMC, Berends FJ, et al. Risk of metformin-associated lactic acidosis (MALA) in patients after gastric bypass surgery. Obesity Surgery. 2018;**28**:1080-1085. DOI: 10.1007/s11695-017-2974-1

[61] Angioi A, Cabiddu G, Conti M, Pili G, Atzeni A, Matta V, et al. Metformin associated lactic acidosis: A case series of 28 patients treated with sustained low-efficiency dialysis (SLED) and long-term follow-up. BMC Nephrology. 2018;**19**:77. DOI: 10.1186/s12882-018-0875-8

[62] Lipska KJ, Flory JH, Hennessy S, Inzucchi SE. Citizen petition to the US food and drug administration to change prescribing guidelines: The metformin experience. Circulation. 2016;**134**:1405-1408. DOI: 10.1161/CIRCULATIONAHA.116.023041

[63] Aroda VR, Edelstein SL, Goldberg RB, Knowler WC, Marcovina SM, Orchard TJ, et al. Long-term metformin use and vitamin B12 deficiency in the diabetes prevention program outcomes study. The Journal of Clinical Endocrinology and Metabolism. 2016;**101**:1754-1761. DOI: 10.1210/jc.2015-3754

[64] Alvarez M, Sierra OR, Saavedra G, Moreno S. Vitamin B12 deficiency and diabetic neuropathy in patients taking metformin: A cross-sectional study. Endocrine Connections. 2019;**8**:1324-1329. DOI: 10.1530/EC-19-0382

[65] Patel JJ, Mundi MS. Metformin for Type 2 Diabetes. Journal of the American Medical Association. 2019;**322**:1312-1313. DOI: 10.1001/jama.2019.11497

[66] Priya G, Kalra S. A review of insulin resistance in type 1 diabetes: Is there a place for adjunctive metformin?

Diabetes Therapy. 2018;**9**:349-361. DOI: 10.1007/s13300-017-0333-9

[67] George P, McCrimmon RJ. Potential role of non-insulin adjunct therapy in type 1 diabetes. Diabetic Medicine. 2013;**30**:179-188. DOI: 10.1111/j.1464-5491.2012.03744.x

[68] Lund SS, Tarnow L, Astrup AS, Hovind P, Jacobsen PK, Alibegovic AC, et al. Effect of adjunct metformin treatment in patients with type-1 diabetes and persistent inadequate glycaemic control. A randomized study. PLoS One. 2008;**3**:e3363. DOI: 10.1371/journal.pone.0003363

[69] Jacobsen IB, Henriksen JE, Beck-Nielsen H. The effect of metformin in overweight patients with type 1 diabetes and poor metabolic control. Basic & Clinical Pharmacology & Toxicology. 2009;**105**:145-149. DOI: 10.1111/j.1742-7843.2009.00380.x

[70] Moon RJ, Bascombe LA, Holt RI. The addition of metformin in type 1 diabetes improves insulin sensitivity, diabetic control, body composition and patient well-being. Diabetes, Obesity & Metabolism. 2007;**9**:143-145. DOI: 10.1111/j.1463-1326.2006.00599.x

[71] Beysel S, Unsal IO, Kizilgul M, Caliskan M, Ucan B, Cakal E. The effects of metformin in type 1 diabetes mellitus. BMC Endocrine Disorders. 2018;**18**:1. DOI: 10.1186/s12902-017-0228-9

[72] Jones KL, Arslanian S, Peterokova VA, Park JS, Tomlinson MJ. Effect of metformin in pediatric patients with type 2 diabetes: A randomized controlled trial. Diabetes Care. 2002;**25**:89-94. DOI: 10.2337/diacare.25.1.89

[73] Group TS, Zeitler P, Epstein L, Grey M, Hirst K, Kaufman F, et al. Treatment options for type 2 diabetes in adolescents and youth: A study of the comparative efficacy of metformin alone or in combination with rosiglitazone or lifestyle intervention in adolescents with type 2 diabetes. Pediatric Diabetes. 2007;**8**:74-87. DOI: 10.1111/j.1399-5448.2007.00237.x

[74] Group TS, Zeitler P, Hirst K, Pyle L, Linder B, Copeland K, et al. A clinical trial to maintain glycemic control in youth with type 2 diabetes. The New England Journal of Medicine. 2012;**366**:2247-2256. DOI: 10.1056/NEJMoa1109333

[75] Nadeau KJ, Chow K, Alam S, Lindquist K, Campbell S, McFann K, et al. Effects of low dose metformin in adolescents with type I diabetes mellitus: A randomized, double-blinded placebo-controlled study. Pediatric Diabetes. 2015;**16**:196-203. DOI: 10.1111/pedi.12140

[76] Cree-Green M, Bergman BC, Cengiz E, Fox LA, Hannon TS, Miller K, et al. Metformin improves peripheral insulin sensitivity in youth with type 1 diabetes. The Journal of Clinical Endocrinology and Metabolism. 2019;**104**:3265-3278. DOI: 10.1210/jc.2019-00129

[77] Anderson JJA, Couper JJ, Giles LC, Leggett CE, Gent R, Coppin B, et al. Effect of metformin on vascular function in children with type 1 diabetes: A 12-month randomized controlled trial. The Journal of Clinical Endocrinology and Metabolism. 2017;**102**:4448-4456. DOI: 10.1210/jc.2017-00781

[78] Bjornstad P, Schafer M, Truong U, Cree-Green M, Pyle L, Baumgartner A, et al. Metformin improves insulin sensitivity and vascular health in youth with type 1 diabetes mellitus. Circulation. 2018;**138**:2895-2907. DOI: 10.1161/CIRCULATIONAHA.118.035525

[79] Sarnblad S, Kroon M, Aman J. Metformin as additional therapy in adolescents with poorly

controlled type 1 diabetes: Randomised placebo-controlled trial with aspects on insulin sensitivity. European Journal of Endocrinology. 2003;**149**:323-329. DOI: 10.1530/eje.0.1490323

[80] Urakami T, Morimoto S, Owada M, Harada K. Usefulness of the addition of metformin to insulin in pediatric patients with type 1 diabetes mellitus. Pediatrics International. 2005;**47**:430-433. DOI: 10.1111/j.1442-200x.2005.02075.x

[81] Libman IM, Miller KM, DiMeglio LA, Bethin KE, Katz ML, Shah A, et al. Effect of metformin added to insulin on glycemic control among overweight/obese adolescents with type 1 diabetes: A randomized clinical trial. JAMA. 2015;**314**:2241-2250. DOI: 10.1001/jama.2015.16174

[82] Soukas AA, Hao H, Wu L. Metformin as anti-aging therapy: Is it for everyone? Trends in Endocrinology and Metabolism. 2019;**30**:745-755. DOI: 10.1016/j.tem.2019.07.015

[83] Anisimov VN, Berstein LM, Egormin PA, Piskunova TS, Popovich IG, Zabezhinski MA, et al. Metformin slows down aging and extends life span of female SHR mice. Cell Cycle. 2008;**7**:2769-2773. DOI: 10.4161/cc.7.17.6625

[84] Anisimov VN, Berstein LM, Popovich IG, Zabezhinski MA, Egormin PA, Piskunova TS, et al. If started early in life, metformin treatment increases life span and postpones tumors in female SHR mice. Aging (Albany NY). 2011;**3**:148-157. DOI: 10.18632/aging.100273

[85] Anisimov VN, Egormin PA, Piskunova TS, Popovich IG, Tyndyk ML, Yurova MN, et al. Metformin extends life span of HER-2/neu transgenic mice and in combination with melatonin inhibits growth of transplantable tumors in vivo. Cell Cycle. 2010;**9**:188-197. DOI: 10.4161/cc.9.1.10407

[86] Pigazzi M, Ricotti E, Germano G, Faggian D, Arico M, Basso G. cAMP response element binding protein (CREB) overexpression CREB has been described as critical for leukemia progression. Haematologica. 2007;**92**:1435-1437. DOI: 10.3324/haematol.11122

[87] Martin-Montalvo A, Mercken EM, Mitchell SJ, Palacios HH, Mote PL, Scheibye-Knudsen M, et al. Metformin improves healthspan and lifespan in mice. Nature Communications. 2013;**4**:2192. DOI: 10.1038/ncomms3192

[88] Konturek PC, Haziri D, Brzozowski T, Hess T, Heyman S, Kwiecien S, et al. Emerging role of fecal microbiota therapy in the treatment of gastrointestinal and extra-gastrointestinal diseases. Journal of Physiology and Pharmacology. 2015;**66**:483-491

[89] Vaiserman AM, Koliada AK, Marotta F. Gut microbiota: A player in aging and a target for anti-aging intervention. Ageing Research Reviews. 2017;**35**:36-45. DOI: 10.1016/j.arr.2017.01.001

[90] Pryor R, Norvaisas P, Marinos G, Best L, Thingholm LB, Quintaneiro LM, et al. Host-microbe-drug-nutrient screen identifies bacterial effectors of metformin therapy. Cell. 2019;**178**:1299-1312.e29. DOI: 10.1016/j.cell.2019.08.003

[91] Kulkarni AS, Brutsaert EF, Anghel V, Zhang K, Bloomgarden N, Pollak M, et al. Metformin regulates metabolic and nonmetabolic pathways in skeletal muscle and subcutaneous adipose tissues of older adults. Aging Cell. 2018;**17**:e12713. DOI: 10.1111/acel.12723

[92] March WA, Moore VM, Willson KJ, Phillips DI, Norman RJ, Davies MJ. The prevalence of polycystic ovary syndrome in a community sample assessed under

contrasting diagnostic criteria. Human Reproduction. 2010;**25**:544-551. DOI: 10.1093/humrep/dep399

[93] Morley LC, Tang T, Yasmin E, Norman RJ, Balen AH. Insulin-sensitising drugs (metformin, rosiglitazone, pioglitazone, D-chiro-inositol) for women with polycystic ovary syndrome, oligo amenorrhoea and subfertility. Cochrane Database of Systematic Reviews. 2017;**11**:CD003053. DOI: 10.1002/14651858.CD003053.pub6

[94] Nandi A, Chen Z, Patel R, Poretsky L. Polycystic ovary syndrome. Endocrinology and Metabolism Clinics of North America. 2014;**43**:123-147. DOI: 10.1016/j.ecl.2013.10.003

[95] Velazquez EM, Mendoza S, Hamer T, Sosa F, Glueck CJ. Metformin therapy in polycystic ovary syndrome reduces hyperinsulinemia, insulin resistance, hyperandrogenemia, and systolic blood pressure, while facilitating normal menses and pregnancy. Metabolism. 1994;**43**:647-654. DOI: 10.1016/0026-0495(94)90209-7

[96] Moghetti P, Castello R, Negri C, Tosi F, Perrone F, Caputo M, et al. Metformin effects on clinical features, endocrine and metabolic profiles, and insulin sensitivity in polycystic ovary syndrome: A randomized, double-blind, placebo-controlled 6-month trial, followed by open, long-term clinical evaluation. The Journal of Clinical Endocrinology and Metabolism. 2000;**85**:139-146. DOI: 10.1210/jcem.85.1.6293

[97] Hirsch A, Hahn D, Kempna P, Hofer G, Nuoffer JM, Mullis PE, et al. Metformin inhibits human androgen production by regulating steroidogenic enzymes HSD3B2 and CYP17A1 and complex I activity of the respiratory chain. Endocrinology. 2012;**153**: 4354-4366. DOI: 10.1210/en.2012-1145

[98] Zheng J, Shan PF, Gu W. The efficacy of metformin in pregnant women with polycystic ovary syndrome: A meta-analysis of clinical trials. Journal of Endocrinological Investigation. 2013;**36**:797-802. DOI: 10.3275/8932

[99] Glueck CJ, Goldenberg N, Pranikoff J, Khan Z, Padda J, Wang P. Effects of metformin-diet intervention before and throughout pregnancy on obstetric and neonatal outcomes in patients with polycystic ovary syndrome. Current Medical Research and Opinion. 2013;**29**:55-62. DOI: 10.1185/03007995.2012.755121

[100] Lautatzis ME, Goulis DG, Vrontakis M. Efficacy and safety of metformin during pregnancy in women with gestational diabetes mellitus or polycystic ovary syndrome: A systematic review. Metabolism. 2013;**62**:1522-1534. DOI: 10.1016/j.metabol.2013.06.006

[101] Ganie MA, Khurana ML, Nisar S, Shah PA, Shah ZA, Kulshrestha B, et al. Improved efficacy of low-dose spironolactone and metformin combination than either drug alone in the management of women with polycystic ovary syndrome (PCOS): A six-month, open-label randomized study. The Journal of Clinical Endocrinology and Metabolism. 2013;**98**:3599-3607. DOI: 10.1210/jc.2013-1040

[102] Costello M, Garad R, Hart R, Homer H, Johnson L, Jordan C, et al. A review of first line infertility treatments and supporting evidence in women with polycystic ovary syndrome. Medical Sciences (Basel). 2019;**7**:1-10. DOI: 10.3390/medsci7090095

[103] Elter K, Imir G, Durmusoglu F. Clinical, endocrine and metabolic effects of metformin added to ethinyl estradiol-cyproterone acetate in non-obese women with polycystic ovarian syndrome: A randomized controlled study. Human Reproduction. 2002;**17**:1729-1737. DOI: 10.1093/humrep/17.7.1729

[104] Di Pietro M, Parborell F, Irusta G, Pascuali N, Bas D, Bianchi MS, et al. Metformin regulates ovarian angiogenesis and follicular development in a female polycystic ovary syndrome rat model. Endocrinology. 2015;**156**:1453-1463. DOI: 10.1210/en.2014-1765

[105] Han Y, Xie H, Liu Y, Gao P, Yang X, Shen Z. Effect of metformin on all-cause and cardiovascular mortality in patients with coronary artery diseases: A systematic review and an updated meta-analysis. Cardiovascular Diabetology. 2019;**18**:96. DOI: 10.1186/s12933-019-0900-7

[106] Rena G, Lang CC. Repurposing metformin for cardiovascular disease. Circulation. 2018;**137**:422-424. DOI: 10.1161/CIRCULATIONAHA.117.031735

[107] Dore FJ, Domingues CC, Ahmadi N, Kundu N, Kropotova Y, Houston S, et al. The synergistic effects of saxagliptin and metformin on CD34+ endothelial progenitor cells in early type 2 diabetes patients: A randomized clinical trial. Cardiovascular Diabetology. 2018;**17**:65. DOI: 10.1186/s12933-018-0709-9

[108] Kooy A, de Jager J, Lehert P, Bets D, Wulffele MG, Donker AJ, et al. Long-term effects of metformin on metabolism and microvascular and macrovascular disease in patients with type 2 diabetes mellitus. Archives of Internal Medicine. 2009;**169**:616-625. DOI: 10.1001/archinternmed.2009.20

[109] Griffin SJ, Leaver JK, Irving GJ. I mpact of metformin on cardiovascular disease: A meta-analysis of randomised trials among people with type 2 diabetes. Diabetologia. 2017;**60**:1620-1629. DOI: 10.1007/s00125-017-4337-9

[110] Boussageon R, Gueyffier F, Cornu C. Metformin as firstline treatment for type 2 diabetes: Are we sure? BMJ. 2016;**352**:h6748. DOI: 10.1136/bmj.h6748

[111] Boussageon R, Supper I, Bejan-Angoulvant T, Kellou N, Cucherat M, Boissel JP, et al. Reappraisal of metformin efficacy in the treatment of type 2 diabetes: A meta-analysis of randomised controlled trials. PLoS Medicine. 2012;**9**:e1001204. DOI: 10.1371/journal.pmed.1001204

[112] Loi H, Boal F, Tronchere H, Cinato M, Kramar S, Oleshchuk O, et al. Metformin protects the heart against hypertrophic and apoptotic remodeling after myocardial infarction. Frontiers in Pharmacology. 2019;**10**:154. DOI: 10.3389/fphar.2019.00154

[113] Bonow RO, Gheorghiade M. The diabetes epidemic: A national and global crisis. The American Journal of Medicine. 2004;**116**(Suppl 5A):2S-10S. DOI: 10.1016/j.amjmed.2003.10.014

[114] Bashier A, Bin Hussain A, Abdelgadir E, Alawadi F, Sabbour H, Chilton R. Consensus recommendations for management of patients with type 2 diabetes mellitus and cardiovascular diseases. Diabetology and Metabolic Syndrome. 2019;**11**:80. DOI: 10.1186/s13098-019-0476-0

[115] Harrington JL, de Albuquerque Rocha N, Patel KV, Verma S, McGuire DK. Should metformin remain first-line medical therapy for patients with type 2 diabetes mellitus and atherosclerotic cardiovascular disease? An alternative approach. Current Diabetes Reports. 2018;**18**:64. DOI: 10.1007/s11892-018-1035-z

[116] Wong AK, Symon R, AlZadjali MA, Ang DS, Ogston S, Choy A, et al. The effect of metformin on insulin resistance and exercise parameters in patients with heart failure. European Journal of Heart Failure. 2012;**14**:1303-1310. DOI: 10.1093/eurjhf/hfs106

[117] Petrie JR, Chaturvedi N, Ford I, Brouwers M, Greenlaw N, Tillin T, et al. Cardiovascular and metabolic effects

of metformin in patients with type 1 diabetes (REMOVAL): A double-blind, randomised, placebo-controlled trial. The Lancet Diabetes and Endocrinology. 2017;**5**:597-609. DOI: 10.1016/S2213-8587(17)30194-8

[118] Jadhav S, Ferrell W, Greer IA, Petrie JR, Cobbe SM, Sattar N. Effects of metformin on microvascular function and exercise tolerance in women with angina and normal coronary arteries: A randomized, double-blind, placebo-controlled study. Journal of the American College of Cardiology. 2006;**48**:956-963. DOI: 10.1016/j.jacc.2006.04.088

[119] Griffin SJ, Bethel MA, Holman RR, Khunti K, Wareham N, Brierley G, et al. Metformin in non-diabetic hyperglycaemia: The GLINT feasibility RCT. Health Technology Assessment. 2018;**22**:1-64. DOI: 10.3310/hta22180

[120] Giovannucci E, Harlan DM, Archer MC, Bergenstal RM, Gapstur SM, Habel LA, et al. Diabetes and cancer: A consensus report. CA: a Cancer Journal for Clinicians. 2010;**60**:207-221. DOI: 10.3322/caac.20078

[121] Evans JM, Donnelly LA, Emslie-Smith AM, Alessi DR, Morris AD. Metformin and reduced risk of cancer in diabetic patients. BMJ. 2005;**330**:1304-1305. DOI: 10.1136/bmj.38415.708634.F7

[122] Hosono K, Endo H, Takahashi H, Sugiyama M, Sakai E, Uchiyama T, et al. Metformin suppresses colorectal aberrant crypt foci in a short-term clinical trial. Cancer Prevention Research (Philadelphia, Pa.). 2010;**3**:1077-1083. DOI: 10.1158/1940-6207.CAPR-10-0186

[123] Hadad S, Iwamoto T, Jordan L, Purdie C, Bray S, Baker L, et al. Evidence for biological effects of metformin in operable breast cancer: A pre-operative, window-of-opportunity, randomized trial. Breast Cancer Research and Treatment. 2011;**128**:783-794. DOI: 10.1007/s10549-011-1612-1

[124] Camacho L, Dasgupta A, Jiralerspong S. Metformin in breast cancer - an evolving mystery. Breast Cancer Research. 2015;**17**:88. DOI: 10.1186/s13058-015-0598-8

[125] Coyle C, Cafferty FH, Vale C, Langley RE. Metformin as an adjuvant treatment for cancer: A systematic review and meta-analysis. Annals of Oncology. 2016;**27**:2184-2195. DOI: 10.1093/annonc/mdw410

[126] Saraei P, Asadi I, Kakar MA, Moradi-Kor N. The beneficial effects of metformin on cancer prevention and therapy: A comprehensive review of recent advances. Cancer Management and Research. 2019;**11**:3295-3313. DOI: 10.2147/CMAR.S200059

[127] Dulskas A, Patasius A, Linkeviciute-Ulinskiene D, Zabuliene L, Urbonas V, Smailyte G. Metformin increases cancer specific survival in colorectal cancer patients-national cohort study. Cancer Epidemiology. 2019;**62**:101587. DOI: 10.1016/j.canep.2019.101587

[128] Vancura A, Bu P, Bhagwat M, Zeng J, Vancurova I. Metformin as an anticancer agent. Trends in Pharmacological Sciences. 2018;**39**:867-878. DOI: 10.1016/j.tips.2018.07.006

[129] Bridges HR, Jones AJ, Pollak MN, Hirst J. Effects of metformin and other biguanides on oxidative phosphorylation in mitochondria. The Biochemical Journal. 2014;**462**:475-487. DOI: 10.1042/BJ20140620

[130] El-Mir MY, Nogueira V, Fontaine E, Averet N, Rigoulet M, Leverve X. Dimethylbiguanide inhibits cell respiration via an indirect effect targeted on the respiratory chain complex I. The Journal of Biological

Chemistry. 2000;**275**:223-228. DOI: 10.1074/jbc.275.1.223

[131] Pernicova I, Korbonits M. Metformin--mode of action and clinical implications for diabetes and cancer. Nature Reviews. Endocrinology. 2014;**10**:143-156. DOI: 10.1038/nrendo.2013.256

[132] Herzig S, Shaw RJ. AMPK: Guardian of metabolism and mitochondrial homeostasis. Nature Reviews. Molecular Cell Biology. 2018;**19**:121-135. DOI: 10.1038/nrm.2017.95

[133] Huang S, Houghton PJ. Targeting mTOR signaling for cancer therapy. Current Opinion in Pharmacology. 2003;**3**:371-377

[134] Vogt PK. PI 3-kinase, mTOR, protein synthesis and cancer. Trends in Molecular Medicine. 2001;**7**:482-484. DOI: 10.1616/s1471-4914(01)0216-x

[135] Schmelzle T, Hall MN. TOR, a central controller of cell growth. Cell. 2000;**103**:253-262. DOI: 10.1016/s0092-8674(00)00117-3

[136] Muller PA, Vousden KH. p53 mutations in cancer. Nature Cell Biology. 2013;**15**:2-8. DOI: 10.1038/ncb2641

[137] Jones RG, Plas DR, Kubek S, Buzzai M, Mu J, Xu Y, et al. AMP-activated protein kinase induces a p53-dependent metabolic checkpoint. Molecular Cell. 2005;**18**:283-293. DOI: 10.1016/j.molcel.2005.03.027

[138] Cerezo M, Tichet M, Abbe P, Ohanna M, Lehraiki A, Rouaud F, et al. Metformin blocks melanoma invasion and metastasis development in AMPK/p53-dependent manner. Molecular Cancer Therapeutics. 2013;**12**:1605-1615. DOI: 10.1158/1535-7163.MCT-12-1226-T

[139] Juan J, Gu QZ, Mavis C, Czuczman MS, Hernandezollizaliturri FJ. Metformin induces p53-dependent mitochondrial stress in therapy-sensitive and -resistant lymphoma pre-clinical model and primary patients sample with B-cell non-Hodgkin lymphoma (NHL). Blood. 2015;**126**:4008. DOI: 10.1181/blood.v126.23.4008.4008

[140] Ben Sahra I, Laurent K, Giuliano S, Larbret F, Ponzio G, Gounon P, et al. Targeting cancer cell metabolism: The combination of metformin and 2-deoxyglucose induces p53-dependent apoptosis in prostate cancer cells. Cancer Research. 2010;**70**:2465-2475. DOI: 10.1158/0008-5472.CAN-09-2782

[141] Yudhani RD, Astuti I, Mustofa M, Indarto D, Muthmainah M. Metformin modulates cyclin D1 and P53 expression to inhibit cell proliferation and to induce apoptosis in cervical cancer cell lines. Asian Pacific Journal of Cancer Prevention. 2019;**20**:1667-1673. DOI: 10.31557/APJCP.2019.20.6.1667

[142] Jeong YK, Kim MS, Lee JY, Kim EH, Ha H. Metformin Radiosensitizes p53-deficient colorectal Cancer cells through induction of G2/M arrest and inhibition of DNA repair proteins. PLoS One. 2015;**10**:e0143596. DOI: 10.1371/journal.pone.0143596

[143] Buzzai M, Jones RG, Amaravadi RK, Lum JJ, DeBerardinis RJ, Zhao F, et al. Systemic treatment with the antidiabetic drug metformin selectively impairs p53-deficient tumor cell growth. Cancer Research. 2007;**67**:6745-6752. DOI: 10.1158/0008-5472.CAN-06-4447

[144] Dotsch V, Bernassola F, Coutandin D, Candi E, Melino G. p63 and p73, the ancestors of p53. Cold Spring Harbor Perspectives in Biology. 2010;**2**:a004887. DOI: 10.1101/cshperspect.a004887

[145] Moses MA, George AL, Sakakibara N, Mahmood K, Ponnamperuma RM, King KE, et al. Molecular mechanisms of p63-mediated

squamous Cancer pathogenesis. International Journal of Molecular Sciences. 2019;**20**:3590. DOI: 10.3390/ijms20143590

[146] Yi Y, Chen D, Ao J, Sun S, Wu M, Li X, et al. Metformin promotes AMP-activated protein kinase-independent suppression of DeltaNp63alpha protein expression and inhibits cancer cell viability. The Journal of Biological Chemistry. 2017;**292**:5253-5261. DOI: 10.1074/jbc.M116.769141

[147] Yoon MK, Ha JH, Lee MS, Chi SW. Structure and apoptotic function of p73. BMB Reports. 2015;**48**:81-90. DOI: 10.5483/bmbrep.2015.48.2.255

[148] Adamovich Y, Adler J, Meltser V, Reuven N, Shaul Y. AMPK couples p73 with p53 in cell fate decision. Cell Death and Differentiation. 2014;**21**:1451-1459. DOI: 10.1038/cdd.2014.60

[149] Schuler KM, Rambally BS, DiFurio MJ, Sampey BP, Gehrig PA, Makowski L, et al. Antiproliferative and metabolic effects of metformin in a preoperative window clinical trial for endometrial cancer. Cancer Medicine. 2015;**4**:161-173. DOI: 10.1002/cam4.353

[150] Cha JH, Yang WH, Xia W, Wei Y, Chan LC, Lim SO, et al. Metformin promotes antitumor immunity via endoplasmic-reticulum-associated degradation of PD-L1. Molecular Cell. 2018;**71**:606-620 .e7. DOI: 10.1016/j.molcel.2018.07.030

[151] Wang YW, He SJ, Feng X, Cheng J, Luo YT, Tian L, et al. Metformin: A review of its potential indications. Drug Design, Development and Therapy. 2017;**11**:2421-2429. DOI: 10.2147/DDDT.S141675

[152] Campbell JM, Stephenson MD, de Courten B, Chapman I, Bellman SM, Aromataris E. Metformin use associated with reduced risk of dementia in patients with Diabetes: A systematic review and meta-analysis. Journal of Alzheimer's Disease. 2018;**65**:1225-1236. DOI: 10.3233/JAD-180263

[153] Moreira RO, Campos SC, Soldera AL. Type 2 Diabetes mellitus and Alzheimer's disease: From physiopathology to treatment implications. Diabetes/Metabolism Research and Reviews. 2013;**71**:365-376. DOI: 10.1002/dmrr.2442

[154] Gudala K, Bansal D, Schifano F, Bhansali A. Diabetes mellitus and risk of dementia: A meta-analysis of prospective observational studies. Journal of Diabetes Investigation. 2013;**4**:640-650. DOI: 10.1111/jdi.12087

[155] Xu W, Caracciolo B, Wang HX, Winblad B, Backman L, Qiu C, et al. Accelerated progression from mild cognitive impairment to dementia in people with diabetes. Diabetes. 2010;**59**:2928-2935. DOI: 10.2337/db10-0539

[156] Hsu CC, Wahlqvist ML, Lee MS, Tsai HN. Incidence of dementia is increased in type 2 diabetes and reduced by the use of sulfonylureas and metformin. Journal of Alzheimer's Disease. 2011;**24**:485-493. DOI: 10.3233/JAD-2011-101524

[157] Shi Q, Liu S, Fonseca VA, Thethi TK, Shi L. Effect of metformin on neurodegenerative disease among elderly adult US veterans with type 2 diabetes mellitus. BMJ Open. 2019;**9**:e024954. DOI: 10.1136/bmjopen-2018-024954

[158] Wahlqvist ML, Lee MS, Hsu CC, Chuang SY, Lee JT, Tsai HN. Metformin-inclusive sulfonylurea therapy reduces the risk of Parkinson's disease occurring with type 2 diabetes in a Taiwanese population cohort. Parkinsonism & Related Disorders. 2012;**18**:753-758. DOI: 10.1016/j.parkreldis.2012.03.010

[159] Ng TP, Feng L, Yap KB, Lee TS, Tan CH, Winblad B. Long-term metformin usage and cognitive function among older adults with diabetes. Journal of Alzheimer's Disease. 2014;**41**:61-68. DOI: 10.3233/JAD-131901

[160] Imfeld P, Bodmer M, Jick SS, Meier CR. Metformin, other antidiabetic drugs, and risk of Alzheimer's disease: A population-based case-control study. Journal of the American Geriatrics Society. 2012;**60**:916-921. DOI: 10.1111/j.1532-5415.2012.03916.x

[161] Moore EM, Mander AG, Ames D, Kotowicz MA, Carne RP, Brodaty H, et al. Increased risk of cognitive impairment in patients with diabetes is associated with metformin. Diabetes Care. 2013;**36**:2981-2987. DOI: 10.2337/dc13-0229

[162] Huang CC, Chung CM, Leu HB, Lin LY, Chiu CC, Hsu CY, et al. Diabetes mellitus and the risk of Alzheimer's disease: A nationwide population-based study. PLoS One. 2014;**9**:e87095. DOI: 10.1371/journal.pone.0087095

[163] Kuhla A, Brichmann E, Ruhlmann C, Thiele R, Meuth L, Vollmar B. Metformin therapy aggravates neurodegenerative processes in ApoE−/− mice. Journal of Alzheimer's Disease. 2019;**68**:1415-1427. DOI: 10.3233/JAD-181017

[164] Curry DW, Stutz B, Andrews ZB, Elsworth JD. Targeting AMPK signaling as a Neuroprotective strategy in Parkinson's disease. Journal of Parkinson's Disease. 2018;**8**:161-181. DOI: 10.3233/JPD-171296

[165] Kickstein E, Krauss S, Thornhill P, Rutschow D, Zeller R, Sharkey J, et al. Biguanide metformin acts on tau phosphorylation via mTOR/protein phosphatase 2A (PP2A) signaling. Proceedings of the National Academy of Sciences of the United States of America. 2010;**107**:21830-21835. DOI: 10.1073/pnas.0912793107

[166] Paseban M, Mohebbati R, Niazmand S, Sathyapalan T, Sahebkar A. Comparison of the neuroprotective effects of aspirin, atorvastatin, captopril and metformin in diabetes mellitus. Biomolecules. 2019;**9**:1-12. DOI: 10.3390/biom9040118

[167] Alzoubi KH, Khabour OF, Al-Azzam SI, Tashtoush MH, Mhaidat NM. Metformin eased cognitive impairment induced by chronic L-methionine administration: Potential role of oxidative stress. Current Neuropharmacology. 2014;**12**:186-192. DOI: 10.2174/1570159X11666131120223201

[168] Jiang T, Yu JT, Zhu XC, Wang HF, Tan MS, Cao L, et al. Acute metformin preconditioning confers neuroprotection against focal cerebral ischaemia by pre-activation of AMPK-dependent autophagy. British Journal of Pharmacology. 2014;**171**:3146-3157. DOI: 10.1111/bph.12655

[169] Venna VR, Li J, Hammond MD, Mancini NS, McCullough LD. Chronic metformin treatment improves post-stroke angiogenesis and recovery after experimental stroke. The European Journal of Neuroscience. 2014;**39**:2129-2138. DOI: 10.1111/ejn.12556

[170] Jin Q, Cheng J, Liu Y, Wu J, Wang X, Wei S, et al. Improvement of functional recovery by chronic metformin treatment is associated with enhanced alternative activation of microglia/macrophages and increased angiogenesis and neurogenesis following experimental stroke. Brain, Behavior, and Immunity. 2014;**40**:131-142. DOI: 10.1016/j.bbi.2014.03.003

Chapter 3

Metformin and Its Benefits in Improving Gut Microbiota Disturbances in Diabetes Patients

Andra Iulia-Suceveanu, Sergiu Ioan Micu, Claudia Voinea, Madalina Elena Manea, Doina Catrinoiu, Laura Mazilu, Anca Pantea Stoian, Irinel Parepa, Roxana Adriana Stoica and Adrian-Paul Suceveanu

Abstract

The human gastrointestinal tract presents a vastly population of microorganisms, called the microbiota. The presence of these microorganisms offers many benefits to the host, through a range of physiological functions. However, there is a potential for these mechanisms to be disrupted condition, known as dysbiosis. Recent results are showing important associations between diabetes and the gut microbiota and how the intestinal flora can influence the prognosis of this illness. Microbial intestinal imbalance has been linked to alterations in insulin sensitivity and in glucose metabolism and may play an important role in the development of diabetes. Metformin is one of the most important and widely used first-line medications for the management of type 2 diabetes (T2D). It is a complex drug with multiple sites of action and multiple molecular mechanisms. In recent years, attention has been directed to other modes of action, other than the classic ones, with increasing evidence of a major key role of the intestine. By analysing the effects of metformin on the homeostasis of the microbiota of diabetes patients, our present topic becomes one of the major importance in understanding how metformin therapy can improve gut microbiota dysbiosis and thus provide a better outcome for this illness.

Keywords: metformin, diabetes mellitus, gut dysbiosis, improvement, microbiota

1. Introduction

The human gastrointestinal tract hosts a complex population of microorganisms. The function and composition of the gut microbiota vary from an individual to another, factors contributing to its differences being various. The mode of birth, the type of diet, exercise, body mass index, different diseases and therapies are factors that influence the gut microbiota composition and function. Type 2 diabetes (T2D), a highly prevalent metabolic disease, is lately characterized as a disease with significant alteration of the composition and function of the gut microbiota. New therapeutic targets are revealed, and researchers are thoroughly exploring these possible pathways and hypotheses to understand the pathogeny of the disease better and also to better manage the treatment options. Metformin, one of the most widely used first-line medication for the management of type 2 diabetes, looks to present other modes of action than the classic ones involving liver metabolism. Studies proved that metformin could modulate the gut microbiota disturbances encountered in type 2 diabetes, in this way improving the outcome of the disease.

1.1 The gut microbiota: definition, development and structure

Among other things, the cohabitation of the man with the environment is at the root of the human evolution, an extraordinary example in this sense being the relationship between humans and microorganisms.

The digestive tract hosts a complex, vast and dynamic community of microorganisms, called the microbiota. Together they form a mutualist relationship, with profound implications for the host both during homeostasis and disease [1].

It is worth mentioning that the gut is not the only place where there is a population of microorganisms with which the human organism is in such a connection (e.g., the skin also harbouring a plethora of bacteria) [2].

The composition of the microbiota varies from individual to another but also from segment to segment of the digestive tract and includes species from all three domains of life: bacteria, Archaea and Eukarya. All of the species are classified into 12 different phyla, of which more than 90% belong to *Actinobacteria*, *Bacteroidetes*, *Firmicutes* and *Proteobacteria* [3].

The process of colonizing the digestive tube with microorganisms is classically believed to begin at birth by "seeding" the newborn with microorganisms originating from the mother's genital area (vaginal passage, mother's areola), the skin, and the microbiota of the contacts in the surrounding environment, and from then the development continues throughout life. In recent years, however, this theory is challenged by a series of studies that have shown the presence of microorganisms in uterine tissues (e.g., the placenta, suggesting that colonization could be initiated before birth, by haematogenous sowing) [4]. At the age of 3–4 years, the core of the microbiota is relatively defined, and its structure is similar to that of the adult but is continuously subject to change depending on various external and internal factors.

Even if the core of the microbiota is established from an early age, several factors contribute to carve its form, explaining its variations from an individual to another [5]:

- Type of birth
- Gestational age
- Diet (starting with breast milk that plays an essential role in the development of the flora)
- Ageing
- Geographic region and cultural habits
- Physical activity
- Diseases
- Drugs (especially antibiotic therapy)

As stated before, the composition also depends on the digestive tract region (biogeography), this being explained by the physiological properties of the digestive segment. For instance, in the small intestine, the pH is lower and the transit time is shorter, which is why only rapidly growing bacteria, with the ability to adhere to the surface, are thought to survive. On the other hand, the colon shows a favourable environment for the development of microorganisms. It is worth mentioning that there are differences in the composition between faecal/luminal and mucosal bacteria [6].

In its final form, this whole microsystem consists of over 2000 species, which make up altogether more than 100 trillion cells, about 10 times more than the cells of the human body, hence the name of "superorganism".

1.2 Functions

The microbiota exerts a significant influence on the host during homeostasis and disease, with profound implications for the proper body's physiological functions, considering the microbiota as a "forgotten organ".

The leading roles of the gut flora are the following:

- Mechanic barrier—strengthening the gut integrity, shaping and regenerating the intestinal epithelium, protecting against pathogens [7]
- Biologic active barrier—consuming the feeding substrates for pathogens [7]
- Key regulators of digestion—involvement in the metabolism of biliary salts, short-chain fatty acids (SCFAs), lipids and glucides [8]
- Harvesting energy [9]
- Regulating host immunity [10]
- Synthesis of vitamins—principal reservoir for B complex vitamins [11]
- Synthesis of dopamine, serotonin and other neurotransmitters [12]

1.3 Dysbiosis: definition, causes and consequences

Any perturbation of the healthy gut microbiota that disrupts the mutualist relationship between the organism and the associated microbes is called dysbiosis. The antagonist term of dysbiosis is eubiosis.

The underlying cause of a gut dysbiosis may be the following [13]:

- Unbalanced diet
- Drug therapy: antibiotics, chemotherapy, antiviral drugs and hormone therapy
- Diseases: cancers, hepatopancreatic diseases and diabetes
- Chronic and acute infections
- Local inflammation
- Presence of intestinal parasites
- Frequent enemas

The effects of dysbiosis are reflected in the processes of the internal environment, contributing to the emergence of numerous pathological conditions such as [14]:

- Autoimmune diseases [15]
- Allergies [16]
- Atherosclerosis [17]
- Obesity
- Diabetes
- Cancers [18]
- Neurological disorders [19]
- Prematurely ageing

2. Dysbiosis: microbiota in type 2 diabetes

The relationship between gut microbiota and diabetes is not fully understood, but changes in its composition and function can contribute to the onset and maintenance of insulin resistance, thus influencing the prognosis of this illness. Both T2D patients and those that are at high risk of developing this disease seem to have an imbalance in the composition and function of the microbiota, just like a "metabolic dysbiosis".

Analysing the literature, the main changes observed in the microbiota composition of diabetic patients are [20–23]:

- Reduced Gram-positive bacteria such as bacteria from phyla *Firmicutes*
- Reduced butyrate-producing bacteria, such as *Roseburia* and *Butyrivibrio*
- Decrease in bacteria that regulate intestinal permeability, such as *Akkermansia muciniphila*
- Increased Gram-negative bacteria, such as *Bacteroides*, *E. coli* and *Proteobacteria*
- Increase in various opportunistic pathogens such as *Clostridium symbiosum* and *Eggerthella lenta*

The Gram-negative bacteria (*E. coli*, *Bacteroidetes* and *Proteobacteria*) present lipopolysaccharides (LPS) at the surface of the membrane. Lipopolysaccharides are also known as endotoxins. They are large molecules consisting of a lipid and a polysaccharide composed of O-antigen with an outer core and an inner core joined by a covalent bond [24]. LPS are found to be elevated in the plasma of diabetic and obese patients by crossing an altered intestinal barrier (leaky gut). Accumulating, they trigger an inflammatory reaction called endotoxinemia. This systemic inflammatory response is associated with dyslipidaemia, increased blood pressure, but also, with insulin resistance and earlier onset of diabetes through a variety of mechanisms such as [25]:

- Activation of pro-inflammatory kinases: mitogen-activated protein kinases and I kappa B kinase complex
- Increased expression of inflammatory proteins: tumour necrosis factor-α (TNFα), monocyte chemotactic protein and interleukin 6
- Impaired insulin signalling at the level of insulin receptor substrate 1
- Inhibition of glucose transport

The passage of LPS through the intestinal mucosa is due to increased intestinal permeability (so-called leaky gut) that can be explained by the diminishing of butyrate and mucin-degrading bacteria such as *Roseburia*, *Butyrivibrio* and *Akkermansia muciniphila*. Furthermore, this epithelial dysfunction can determine an important translocation of intestinal bacteria into the adipose tissue, which maintains a low-grade inflammation and insulin resistance, process called "metabolic infection" [26, 27].

2.1 Dysbiosis: microbiota in type 1 diabetes (T1D)

At the moment, the amount of information regarding an alleged link between gut microbiota and T1D is modest. Several studies showed similarities between the disturbances of the microbiota found in T2D and T1D patients: reduced population of *Firmicutes* and increased the population of *Bacteroidetes* and increased in intestinal permeability. Increased gut permeability might contribute to pancreatic β-cell damage due to the increased absorption of exogenous antigens such as Streptomyces toxin—streptozotocin—that has tropism for pancreatic tissue and can cause lesions at its level [28].

2.1.1 Dysbiosis: protective anti-inflammatory- and anti-insulin-resistant mechanisms

There are also mechanisms mediated by the gut microbiota such as the production of short-chain fatty acids and secondary bile acids (SBA) that counteract those pro-inflammatory- and insulin-resistant effects. These mechanisms can be affected in the case of dysbiosis.

SCFAs are produced from dietary fibres that are fermented by the intestinal bacteria. Acetate, butyrate and propionate are the three most common SCFAs. They exert an essential role in the metabolism of carbohydrates, lipids, in maintaining the integrity of the intestinal barrier and in modulating inflammatory reactions through a variety of functions [29]:

- Maintaining the integrity of the colon epithelium: Butyric acid is the primary energy source of the colon's epithelial cells. It stimulates the proliferation but also the differentiation and apoptosis of the colonocyte, thus participating in the coordination of its life cycle. It also participates in the regulation of tight junction proteins (claudin 1 and zonula occludens).
- Improves carbohydrate metabolism: Propionate lowers the accumulation of lipids in the adipose tissue and reduces hepatic lipogenesis thus decreases the

insulin resistance. Propionate and acetate also stimulate the production of glucagon-like peptide-1.

- Anti-inflammatory role: Butyric acid plays an essential role in maintaining the integrity of the intestinal mucosa, preventing endotoxemia and metabolic infection. Butyric acid also inhibits the nuclear factor kappa-beta from the macrophages that cause a suppression of TNF-alpha, IL-6 and myeloperoxidase activity.

At the intestinal level, bacteria metabolize primary bile acids (cholic and chenodeoxycholic acids) to secondary bile acids (deoxycholic and lithocholic acids). Bile acids are involved in multiple metabolic pathways, research over the last decades, demonstrating an essential role against inflammation and insulin resistance. Secondary bile acids contribute to a decrease in insulin resistance through:

- Stimulating the production of glucagon-like peptide-1 by binding to G-protein-coupled receptor 1 [30]

- Modulating glucose absorption through interaction with farnesoid X receptor (FXR)

- Modulating energy expenditure: increase energy expenditure in brown adipose tissue by activating enzyme type 2 iodothyronine deiodinase and oxygen consumption, thus contributing to the prevention of obesity [31]

- Increasing triglyceride clearance

- Bile acids are the major pathway for catabolism of cholesterol, thus regulating the metabolism of lipids

In terms of their anti-inflammatory role, lithocholic acid inhibits the release of pro-inflammatory cytokines TNF-alpha, IL1 and IL6 from colon epithelium [32].

3. Metformin and the gut

Metformin presents as a sophisticated drug having multiple sites of action and various molecular mechanisms. Lately, attention has been directed to other modes of action, different than the classic ones. Its action at the intestinal level was suggested by the results of several studies that showed the following:

- A delayed-release formula is retained almost entirely in the gut, with minimal systemic absorption. It is effective at lowering blood glucose as the standard immediate-release formulation in individuals with type 2 diabetes [33].

- In diabetic rats, intravenous administration of metformin is less effective than intra-duodenal administration for lowering blood glucose levels [34].

- Human genetic studies proved that variants in SLC22A1 gene (the gene encoding OCT1), which reduce hepatic uptake of metformin, do not impact upon the efficacy of metformin to lower HbA1c in individuals with type 2 diabetes [35].

Regarding the effects of metformin on the gut microbiota, studies have shown that administration of metformin produced several changes in the composition of the intestinal flora such as the following [36]:

- Increase microbes from *Verrucomicrobiaceae*, *Porphyromonadaceae*, *Rikenellaceae*, *Akkermansia muciniphila*, and *Prevotellaceae* spp. moreover, species from *Escherichia-Shigella* sp.

- Decrease of the *Lachnospiraceae*, *Rhodobacteraceae* spp., *Peptostreptococcaceae* and *Clostridiaceae*

Furthermore by comparing the modified microbiome profile by metformin treatment, with the microbiome profiles under various disease situations, these changes have been negatively correlated with multiple diseases that have an inflammatory pathogenic substrate such as colitis, chronic diarrhoea and irritable bowel syndrome, suggesting that its anti-inflammatory proprieties can be determined through regulation of the microbiota homeostasis.

The main side effects of metformin are gastrointestinal: nausea, vomiting, diarrhoea and abdominal pain. These side effects occur most frequently at the beginning of treatment, and in most cases, they disappear spontaneously. The cause of these side effects is not fully understood and may be due to the growth of opportunistic pathogenic bacteria from *Escherichia* to *Shigella* spp. which are shown to increase at the beginning of treatment. If we relate to the increase of these opportunistic pathogens, the further reduction of side effects can be caused by a reduction of the substrate to which these microorganisms are dependent (substrates provided by polysaccharide-degrading anaerobes) through diet and an increase of anaerobic mucus-associated bacteria such as *Akkermansia muciniphila* [37].

4. Metformin and the microbiota of type 2 diabetes

As stated before, the gut microbiota profile is profoundly modified in T2D patients in terms of its structure and composition. Administration of metformin results in improved glucose metabolism, but the way this is achieved is not fully understood, and its implications upon the intestinal flora are incompletely discovered. Analysing data from the literature, administration of metformin causes the composition to change and, therefore, the physiology of the microbiota as well.

5. Metformin and *Bacteroides fragilis*

Administration of metformin is associated with an essential decrease in *Bacteroides fragilis* [38].

Bacteroides fragilis is an obligately anaerobic, Gram-negative, rod-shaped bacteria, whose essential feature in metabolic pathology is the presence of capsular lipopolysaccharides. LPS are found to be elevated in the plasma of diabetic and obese patients and are associated with dyslipidaemia and increased blood pressure but also with insulin resistance and earlier onset of diabetes through a plenty of mechanisms that have been described previously. Colonizing mice with *Bacteroides fragilis* by transferring stool samples enriched with these bacteria determines an increase in body weight, impaired glucose tolerance and a decrease in insulin sensitivity.

Mechanisms by which metformin has determined the decrease of this species have not been elucidated but have been assumed since *Bacteroides fragilis* were reduced in mice that received stool samples from patients who had been given metformin.

Besides reducing *Bacteroides fragilis*, the bile acid glycoursodeoxycholic (GUDCA) is increased through decreasing the bacteria's bile salt hydrolase activity. GUDCA is a glycine-conjugated form of the secondary bile acid deoxycholic acid, which has been known to have anti-inflammatory proprieties by reducing the levels of pro-inflammatory cytokines. Another biological function of GUDCA is to antagonize the farnesoid X receptor.

The FXR is predominantly found at the intestinal and hepatic tissue. Bile acids are the major ligands (activators) of this receptor. It is mainly involved in the metabolism of bile acids but also of carbohydrates and lipids.

The primary functions of FXR activation is the suppression of cholesterol 7 alpha-hydroxylase (CYP7A1), which reduces the synthesis of bile acids (via the feedback mechanism, FXR is activated by bile acids and further determines the suppression of this enzyme, thus reducing the synthesis of bile acids). FXR inhibition produces an increase in bile acids improving metabolic endpoints due to their anti-inflammatory and insulin sensitivity effects [39].

6. Metformin and *Akkermansia muciniphila*

As stated before, the epithelial barrier of T2D patients is affected by an increase in its permeability (so-called leaky gut) followed by a migration of different toxins such as LPS in the systemic circulation causing inflammatory responses, insulin resistance and impaired glucose tolerance. In addition to these changes, a decrease in the *Akkermansia muciniphila* population was observed.

Akkermansia muciniphila is a mucin-degrading bacterium of the phylum *Verrucomicrobia* that resides predominantly in the mucus layer of the colon, where it is involved in maintaining intestinal integrity by promoting mucus secretion and making the barrier mechanism more stable and therefore decreasing its epithelial permeability. Oral supplementation with this bacterial population was shown to reduce intestinal permeability and improve glucose metabolism [40, 41].

A significant change in the composition of the microbiota under metformin treatment regarding intestinal permeability is represented by an increase in the population of *Akkermansia muciniphila*. The mechanism by which this process is accomplished is not fully understood, but it seems that these bacteria metabolise unabsorbable carbohydrates and mucin in short-chain fatty acids, which in turn will be used as fuel for goblet cells. Stimulated goblet cells will further produce mucin, in this way leading to the thickening of the mucus layer and thus to a decrease in the epithelial permeability. Besides increasing the population of *A. muciniphila*, administration of metformin is associated with an increase in the density of mucin-producing goblet cells probably through the indirect mechanism stated above [42, 43] **Figure 1**.

6.1 Metformin and SCAF-producing bacteria

One of the main features of the dysbiosis found in T2D patients is the decrease in butyrate-producing bacteria such as *Roseburia* and *Butyrivibrio*.

Butyrivibrio is a Gram-negative, anaerobic bacteria belonging to the *Clostridia* class, which was first described in the mid-twentieth century [44].

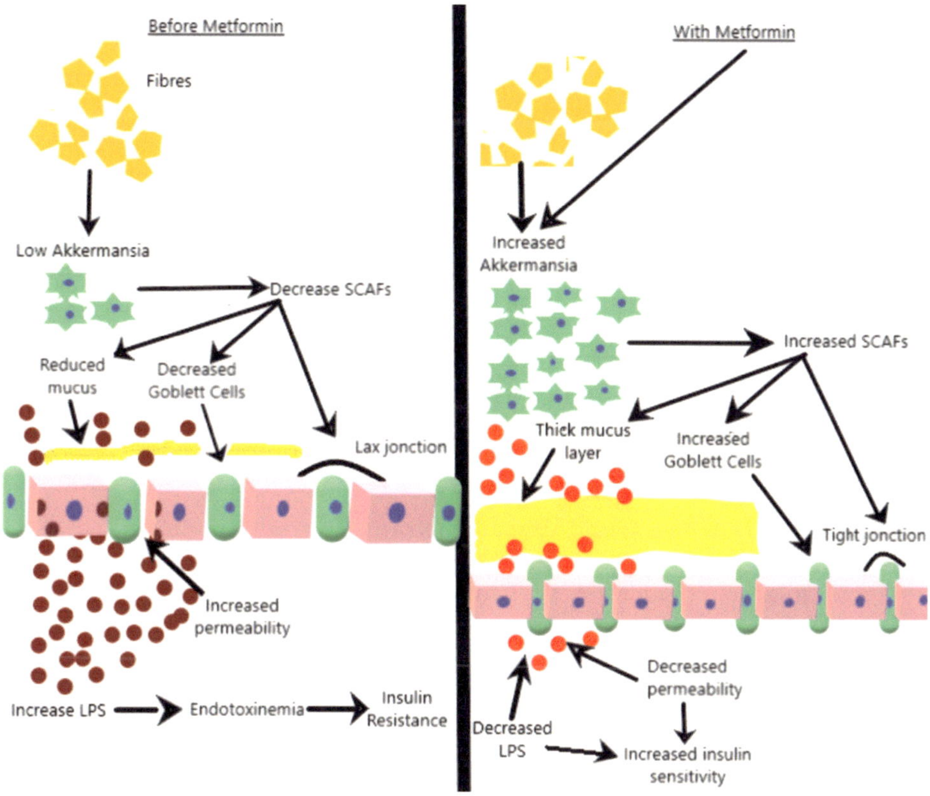

Figure 1.
Akkermansia muciniphila *mode of action [42, 43].*

Roseburia is a Gram-positive anaerobic bacteria member of the *Firmicutes* phyla named in honour of distinguished microbiologist Theodor Rosebury [45].

As stated above, short-chain fatty acids such as butyrate, propionate, and acetate are the product of gut microbiota activity, resulting from the fermentation of the carbohydrates that escapes the absorption process, playing an essential role in the process of enhancing intestinal integrity, reducing inflammation and improving the metabolism of glucose and lipids.

Significant increase of butyrate-producing bacteria, especially *Butyrivibrio* and *Roseburia*, is observed in T2D patients treated with metformin [43].

6.2 Metformin and probiotics

The genus *Bifidobacterium* is a Gram-positive microorganism, member of the *Bifidobacteriaceae* family, belonging to the great *Actinobacteria* phylum, one of the most abundant species of the gut microbiota.

Lactobacillus is a Gram-positive, facultative anaerobic or microaerophilic, rod-shaped, non-spore-forming bacteria that produces lactic acid from converting carbohydrates.

Oral supplementation of *L. casei* and *B. bifidum*, which are frequently used as a probiotic treatment option, alone and in combination, has been shown to improve insulin resistance (decreased fasting blood glucose, decrease HbA1C) and lower the serum lipid levels by enhancing short-chain fatty acids production, and thus improving the outcome of T2D patients [46].

Administration of metformin has been shown to increase the population of *Bifidobacterium adolescentis*, *Bifidobacterium bifidum*, and also *Lactobacillus* [47].

6.3 Metformin and *Adlercreutzia*

The soybean, a legume species native from East Asia, is widely grown for its edible bean, which has numerous uses. It has been assumed that soy foods contribute to reducing the risk of T2D and the progression of this disease in diabetic patients although opinions are divided by the results of studies which inform this theory or rather confirm it [48].

At the gut level, the main species that metabolizes soybean isoflavonoids to equol are the ones from *Adlercreutzia*. It is worth mentioning that not in all people isoflavonoids are metabolized to equol (so-called equol producers). It was speculated that the health benefits of soy-based diets might be higher in equol producers than in equol nonproducers [49].

It seems that metformin treatment increases the population of *Adlercreutzia* in diabetic patients and therefore stimulating the production of equol, thus enhancing soy-based diet health benefits [50].

6.4 Summary of changes found after and before metformin treatment

These tables help summarise the changes found in the gut microbiota both before and after metformin treatment in T2D patients **Tables 1** and **2**.

Structure before metformin treatment	Structure after metformin treatment
Reduced Gram-positive bacteria, such as bacteria from phyla *Firmicutes*	Increased *Firmicutes*
Reduced butyrate-producing bacteria, such as *Roseburia* and *Butyrivibrio*	Increased *Roseburia* and *Butyrivibrio*
Decrease in bacteria that regulate intestinal permeability, such as *Akkermansia muciniphila*	Significant increase of *Akkermansia muciniphila*
Increased Gram-negative bacteria, such as *Bacteroides*, *E. coli* and *Proteobacteria*	Significant decrease of *Bacteroides fragilis*
Increase in various opportunistic pathogens, such as *Clostridium symbiosum* and *Eggerthella lenta*	Increased probiotic bacteria, such as *Bifidobacterium* and
	Increase *Adlercreutzia*

Table 1.
Summary of changes in microbiota composition before and after metformin treatment of T2D.

Mechanisms before metformin	Mechanisms after metformin
Decrease production of SCFAs	Increased production of SCFAs
Decrease production of bile acids	Increased bile acid production, especially GUDCA Inhibition of farnesoid X receptor
Epithelial dysfunction and increased intestinal permeability	Enhancing the intestinal barrier, decreasing its permeability
Increased systemic LPS	Decreased in LPS migration, reduced systemic LPS
Endotoxemia and metabolic infection	Reduced endotoxemia
Inflammation	Decreased inflammation
Insulin resistance	Increased insulin sensitivity
	Increased production of equol

Table 2.
Summary of changes in the functions of microbiota before and after metformin treatment.

7. Conclusions

Alterations of the intestinal microbiota are a key element in understanding the pathophysiology of diabetes and maybe to explain the variability in terms of its therapeutic response and complications occurrence in different patients.

Metformin exerts a significant influence on the bacterial constellation found in the gut, bringing a significant contribution to restoring its balance.

With changes in both composition and function, modulation of the intestinal flora of patients with type 2 diabetes mellitus, obtained by various methods, can bring a better outcome of diabetes patients and can improve the morbidity and mortality rates of this widely present metabolic disease.

Author details

Andra Iulia-Suceveanu[1*], Sergiu Ioan Micu[1], Claudia Voinea[2], Madalina Elena Manea[3], Doina Catrinoiu[3], Laura Mazilu[4], Anca Pantea Stoian[5], Irinel Parepa[6], Roxana Adriana Stoica[5] and Adrian-Paul Suceveanu[1]

1 Internal Medicine—Gastroenterology Department, Faculty of Medicine, "Ovidius" University, Constanta, Romania

2 Endocrinology Department, Faculty of Medicine, "Ovidius" University, Constanta, Romania

3 Diabetes Mellitus and Nutritional Diseases Department, Faculty of Medicine, "Ovidius" University, Constanta, Romania

4 Oncology Department, Faculty of Medicine, "Ovidius" University, Constanta, Romania

5 Diabetes Mellitus and Nutritional Diseases Department, University of Medicine and Pharmacy "Carol Davila", Bucharest, Romania

6 Cardiology Department, Faculty of Medicine, "Ovidius" University, Constanta, Romania

*Address all correspondence to: andrasuceveanu@yahoo.com

References

[1] Boucher DH, James S, Keeler KH. The ecology of mutualism. Annual Review of Ecology, Evolution, and Systematics 1982;**13**:315-347

[2] Chen YE, Fischbach MA, Belkaid Y. Skin microbiota-host interactions. Nature. 2018;**555**(7697):543. DOI: 10.1038/nature25177.

[3] Thursby E, Juge N. Introduction to the human gut microbiota. Biochemical Journal. 2017;**474**(11):1823-1836. DOI: 10.1042/BCJ20160510

[4] Aagaard K, Ma J, Antony KM, Ganu R, Petrosino J, Versalovic J. The placenta harbors a unique microbiome. Science Translational Medicine. 2014;**6**(237):237ra65. DOI: 10.1126/scitranslmed.3008599

[5] Jandhyala SM, Talukdar R, Subramanyam C, Vuyyuru H, Sasikala M, Nageshwar Reddy D. Role of the normal gut microbiota. World Journal of Gastroenterology. 2015;**21**(29):8787-8803. DOI: 10.3748/wjg.v21.i29.8787

[6] Donaldson GP, Lee SM, Mazmanian SK. Gut biogeography of the bacterial microbiota. Nature Reviews. Microbiology. 2016;**14**(1): 20-32. DOI: 10.1038/nrmicro3552

[7] Vancamelbeke M, Vermeire S. The intestinal barrier: A fundamental role in health and disease. Expert Review of Gastroenterology & Hepatology. 2017;**11**(9):821-834. DOI: 10.1080/17474124.2017.1343143

[8] Rowland I, Gibson G, Heinken A, Scott K, Swann J, Thiele I, et al. Gut microbiota functions: Metabolism of nutrients and other food components. European Journal of Nutrition. 2018;**57**(1):1-24. DOI: 10.1007/s00394-017-1445-8

[9] Blaut M. Gut microbiota and energy balance: Role in obesity. The Proceedings of the Nutrition Society. 2015;**74**(3):227-234. DOI: 10.1017/S0029665114001700

[10] Lazar V, Ditu L-M, Pircalabioru GG, Gheorghe I, Curutiu C, Holban AM, et al. Aspects of gut microbiota and immune system interactions in infectious diseases, immunopathology, and Cancer. Frontiers in Immunology. 2018;**9**:1830. DOI: 10.3389/fimmu.2018.01830

[11] LeBlanc JG, Milani C, de Giori GS, Sesma F, van Sinderen D, Ventura M. Bacteria as vitamin suppliers to their host: A gut microbiota perspective. Current Opinion in Biotechnology. 2013;**24**(2):160-168. DOI: 10.1016/j.copbio.2012.08.005

[12] Yano JM, Yu K, Donaldson GP, Shastri GG, Ann P, Ma L, et al. Indigenous bacteria from the gut microbiota regulate host serotonin biosynthesis. Cell. 2015;**161**(2):264-276. DOI: 10.1016/j.cell.2015.02.047

[13] Hawrelak JA, Myers SP. The causes of intestinal dysbiosis: A review. Alternative Medicine Review. 2004;**9**(2):180-197

[14] Carding S, Verbeke K, Vipond DT, Corfe BM, Owen LJ. Dysbiosis of the gut microbiota in disease. Microbial Ecology in Health and Disease. 2015;**26**:26191. Feb 2 Published 2015. DOI: 10.3402/mehd.v26.26191

[15] De Luca SY. The microbiome in autoimmune diseases. Clinical and Experimental Immunology. 2019;**195**(1):74-85. DOI: 10.1111/cei.13158

[16] Pascal M, Perez-Gordo M, Caballero T, et al. Microbiome and allergic

diseases. Frontiers in Immunology. 2018;**9**:1584. 17 Jul 2018. DOI: 10.3389/fimmu.2018.01584

[17] Ma J, Li H. The role of gut microbiota in atherosclerosis and hypertension. Frontiers in Pharmacology. 2018;**9**:1082. 25 Sep 2018. DOI: 10.3389/fphar.2018.01082

[18] Dahmus JD, Kotler DL, Kastenberg DM, Andrew Kistle C. The gut microbiome and colorectal cancer: A review of bacterial pathogenesis. Journal of Gastrointestinal Oncology. 2018;**9**(4):769-777. DOI: 10.21037/jgo.2018.04.07

[19] Kowalski K, Mulak A. Brain-gut-microbiota axis in Alzheimer's disease. Journal of Neurogastroenterology and Motility. 2019;**25**(1):48-60. DOI: 10.5056/jnm18087

[20] Tilg H, Moschen AR. Microbiota and diabetes: An evolving relationship. Gut. 2014;**63**:1513-1521

[21] Munro N. Gut microbiota: Its role in diabetes and obesity. Diabetes & Primary Care. 2016;**18**:1-6

[22] Harsch IA, Konturek PC. The role of gut microbiota in obesity and type 2 and type 1 diabetes mellitus: New insights into "old" diseases. Medical Science. 2018;**6**(2):32. DOI: 10.3390/medsci6020032

[23] Aw W, Fukuda S. Understanding the role of the gut ecosystem in diabetes mellitus. Journal of Diabetes Investigation. 2018;**9**(1):5-12. DOI: 10.1111/jdi.12673

[24] https://en.wikipedia.org/wiki/Lipopolysaccharide

[25] Liang H, Hussey SE, Sanchez-Avila A, Tantiwong P, Musi N. Effect of lipopolysaccharide on inflammation and insulin action in human muscle. PLoS ONE. 2013;**8**(5):e63983. 21 May 2013. DOI: 10.1371/journal.pone.0063983

[26] Amar J, Serino M, Lange C, Chabo C, Iacovoni J, Mondot S, et al. Involvement of tissue bacteria in the onset of diabetes in humans: Evidence for a concept. Diabetologia. 2011;**54**:3055-3061. DOI: 10.1007/s00125-011-2329-8

[27] Burcelin R, Serino M, Chabo C, Garidou L, Pomié C, Courtney M, et al. Metagenome and metabolism: The tissue microbiota hypothesis. Diabetes, Obesity & Metabolism. 2013;**15**(Suppl. 3):61-70. DOI: 10.1111/dom.12157

[28] Zheng P, Li Z, Zhou Z. Gut microbiome in type 1 diabetes: A comprehensive review. Diabetes/Metabolism Research and Reviews. 2018;**34**(7):e3043. DOI: 10.1002/dmrr.3043

[29] Tan J, McKenzie C, Potamitis M, Thorburn AN, Mackay CR, Macia L. The role of short-chain fatty acids in health and disease. Advances in Immunology. 2014;**121**:91-119. DOI: 10.1016/B978-0-12-800100-4.00003-9

[30] Albaugh VL, Banan B, Antoun J, Xiong Y, Guo Y, Ping J, et al. Role of bile acids and GLP-1 in mediating the metabolic improvements of bariatric surgery. Gastroenterology Journal. 2019;**156**(4):1041-1051.e4. DOI: 10.1053/j.gastro.2018.11.017

[31] Watanabe M et al. Bile acids induce energy expenditure by promoting intracellular thyroid hormone activation. Nature. 2006;**439**(7075):484-489

[32] Ward BJ, Lajczak-Mc GJ, Kelly N, O'Dwyer OM, Giddam AK, et al. Ursodeoxycholic acid and lithocholic acid exert anti-inflammatory actions in the colon. AJP Gastrointestinal

and Liver Physiology. 2017;**312**. DOI: 10.1152/ajpgi.00256.2016

[33] DeFronzo RA, Buse JB, Kim T, et al. Once-daily delayed-release metformin lowers plasma glucose and enhances fasting and postprandial GLP-1 and PYY: Results from two randomised trials. Diabetologia. 2016;**59**:1645. DOI: 10.1007/s00125-016-3992-6

[34] Bonora E, Cigolini M, Bosello O, Zancanaro C, Capretti L, Zavaroni I, et al. Lack of effect of intravenous metformin on plasma concentrations of glucose, insulin, C-peptide, glucagon and growth hormone in non-diabetic subjects. Current Medical Research and Opinion. 1984;**9**(1):47-51

[35] Sundelin E, Gormsen LC, Jensen JB, Vendelbo MH, Jakobsen S, Munk OL, et al. Genetic polymorphisms in organic cation transporter 1 attenuates hepatic metformin exposure in humans. Clinical Pharmacology and Therapeutics. 2017;**102**(5):841-848. DOI: 10.1002/cpt.701

[36] Ma W, Chen J, Meng Y, Yang J, Cui Q, Zhou Y. Metformin alters gut microbiota of healthy mice: Implication for its potential role in gut microbiota homeostasis. Frontiers in Microbiology. 2018;**9**:1336. DOI: 10.3389/fmicb.2018.01336

[37] Elbere I et al. Association of metformin administration with gut microbiome dysbiosis in healthy volunteers. PLoS ONE. 2018;**13**(9):e0204317. DOI: 10.1371/journal.pone.0204317

[38] Sun L et al. Gut microbiota and intestinal FXR mediate the clinical benefits of metformin. Nature Medicine. 2018;**24**(12):1919-1929. DOI: 10.1038/s41591-018-0222-4

[39] Fernandes A, Vaz AR, Falcao AS, et al. Glycoursodeoxycholic acid and interleukin-10 modulate the reactivity of rat cortical astrocytes to unconjugated bilirubin. Journal of Neuropathology and Experimental Neurology. 2007;**66**(9):789-798

[40] Geerlings SY, Kostopoulos I, de Vos WM, Belzer C. *Akkermansia muciniphila* in the human gastrointestinal tract: When, where, and how?. Microorganisms 2018;**6**(3): pii E75. DOI: 10.3390/microorganisms6030075.

[41] Naito Y, Uchiyama K, Takagi T. A next-generation beneficial microbe: *Akkermansia muciniphila*. Journal of Clinical Biochemistry and Nutrition. 2018;**63**(1):33-35. DOI: 10.3164/jcbn.18-57

[42] Shin NR, Lee JC, Lee HY, Kim MS, Whon TW, Lee MS, et al. An increase in the *Akkermansia* spp. population induced by metformin treatment improves glucose homeostasis in diet-induced obese mice. Gut. 2014;**63**(5):727-735. DOI: 10.1136/gutjnl-2012-303839

[43] de la Cuesta-Zuluaga MNT, Corrales-Agudelo V, Velásquez-Mejía EP, Carmona JA, Abad JM, Escobar JS. Metformin is associated with higher relative abundance of mucin-degrading *Akkermansia muciniphila* and several short-chain fatty acid-producing microbiota in the gut. Diabetes Care. 2017;**40**(1):54-62. DOI: 10.2337/dc16-1324

[44] https://en.wikipedia.org/wiki/Butyrivibrio

[45] https://en.wikipedia.org/wiki/Roseburia

[46] Sharma P, Bhardwaj P, Singh R. Administration of *Lactobacillus casei* and *Bifidobacterium bifidum* ameliorated hyperglycemia, dyslipidemia, and oxidative stress in diabetic rats. International Journal of Preventive Medicine. 2016;7:102. DOI: 10.4103/2008-7802.188870

[47] Rodriguez J, Hiel S, Delzenne NM. Metformin: Old friend, new ways of action-implication of the gut microbiome? Current Opinion in Clinical Nutrition and Metabolic Care. 2018;**21**(4):294-301. DOI: 10.1097/MCO.0000000000000468

[48] Mueller NT, Odegaard AO, Gross MD, Koh W-P, Yu MC, Yuan J-M, et al. Soy intake and risk of type 2 diabetes mellitus in Chinese Singaporeans. European Journal of Nutrition. 2012;**51**(8):1033-1040. DOI: 10.1007/s00394-011-0276-2

[49] Hong K-W et al. Epidemiological profiles between equol producers and nonproducers: A genome wide association study of the equol-producing phenotype. Genes & Nutrition. 2012;**7**(4):567-574. DOI: 10.1007/s12263-012-0292-8

[50] Lv Y, Zhao X, Guo W, Gao Y, Yang S, Li Z, et al. The relationship between frequently used glucose-lowering agents and gut microbiota in type 2 diabetes mellitus. Journal Diabetes Research. 2018;**2018**:1890978. DOI: 10.1155/2018/1890978

Chapter 4

Potential Protective Effects of Metformin on Ocular Complications in Patients with Type 2 Diabetes

Jasna Kusturica, Aida Kulo, Maida Rakanović-Todić, Lejla Burnazović-Ristić and Sanita Maleškić

Abstract

Diabetes mellitus (DM) as a chronic condition is a growing global problem. Its numerous complications, including ocular diseases, affect patients' quality and length of life. Metformin is an effective, safe, and inexpensive first-line pharmacotherapy for type 2 diabetes (T2D). The current evidence indicates metformin's multiple sites of action and multiple molecular mechanisms leading to its beneficial impact on metabolism, inflammation, oxidative stress, aging, as well as to its cardiovascular, neurological, bone, and antiproliferative properties. These impacts are the result of its acting on adenosine monophosphate-activated protein kinase (AMPK)-dependent and AMPK-independent pathways. Limited data suggest the protective role of metformin on microvascular ocular complications, including retinopathy, glaucoma, and age-related macular degeneration in patients with T2D. However, to confirm its mentioned protective and therapeutic effects, more large, randomized, double-blind, and placebo-controlled clinical studies are needed.

Keywords: type 2 diabetes, metformin, molecular mechanisms, ocular complications

1. Introduction

Diabetes mellitus (DM) is a chronic systemic disease accompanied by impaired metabolism of carbohydrates, proteins, and fats. The American Diabetes Association (ADA) [1] distinguishes two basic types of diabetes mellitus, type 1 (T1D) and type 2 (T2D), while, in addition, gestational diabetes and specific forms of the disease are also recognized. The main pathophysiologic events in DM are insulin deficiency and insulin resistance. The most significant event is insulin resistance that develops in target tissues of action of insulin (muscle, fat tissues, and liver). In T1D, autoimmune destruction of β cells of the pancreatic islets (Langerhans islets) leads to deficient production and absolute insulin deficiency, while in T2D, insulin secretion is considered insufficient to overcome insulin resistance in peripheral tissues (relative insulin deficiency).

T1D is commonly diagnosed in childhood and early adolescence, affects men and women equally, and shows the highest prevalence in the white race. T2D occurs in older life, while an increase in incidence is associated with poorer socioeconomic status, and an increase in risks is associated with lower economic income, education levels, and unemployment. Overall, DM prevalence is expected to increase to 10.1% in the coming decades [2]. The global trend of the increasing prevalence of both types of DM implies a significant influence of environmental factors on the development of the disease.

The polygenic inheritance of DM has been suggested, with different gene variants that contribute to the overall risk of disease [3, 4]. The risk of developing the disease in the offspring is higher if one parent has T2D (~40%) and T1D (~5%). Gene variants that associate with type 1 and type 2 diseases have a different genetic basis. A limited number of specific gene variants characterize a small subset of patients with Maturity-onset diabetes of the young, a monogenic disease with autosomal dominant transmission [4].

A fundamental pathogenic event in the etiology of T1D is an aberrant immune response and production of autoantibodies to β cells. In children and adolescents with T1D, the polyendocrine autoimmune syndrome has also been described, which involves the expression of autoimmune activity against more than one endocrine organ. T1D is associated with the incidence of autoimmune thyroiditis, celiac and autoimmune gastric disease, and other rare autoimmune conditions [5, 6]. Molecular mimicry and viral infections have been investigated the longest, while recently the focus of research is covering deficiencies in immunoregulation that have been identified in patients with T1D [4]. The interaction of genetic and environmental factors may be important for triggering autoimmune events and the onset of T1D [3]. Association was established between the occurrence of T1D and the consumption of foods rich in nitrates or nitrites, low serum vitamin D levels, or early exposure to enteroviral and other infections. The timing of the introduction of cereals and gluten into the diet and alterations of the gut microbiome were suggested to affect the β-cell autoimmune response with autoantibody production [7]. Consistently, a pattern of assimilation of the local incidence rate of T1D has been observed in persons who migrated from lower geographical areas to a higher incidence area [3].

The increase in T2D prevalence has been particularly linked to obesity, sedentary lifestyles, and unhealthy diets. One of the major risk factors for T2D is obesity. Insulin resistance is thought to develop with increasing fat deposition in the liver and muscle. Visceral obesity contributes to the development of insulin resistance and possibly independently contributes to the development of T2D [8]. In prediabetes and early-stage T2D, partial reversibility of insulin secretion disorders has been observed after the restriction in the high-calorie intake and weight loss [9].

Three symptoms characterize the early onset of DM, i.e., hyperglycemia, polyuria, and increased thirst. The recommended diagnostic criteria and therapeutic monitoring of DM are based on impaired fasting glucose levels, impaired glucose tolerance test, and measuring glycosylated hemoglobin Type A1C (HbA1C). HbA1C is an indicator of long-term glycemic control (over the period of past 2–3 months), as it reflects the average level of glucose to which the erythrocytes were exposed to. In the treatment of DM, special attention is given to a balanced diet and physical activity. Administrations of exogenous insulin and insulin analogs are the first-line treatments for T1D. Insulin therapy requires an individualized approach and involves maintaining blood glucose levels as close as possible to reference levels while avoiding hypoglycemia, which is the most significant side effect of this treatment. Glycemia regulation in T2D is being attempted by oral antidiabetic agents, and if adequate control of the disease cannot be established, insulin therapy is initiated. Antidiabetics usually work by increasing the secretion of insulin from the pancreatic β cells or by reducing the insulin resistance. Also, drugs have been developed both to reduce the postprandial glycemia by slowing and reducing the absorption of food from the gut and to reduce the production and release of glucose from the liver.

Complications of the disease significantly influence the quality of life of patients with DM. Acute complications of diabetes are metabolic and, in their extreme form, include diabetic ketoacidosis and nonketotic hyperosmolar coma. While those acute complications can directly endanger the patient's life, late chronic complications are significant due to the impact on the quality of life and morbidity and mortality associated with the disease itself. Both, acute and chronic complications are in inverse onset with the degree of metabolic control of the disease [4]. HbA1C level showed association with risks of cardiovascular disease [10] and is considered to be associated with microvascular disease [11].

2. Chronic complications of the disease

Chronic DM complications can be a cause of cardiovascular events, renal failure, blindness, or lower limb amputation. They are classified as macrovascular and microvascular. Coronary disease and myocardial infarction arise as macrovascular complications of DM. It is estimated that 80% of patients with T2D develop cardiovascular complications [12]. Microvascular complications of DM include diabetic retinopathy (DR), nephropathy, and neuropathy. Retinal capillary endothelial cells, mesangial cells of the renal glomeruli, glial cells, and Schwann cells of the peripheral nerves are particularly exposed as they lack the ability to inhibit glucose transport to the cell under hyperglycemia conditions [13].

The impact of glycemic control on the development of microvascular complications of T2D has been documented in large prospective studies [12, 14–16]. The DISCOVER study was conducted in 38 countries and included 16,000 patients with T2D, with an average disease duration of 4.1 years [12]. The results of this study indicated that the prevalences of microvascular and macrovascular complications were 18.8 and 12.7%, respectively. The most common microvascular complications included peripheral neuropathy (7.7%), chronic kidney disease (5.0%), and albuminuria (4.3%). Coronary artery disease (8.2%), heart failure (3.3%), and stroke (2.2%) were the most commonly reported macrovascular complications. An association was observed for the following factors of risk: age, male gender, diabetes duration, and history of hypoglycemia.

In the development of diabetic neuropathy, the changes in cellular metabolism that result from hyperglycemia and dyslipidemia are leading to oxidative stress as a leading causative factor [17]. Hyperglycemia also exerts a negative effect on the β cells themselves, due to the increased formation of reactive oxygen species (ROS). β cells have reduced amounts of catalase enzyme and superoxide dismutase that metabolize ROS under normal conditions, and an increased amount of ROS activates proapoptotic nuclear factor kappa B (NF-κB).

Several mechanisms underlie the onset of microvascular complications, and their common feature is the formation of excess oxygen radicals that cause DNA damage. In hyperglycemia, an accumulation of advanced glycation end (AGE) product and increases in the activity of the hexosamine biosynthesis pathway, polyol pathway, and protein kinase C (PKC) are described [13, 17, 18]. High plasma glucose concentrations cause glycation of amine groups in proteins, and consequently, AGE is formed. AGE causes changes in the signaling pathway of macrophages or vascular endothelial cells with the release of various cytokines and increases the expression of vascular endothelial growth factor (VEGF), which causes increased vascular permeability and retinal angiogenesis [19]. Also, AGE-mediated ROS generation is considered as a pathogenesis factor [17].

In addition, hyperglycemia increases the activity of the hexosamine pathway, the synthesis of diacylglycerol (DAG), and the activity of aldose reductase within the polyol pathway. Fructose-6-phosphate synthesis of glucosamine-6-phosphate is the first step in the hexosamine biosynthesis pathway. Activation of the hexosamine pathway increases the formation of uridine diphosphate N-acetylglucosamine, which is a substrate donor and catalyzes the binding of monosaccharide GlcNAc to serine and threonine residues of cytosolic and nuclear proteins, including the transcription factor NF-κB. DAG activates PKC isoforms, while basal membrane thickening, increased permeability, coagulation and contractility abnormalities, increased angiogenesis, and cardiomyopathy are all considered to be related to PKC activation. Increased activity of the polyol pathway leads to increased sorbitol formation. When converting glucose to sorbitol, nicotinamide adenine dinucleotide phosphate is consumed, and the production of reduced glutathione as a key antioxidant in the cell is reduced. All these cause the cell to be more susceptible to oxidative stress. Finally, the interaction of metabolic and vascular disorders leads to impaired cellular function and, over the long term, can mediate cell damage and apoptosis.

2.1 Ocular complications of DM

Ocular complications of DM include DR, glaucoma, and cataracts.

The most common ocular complication is DR. Its occurrence is associated with patient age, duration of DM, and hyperglycemia [20]. The contribution of inflammation-mediated pathways and angiogenesis to the progression of DR has been documented [21, 22]. One of the first clinical features of DR is proliferation of endothelial cells and forming of the microaneurysms in retinal capillaries [23]. Capillary damage of ischemia gradually leads to neovascularization. Newly formed capillaries are prone to microhemorrhages. The VEGF signaling is considered to have a significant role in the regulation of neovascularization in retina and pathogenesis of DR [23–25]. Recent advances in treatment of DR include developments in anti-VEGF therapy, which is associated with significant reductions in vision loss due to DR [23].

VEGF levels could be influenced by oxidative stress and formation of ROS, and it has been suggested that exposition of retinal cells to H_2O_2 might be important in stimulation of VEGF-dependent angiogenesis. Imbalance of VEGF isoforms in retinal cells has been observed *in vivo* [24]. Nevertheless, altered expression of VEGF in retinal pigment epithelial (RPE) cells of normoglycemic and diabetic mice was not observed, whereas expression of antiangiogenic VEGF165b isoform was significantly reduced in diabetic retina. Authors suggested that both hyperglycemia and oxidative stress contribute to the changes in balance of pro- and antiangiogenic factors in the retina.

Along with DR, ocular complications of DM include glaucoma and cataracts. Although age is the most significant risk factor in glaucoma development, DM has been confirmed as an etiological factor for neovascular glaucoma, while there are controversial opinions regarding open-angle glaucoma (OAG) and angle-closure glaucoma (ACG) [26]. The association of T2D and cataract has been demonstrated [26, 27], and assumed underlying mechanisms are compiled of increased oxidative stress, activation of the polyol pathway leading to an increase in the osmotic stress, and glycation of lens proteins [26, 28].

3. Method

We performed a short review to assess and discuss potential protective effects of metformin on ocular complications in patients with T2D.

4. Metformin: protective effects on ocular complications

Apart from glycemic control, metformin has shown to have antiinflammatory, antiangiogenic, and calorie restriction-related antiaging activity. Limited data suggest the protective role of metformin on microvascular ocular complications in patients with T2D. The list of studies regarding the link between metformin and ocular involvements in diabetes is presented in **Table 1**.

4.1 Link between metformin and VEGF-A

Changed levels of not only VEGF-A, one of the most potent members of angiogenic factor family, but also of its isoforms such as VEGF120, VEGF164, and VEGF188 are results of hyperglycemia and oxidative stress in mice [24, 25]. Previous studies have shown that angiogenesis and neovascularization in the eyes of diabetic patients, including DR, are result of increased level of VEGFs [29, 30]. Metformin was shown to mediate the reduction of the VEGF-A expression and angiogenic inhibitors in CD34+ cells under the state of hyperglycemia-hypoxia [31]. Other preliminary study reports that compared to significantly increased plasma VEGF levels in patients treated with pioglitazone, no change in VEGF levels was detected in patients treated with metformin [32]. It is interesting that change of VEGF-A during metformin therapy is independent of metformin-associated effects regarding BMI, HbA1C levels, and waist circumference of fat percentage. Even when the blood glucose and HbA1C levels were not in the recommended range, patients treated with metformin had a lower incidence of ocular complications than patients in the nonmetformin group [33].

4.2 Protective effect on diabetic retinopathy

The beneficial effects of metformin were detected in patients with DR [25, 33]. It was documented that 45.5% of patients from the nonmetformin group developed DR compared to 27.3% of patients from the group treated with metformin [34]. However, metformin protective effects on DR are not purely clear. Several studies investigated its effects on vascular endothelium of retina, mainly focusing on pathological background and features of angiogenesis and inflammation. There is evidence that metformin could potently protect endothelial cells via antiangiogenic, antiinflammatory, and antioxidant mechanisms [35, 36].

Han et al. [37] in their *in vitro* study found that metformin directly inhibits angiogenesis of human retinal vascular endothelial cells (hRVECs) and has prevented tumor necrosis factor alpha (TNFα)-induced upregulation of multiple inflammatory cytokines in hRVECs.

Retinal degenerations are characterized by a progressive loss of photoreceptors or their support cells, the retinal pigmented epithelium (RPE). Xu et al. [38] used metformin to determine whether stimulation of the adenosine monophosphate-activated protein kinase (AMPK) pathway protects the photoreceptors and the RPE from retinal degeneration (**Table 1**). Metformin was able to protect the photoreceptors from light damage, delay rod, and cone degeneration in the Rd10 model and to increase the resistance of the RPE to the injury. Also, authors concluded that metformin's mechanism of protection was associated with increased mitochondrial biogenesis and reduced oxidative stress.

The long-term oral metformin was associated with significantly reduced severity of DR in patients with T2D [39]. It could be explained by metformin-induced restoration of energy balance in the retina through activation of AMPK [25]. AMPK

Authors, Year	Study title	Study design	Study outcome	Ref.
Brown EE et al., 2019	The Common Antidiabetic Drug Metformin Reduces Odds of Developing Age-Related Macular Degeneration	Retrospective case-control study with medical records from patients ˃55 years. Three controls were matched for every AMD case, defined by Int. Class. of Diseases, 9th Revision code, based on Charlson Comorbidity Index.	Patients treated with metformin had decreased odds of developing AMD suggesting its therapeutic role in development or progression of AMD in patients at risk.	[47]
Chen YY et al., 2019	Association Between Metformin and a Lower Risk of Age-Related Macular Degeneration in Patients with Type 2 Diabetes	Population-based retrospective cohort study with 68,205 patients with T2D.	Metformin use, especially in higher doses, was associated with significantly lower risk of development of AMD.	[48]
Li Y et al., 2018	Association of Metformin Treatment with Reduced Severity of Diabetic Retinopathy in Type 2 Diabetic Patients	Retrospective chart review study with 335 patients with DR and with T2D ≥15 years. The severity of DR was determined by Early Treatment Diabetic Retinopathy Study scale.	Long-term use of metformin was independently associated with significant lower rate of severe nonproliferative DR or proliferative DR in patients with T2D ≥15 years.	[41]
Han J et al., 2018	Metformin Suppresses Retinal Angiogenesis and Inflammation In Vitro and In Vivo	Metformin effects and mechanism were tested in vitro in hRVEC culture and in vivo in vldlr−/− mice.	Metformin showed potent antiangiogenic and antiinflammatory effects on hRVECs, reduced retinal neovascularization in vldlr−/− mice, and suppressed leukostasis in STZ-induced diabetic mice, suggesting its potential to target key pathogenic components in DR.	[37]
Xu L et al., 2018	Stimulation of AMPK Prevents Degeneration of Photoreceptors and the Retinal Pigment Epithelium	In vivo study with metformin tested in three different mouse models of retinal degeneration: a light-induced degenerative model, the Pde6brd10 inherited retinal degeneration model, and a model of sodium iodate-induced RPE and retinal injury, as well as in AMPK retinal knockout mice.	By stimulation of AMPK metformin protected photoreceptors and the RPE in three different mouse models of retinal degeneration, including acute bright light damage, Pde6brd10 inherited retinitis pigmentosa, and sodium iodate-induced RPE injury. Local expression of AMPK catalytic subunit α2 was required for those effects.	[38]
Maleskic S et al., 2017	Metformin Use Associated with Protective Effects for Ocular Complications in Patients with Type 2 Diabetes – Observational Study	Observational study with medical records from 234 patients with T2D (190 patients using metformin and 44 using other oral antihyperglycemic agents).	Metformin use was associated with fewer ocular complications with decreased odds of both glaucoma and DR compared to other oral antihyperglycemic agents.	[33]

Authors, Year	Study title	Study design	Study outcome	Ref.
Yi QY et al., 2016	Metformin Inhibits the Development of Diabetic Retinopathy through Inducing Alternative Splicing of VEGF-A	Metformin effects on the development of DR were tested in STZ-induced diabetic model in mice.	Metformin inhibited VEGF signaling by inducing VEGF-A mRNA splicing to VEGF120 isoform, creating a potential for new treatment option for DR.	[25]
Simão S et al., 2016	Oxidative Stress Modulates the Expression of VEGF Isoforms in the Diabetic Retina	Retinal tissue and D407 RPE cells from wild-type and Ins2Akita mouse model of diabetes were used as experimental models.	Both hyperglycemia and oxidative stress disrupted the equilibrium between pro- and antiangiogenic factors in the retina. Hyperglycemia contributed to deregulation of the expression of VEGF proteins and the production of ROS in RPE cells. Pathological H2O2 levels downregulated the VEGF165b.	[24]
Lin H-C et al., 2015	Association of Geroprotective Effects of Metformin and Risk of Open-Angle Glaucoma in Persons with Diabetes Mellitus	Retrospective cohort study with patients with T2D aged ≥40 years and with no preexisting record of OAG.	Metformin use was associated with reduction in risk of developing OAG. Proposed mechanisms involved improved glycemic control or effects involving neurogenesis, inflammatory systems, or longevity pathways.	[43]
Richards JE et al., 2014	Targeting aging: Geroprotective Medication Metformin Reduces Risk of Adult-onset Open-angle Glaucoma	Longitudinal data from a large database were used, and patients with diabetes, aged ≥40 with no preexisting OAG, were monitored for incident OAG.	Metformin use was associated with reduced risk of OAG, on a dose-dependent manner. Proposed mechanisms involved neurogenesis, longevity pathways, and/or reduced inflammation.	[46]

AMD: Age-Related Macular Degeneration; DR: Diabetic Retinopathy; hRVEC: human retinal vascular endothelial cell; vldlr-/-mice: very-low-density lipoprotein receptor knockout mutant mouse; STZ: streptozotocin; AMPK: adenosine monophosphate-activated protein kinase; RPE: retinal pigmented epithelium; VEGF-A: vascular endothelial cell growth factor A; OAG: Open-Angle Glaucoma; POAG: primary open-angle glaucoma.

Table 1.
List of studies regarding the link between metformin and ocular involvements in diabetes.

activation was suggested to be protective for the tissues that are undergoing metabolic stress. However, the regulation on endothelial inflammatory and angiogenic responses by metformin also has been shown through both AMPK-dependent and AMPK-independent mechanisms [37, 40].

According to a retrospective study [41], there is a correlation between the long-term metformin treatment and reduced severity of DR in patients with T2D regardless of their HbA1c level, gender, race or treatment with sulfonylurea or insulin.

In summary, metformin might be used for the purpose of reducing DR progression in patients with long history of T2D.

4.3 Protective effect on glaucoma

Glaucoma is a type of neuropathy, and association with DM was identified – it could cause optic neuropathy [42]. The thicker central cornea in patients with DM than in healthy subjects could be a cause of higher intraocular pressure in those patients [26]. A retrospective cohort study showed that metformin use is associated with reduced risk of developing open-angle glaucoma and suggested that metformin could have an impact on glaucoma risk on multiple levels including glycemic control and calorie restriction (CR) [43]. As previous studies suggested that age-related tissue changes significantly contribute to glaucoma development [44], the antiaging effect of metformin as a CR mimetic drug could delay the progression of tissue damage [45].

Risk reduction of glaucoma was shown to be dose-dependent for metformin and independent of glycemic control in the population with DM [46]. In the observational study, patients treated with metformin had a lower prevalence of glaucoma than patients treated with other oral antidiabetic medications, 3.2 vs. 11.4%, respectively [33].

4.4 Protective effect on age-related macular degeneration

Recently, the first studies on this topic indicated an association between metformin use and the reduction of age-related macular degeneration (AMD) development [47, 48]. Those authors assumed metformin's protective role in development or progression of AMD based on both its antiinflammatory and antioxidative properties and on AMD pathogenesis. Namely, besides environmental and genetic factors, AMD pathogenesis involves inflammation and oxidative stress, which can lead to choroidal neovascularization and geographic atrophy with potential loss of vision [47–50].

In study Chen et al., both the incidence of AMD (3.4 vs. 6.6%) and cumulative hazard for AMD were significantly lower among metformin users than nonusers. Lower hazard ratios for AMD were shown to be associated with higher dose of metformin and longer duration of therapy, and they remained even after adjustment for the patients' age, gender, and comorbidities [48].

Similar results were found in the study by Brown et al., where decreased odds of developing AMD, except for metformin, were not associated with dipeptidyl peptidase 4 inhibitors, selective serotonin reuptake inhibitors, tetracyclic antidepressants, and statins [47].

Almost 8.4 million people worldwide are affected by AMD [51]. It is the most common cause of vision impairment in the developed countries, and the third one, after uncorrected refractive errors and cataract, globally [52–54]. Estimated blindness prevalence related to AMD is 8.7% [55]. However, it is projected that due to the extended life expectancy, the number of people with AMD will increase [52–54]. Current AMD therapy with anti-VEGF drugs is costly, i.e., the cost of an injection of anti-VEGF is up to £800, and usually eight injections per year are recommended [51]. Therefore, as metformin is well-known cheap drug, its potentially protective effect on AMD is promising, especially for countries with limited health care resources.

5. Conclusion

Metformin is effective, well-tolerated, and inexpensive first-line pharmacotherapy for T2D. Its additional potential protective effects on ocular complications in patients with T2D may have a major beneficial impact on the disease course and quality and length of their life. Well-designed randomized controlled clinical trials should be conducted to evaluate the effects of metformin either on the prevention of ocular complication or on the therapy of already developed ocular complications in patients with T2D.

Conflict of interest

The authors declare no conflict of interest.

Author details

Jasna Kusturica*, Aida Kulo, Maida Rakanović-Todić, Lejla Burnazović-Ristić and Sanita Maleškić
Institute of Pharmacology, Clinical Pharmacology and Toxicology, Medical Faculty, University of Sarajevo, Sarajevo, Bosnia and Herzegovina

*Address all correspondence to: jasna.kusturica@mf.unsa.ba

References

[1] American Diabetes Association (ADA). Classification and diagnosis of diabetes. Diabetes Care. 2019;**42**(1):S13-S28

[2] International Diabetes Federation. IDF Diabetes Atlas. 6th ed. Brussels, Belgium: International Diabetes Federation; 2013. Available from: http://www.idf.org/diabetesatlas [Accessed: 15 December 2019]

[3] Skyler SJ, George L, Bakris LG, Bonifacio E, Darsow T, Eckel HR, et al. Differentiation of diabetes by pathophysiology, natural history, and prognosis. Diabetes. 2017;**66**:241-255. DOI: 10.2337/db16-0806

[4] Yau M, Maclaren NK, Sperling M. Etiology and pathogenesis of diabetes mellitus in children and adolescents. [Updated 13 February 2018]. In: Feingold KR, Anawalt B, Boyce A, et al., editors. Endotext. South Dartmouth (MA): MDText.com, Inc.; 2000. Available from: https://www.ncbi.nlm.nih.gov/books/NBK498653/ [Accessed: 15 December 2019]

[5] Hansen PM, Matheis N, Kahaly JG. Type 1 diabetes and polyglandular autoimmune syndrome: A review. World Journal of Diabetes. 2015;**6**(1):67-79. DOI: 10.4239/wjd.v6.i1.67

[6] Kakleas K, Soldatou A, Karachaliou F, Karavanaki K. Associated autoimmune diseases in children and adolescents with type 1 diabetes mellitus (T1DM). Autoimmunity Reviews. 2015;**14**(9):781-797. DOI: 10.1016/j.autrev.2015.05.002

[7] Serena G, Camhi S, Sturgeon C, Yan S, Fasano A. The role of gluten in celiac disease and type 1 diabetes. Nutrients. 2015;7(9):7143-7162. DOI: 10.3390/nu7095329

[8] Boyko EJ, Fujimoto WY, Leonetti DL, Newell-Morris L. Visceral adiposity and risk of type 2 diabetes. A prospective study among Japanese Americans. Diabetes Care. 2000;**23**(4):65-71. DOI: 10.1371/journal.pone.0043502

[9] McCaffery JM, Jablonski KA, Franks PW, Dagogo-Jack S, Wing RR, Knowler WC, et al. Diabetes prevention program research group. TCF7L2 polymorphism, weight loss and proinsulin: Insulin ratio in the diabetes prevention program. PLoS One. 2011;**6**:e21518. DOI: 10.1371/journal.pone.0021518

[10] Selvin E, Michael W, Steffes MW, Zhu H, Matsushita K, Wagenknecht L, et al. Glycated hemoglobin, diabetes, and cardiovascular risk in nondiabetic adults. The New England Journal of Medicine. 2010;**362**:800-811. DOI: 10.1056/NEJMoa0908359

[11] American Diabetes Association (ADA). Diagnosis and classification of diabetes mellitus. Diabetes Care. 2010;**33**(1):S62-S69. DOI: 10.2337/dc10-S062

[12] Kosiborod M, Gomes MB, Nicolucci A, Pocock S, Rathmann W, Shestakova MV, et al. DISCOVER investigators: Vascular complications in patients with type 2 diabetes: Prevalence and associated factors in 38 countries (the DISCOVER study program). Cardiovascular Diabetology. 2018;**17**:150. DOI: 10.1186/s12933-018-0787-8

[13] Brownlee M. The pathobiology of diabetic complications: A unifying mechanism. Diabetes. 2005;**54**(6):1615-1625. DOI: 10.2337/diabetes.54.6.1615

[14] Casanova F, Adingupu DD, Adams F, Gooding KM, Looker HC, Aizawa K, et al. The impact of cardiovascular co-morbidities and duration of diabetes on the association between microvascular function and

glycaemic control. Cardiovascular Diabetology. 2017;**16**:114. DOI: 10.1186/s12933-017-0594-7

[15] Mohammedi K, Woodward M, Marre M, Colagiuri S, Cooper M, Harrap S, et al. Comparative effects of microvascular and macrovascular disease on the risk of major outcomes in patients with type 2 diabetes. Cardiovascular Diabetology. 2017;**16**:95. DOI: 10.1186/s12933-017-0574-y

[16] Holman RR, Paul SK, Bethel MA, Matthews DR, Neil HA. 10-year followup of intensive glucose control in type 2 diabetes. The New England Journal of Medicine. 2008;**359**:1577-1589. DOI: 10.1056/NEJMoa0806470

[17] Babizhayev MA, Strokov IA, Nosikov VV, Savel'yeva EL, Sitnikov VF, Yegorov YE, et al. The role of oxidative stress in diabetic neuropathy: Generation of free radical species in the glycation reaction and gene polymorphisms encoding antioxidant enzymes to genetic susceptibility to diabetic neuropathy in population of type I diabetic patients. Cell Biochemistry and Biophysics. 2015;**71**(3):1425-1443. DOI: 10.1007/s12013-014-0365-y

[18] Nishikawa T, Edelstein D, Du XL, Yamagishi S, Matsumura T, Kaneda Y, et al. Normalizing mitochondrial superoxide production bloks three pathways of hyperglycaemic damage. Nature. 2000;**404**:787-790. DOI: 10.1038/35008121

[19] Aiello LP, Avery RL, Arrigg PG, Keyt BA, Jampel HD, Shah ST, et al. Vascular endothelial growth factor in ocular fluid of patients with diabetic rethinopathy and other renal disorders. The New England Journal of Medicine. 1994;**331**:1480-1487. DOI: 10.1007/978-1-59259-979-0_5

[20] Del Canizo Gomez FJ, Perez CF, Ruiz IM, de Gorospe Perez-Jauregui C, Rodriguez SB, Losada TG. Microvascular complications and risk factors in patients with type 2 diabetes. Endocrinología y Nutrición. 2011;**58**(4):163-168. DOI: 10.1016/j.endonu.2011.01.006

[21] Fong DS, Aiello L, Gardner TW, King GL, Blankenship G, Cavallerano JD, et al. American Diabetes Association: Retinopathy in diabetes. Diabetes Care. 2004;**27**(1):84-87. DOI: 10.2337/diacare.27.2007.s84

[22] Kern TS. Contributions of inflammatory processes to the development of the early stages of diabetic retinopathy. Experimental Diabetes Research. 2007;**2007**:95103. DOI: 10.1155/2007/95103

[23] Lasker/IRRF Initiative for Innovation in Vision Science. Diabetic retinopathy: Where we are and a path to progress. 2012. Available from: http://www.laskerfoundation.org/media/filer_public/90/da/90dac4e3-af6f-4602-b479-df75837c6a5a/irrf_12.pdf

[24] Simão S, Bitoque D, Calado S, Silva GA. Oxidative stress modulates the expression of VEGF isoforms in the diabetic retina. New Frontiers in Ophthalmology. 2016;**2**(2):77-83. DOI: 10.15761/NFO.1000119

[25] Yi QY, Deng G, Chen N, Bai ZS, Yuan JS, Wu GH, et al. Metformin inhibits the development of diabetic retinopathy through inducing alternative splicing of VEGF-A. American Journal of Translational Research. 2016;**8**(9):3947-3954

[26] Sayin N, Kara N, Pekel G. Ocular complications of diabetes mellitus. World Journal of Diabetes. 2015;**6**(1):92-108. DOI: 10.4239/wjd.v6.i1.92

[27] Pascolini D, Mariotti SP. Global estimates of visual impairment: 2010.

The British Journal of Ophthalmology. 2012;**96**(5):614-618. DOI: 10.1136/bjophthalmol-2011-300539

[28] Jeganathan VS, Wang JJ, Wong TY. Ocular association of diabetes other than diabetic retinopathy. Diabetes Care. 2008;**31**(9):1905-1912. DOI: 10.2337/dc08-0342

[29] Caldwell RB, Bartoli M, Behzadian MA, El-Remessy AE, Al-Shabrawey M, Platt DH, et al. Vascular endothelial growth factor and diabetic retinopathy: Pathophysiological mechanisms and treatment perspectives. Diabetes/Metabolism Research and Reviews. 2003;**19**:442-455. DOI: 10.1002/dmrr.415

[30] Wang X, Wang G, Wang Y. Intravitreous vascular endothelial growth factor and hypoxia-inducible factor 1a in patients with proliferative diabetic retinopathy. American Journal of Ophthalmology. 2009;**148**:883-889. DOI: 10.1016/j.ajo.2009.07.007

[31] Bakhashab S, Ahmed FW, Schulten HJ, Bashir A, Karim S, Al-Malki AL, et al. Metformin improves the angiogenic potential of human CD34+ cells co-incident with downregulating CXCL10 and TIMP1 gene expression and increasing VEGFA under hyperglycemia and hypoxia within a therapeutic window for myocardial infarction. Cardiovascular Diabetology. 2016;**15**:27. DOI: 10.1186/s12933-016-0344-2

[32] Baba T, Shimada K, Neugebauer S, Yamada D, Hashimoto S, Watanabe T. The oral insulin sensitizer, thiazolidinedione, increases plasma vascular endothelial growth factor in type 2 diabetic patients. Diabetes Care. 2001;**24**:953-954. DOI: 10.2337/diacare.24.5.953

[33] Maleškić S, Kusturica J, Gušić E, Rakanović-Todić M, Šečić D, Burnazović-Ristić L, et al. Metformin use associated with protective effects for ocular complications in patients with type 2 diabetes - observational study. Acta Medica Academica. 2017;**46**(2):116-123. DOI: 10.5644/ama2006-124.196

[34] Ryu C, Munie M, Noorulla S, Edwards P, Qiso X, Gao H. Effect of metformin on the development of diabetic retinopathy. Investigative Ophthalmology & Visual Science. 2013;**54**:2449

[35] Tan BK, Adya R, Chen J, Farhatullah S, Heutling D, Mitchell D, et al. Metformin decreases angiogenesis via NF-kappaB and Erk1/2/Erk5 pathways by increasing the antiangiogenic thrombospondin-1. Cardiovascular Research. 2009;**83**:566-574. DOI: 10.1093/cvr/cvp131

[36] Albini A, Tosetti F, Li VW, Noonan DM, Li WW. Cancer prevention by targeting angiogenesis. Nature Reviews Clinical Oncology. 2012;**9**:498-509. DOI: 10.1038/nrclinonc.2012.120

[37] Han J, Li Y, Liu X, Zhou T, Sun H, Edwards P, et al. Metformin suppresses retinal angiogenesis and inflammation in vitro and in vivo. PLoS One. 2018;**13**(3):e0193031. DOI: 10.1371/journal.pone.0193031

[38] Xu L, Kong L, Wang J, Ash JD. Stimulation of AMPK prevents degeneration of photoreceptors and the retinal pigment epithelium. Proceedings of the National Academy of Sciences of the United States of America. 2018;**115**(41):10475-10480. DOI: 10.1073/pnas.1802724115

[39] Munie M, Ryu C, Noorulla S, Rana S, Malach D, Qiao X, et al. Effect of metformin on the development and severity of diabetic retinopathy. ARVO Annual Meeting Abstract. Investigative Ophthalmology & Visual Science. 2014;**55**:1069

[40] Dallaglio K, Bruno A, Cantelmo AR, Esposito AI, Ruggiero L, Orecchioni S, et al. Paradoxic effects of metformin on endothelial cells and angiogenesis. Carcinogenesis. 2014;**35**(5):1055-1066. DOI: 10.1093/carcin/bgu001

[41] Li Y, Ryu C, Munie M, Noorulla S, Rana S, Edwards P, et al. Association of metformin treatment with reduced severity of diabetic retinopathy in type 2 diabetic patients. Journal of Diabetes Research. 2018;**2018**:2801450. DOI: 10.1155/2018/2801450

[42] Zhou M, Wang W, Huang W, Zhang X. Diabetes mellitus as a risk factor for open-angle glaucoma: A systematic review and meta-analysis. PLoS One. 2014;**9**(8):e102972. DOI: 10.1371/journal.pone.0102972

[43] Lin H-C, Stein JD, Nan B, Childers D, Newman-Casey PA, Thompson DA, et al. Association of Geroprotective effects of metformin and risk of open-angle glaucoma in persons with diabetes mellitus. JAMA Ophthalmology. 2015;**133**(8):915-923. DOI: 10.1001/jamaophthalmol.2015.1440

[44] Guedes G, Tsai JC, Loewen N. Glaucoma and aging. Current Aging Science. 2011;**4**(2):110-117. DOI: 10.2174/1874609811104020110

[45] Anisimov VN. Metformin: Do we finally have an anti-aging medication? Cell Cycle. 2013;**12**(22):3483-3489. DOI: 10.4161/cc.26928

[46] Richards JE, Lin HC, Nan B, Talwar N, Childers D, Newman-Casey PA, et al. Targeting aging: Geroprotective medication metformin reduces risk of adult-onset open-angle glaucoma. Investigative Ophthalmology & Visual Science. 2014;**55**:1668

[47] Brown EE, Ball JD, Chen Z, Khurshid GS, Prosperi M, Ash JD. The common antidiabetic drug metformin reduces odds of developing age-related macular degeneration. Investigative Ophthalmology & Visual Science. 2019;**60**(5):1470-1477. DOI: 10.1167/iovs.18-26422

[48] Chen Y-Y, Shen Y-C, Lai Y-J, Wang C-Y, Lin K-H, Feng S-C, et al. Association between metformin and a lower risk of age-related macular degeneration in patients with type 2 diabetes. Journal of Ophthalmology. 2019:1649156. DOI: 10.1155/2019/1649156

[49] Lambert NG, ElShelmani H, Singh MK, Mansergh FC, Wride MA, Padilla M, et al. Risk factors and biomarkers of age-related macular degeneration. Progress in Retinal and Eye Research. 2016;**54, 54**:64-102. DOI: 10.1016/j.preteyeres.2016.04.003

[50] Moschos MM, Nitoda E, Chatziralli IP, Demopoulos CA. Age-related macular degeneration: Pathogenesis, genetic background, and the role of nutritional supplements. Journal of Chemistry. 2014;**9**:317536. DOI: 10.1155/2014/317536

[51] The Lancet Editorial. Age-related macular degeneration: Treatment at what cost? The Lancet. 2018;**392**(10153):1090. DOI: 10.1016/S0140-6736(18)32291

[52] Friedman DS, O'Colmain BJ, Muñoz B, Tomany SC, McCarty C, de Jong PT, et al. Prevalence of age-related macular degeneration in the United States. Archives of Ophthalmology. 2004;**122**(4):564-572. DOI: 10.1001/archopht.122.4.564

[53] Colijn JM, Buitendijk GHS, Prokofyeva E, Alves D, Cachulo ML, Khawaja AP, et al. Prevalence of age-related macular degeneration in Europe: The past and the future. Journal of Ophthalmology. 2017;**124**(12):1753-1763. DOI: 10.1016/j.ophtha.2017.05.035

[54] Bourne RRA, Flaxman SR, Braithwaite T, Cicinelli MV, Das A, Jonas JB, et al. Magnitude, temporal trends, and projections of the global prevalence of blindness and distance and near vision impairment: a systematic review and meta-analysis. The Lancet Global Health. 2017;5(9):e888-e897. DOI: 10.1016/S2214-109X(17)30293-0

[55] WHO. Blindness and vision impairment. Available from: https://www.who.int/news-room/fact-sheets/detail/blindness-and-visual-impairment [Accessed: 8 October 2019]

Chapter 5

Galega officinalis L. and Immunological Status in Diabetes Mellitus

Mariia Nagalievska, Halyna Hachkova and Nataliia Sybirna

Abstract

Under diabetes mellitus, the administration of *Galega officinalis* promotes restoration of leukocyte precursors' bone marrow pool and normalizes their proliferative activity. This plant protects the functional state of leukocytes by modulating actin cytoskeleton formation and through quantitative redistribution of leukocyte membrane glycoconjugates. *Galega officinalis* prevents the development of diabetes-associated oxidative stress which results in antiapoptotic activity. The normalization of leukocytes' proliferative and functional capacity by *Galega officinalis*, along with its antiapoptotic and hypoglycemic effects, can improve the course of the disease and may prevent the development of complications of diabetes.

Keywords: *Galega officinalis*, diabetes mellitus, leukocytes, immune system

1. Introduction

Diabetes mellitus belongs to a group of metabolic diseases accompanied by chronic inflammation and attenuation of the immune response, which subsequently contributes to the development of a number of complications [1]. Cells that are most affected by glycemic status and insulin level are leukocytes, which play major roles in inflammation and immune responses [2]. Constant high glucose levels result in the formation of cytotoxic compounds, leading to lower viability of peripheral blood leukocytes. This is mediated by enhanced reactive species production, activation of mitogen-activated protein kinase (MAPK) pathway, high levels of pro-inflammatory and poly (adenosine diphosphate [ADP]-ribose) polymerase (PARP) transcription factors, as well as inactivation of pro-survival pathways which altogether leads to increased apoptosis rate. The alterations in these molecular pathways are usually associated with increased leukocyte mobilization, which causes changes in their morphology and functional state [1, 3].

The multitude of diabetes mellitus complications creates the need for drugs with a wide spectrum of action, which would not only provide effective reduction of blood glucose but would also exhibit cytoprotective properties. The most commonly used anti-diabetes drug globally is metformin. Metformin shows a pleiotropic effect mediated by its hypoglycemic function, as well as inhibitory effect on oxidative stress and inflammation.

In many cases medicinal plants can be safe and effective alternatives to synthetic compounds in disease management, since they possess a unique composition of biologically active substances [4].

IntechOpen

Galega officinalis (*Galega*, goat's rue, French lilac) is a promising plant that can be used for treatment of a wide range of inflammatory diseases, including diabetes mellitus. *G. officinalis* is well-known for its hypoglycemic action, and it has been long used as part of a plant mixture for treatment of diabetes mellitus [5]. For a long time, the antidiabetic effect of *G. officinalis* was associated with high content of alkaloid galegine, which is one of the main components of this plant's leaves. In fact, metformin, discussed above, is a synthetic form of galegine, which was originally used to treat diabetes mellitus type 2 [5]. The toxicity of *G. officinalis'* alkaloids decreased its attractiveness as a hypoglycemic drug. However, it was found that even the non-alkaloid extract has a hypoglycemic effect and is potentially nontoxic [6, 7]. Based on such historical use and a large number of recent scientific studies, *G. officinalis* is a source of potent biologically active substances for the prevention and treatment of diabetes mellitus [8].

2. Effects of metformin on the immune system

Metformin (N,N-dimethylbiguanide) is an oral antihyperglycemic agent, which from a chemical point of view is a synthetic derivative of guanidine. The hypoglycemic effect of this drug is realized through the inhibition of hepatic glucose production, reducing intestinal glucose absorption and improving glucose uptake and utilization by peripheral tissues. Recent research has shed light on the pleiotropic effect of metformin, ranging from hypoglycemic function to cardio- and nephroprotection, as well as inhibitory effects on oxidative stress and inflammation [9–11].

The scientific data concerning the influence of metformin on the immune system is controversial, and its effect strongly depends on the pathology in which it is used. For example, metformin enhances antitumor immunity, but in other contexts, it can act as an anti-inflammatory or immunosuppressive agent [8]. Metformin can suppress senescence- and cancer-related inflammation. The majority of experimental data indicates that metformin modulates leukocytes' functional activity by activating 5′ adenosine monophosphate-activated protein kinase (AMPK). Metformin can activate AMPK in multiple cell populations, including macrophages and neutrophils [12, 13]. It has also been demonstrated that metformin inhibits innate immune response to fungal infection in an AMPK-dependent manner and lessens central nervous system inflammation [14].

Considering the significant modulating effect of metformin on the immune system, it is unsurprising that it has a strong effect on immunocompetent blood cells, which we discuss below.

2.1 Metformin influence on defective hematopoiesis

Studies conducted on Fanconi anemia mice showed the unique property of metformin to improve hematopoiesis by restoring hematopoietic stem cell (HSC) numbers. It also delays tumor formation, presumably via reduction of DNA damage induced by aldehydes [15]. An important part of metformin protective effect may be conferred by aldehyde detoxification. Other mechanisms by which metformin may act to protect the cell's DNA are reducing the activity of mitochondrial complex 1 activity, thus potentially reducing oxidative DNA damage. It is also possible that metformin can switch the metabolic balance between oxidative phosphorylation and anaerobic glycolysis and downregulate inflammatory pathways which are thought to contribute to bone marrow failure [15]. Another study demonstrates that metformin treatment significantly inhibited the total-body irradiation-induced increase in the levels of DNA double-strand breaks and reactive oxygen species

(ROS) by attenuation of NOX4 expression in HSCs. Furthermore, metformin modulates the expression of antioxidant enzymes in HSCs [16].

2.2 Influence of metformin on functional state of leukocytes

Many diabetic patients who receive metformin show significantly reduced neutrophil-to-lymphocyte ratio [9]. Metformin is able to reduce hyperneutrophilia in girls with hyperinsulinemic hyperandrogenism and improves white blood cell count in women with polycystic ovary syndrome, two conditions characterized by a pronounced systemic inflammatory state [17]. Metformin increased the number of CD8-positive tumor-infiltrating lymphocytes. Normalizing effect of metformin on the number of immunocompetent cells is associated with its ability to upregulate AMPK and as a consequence of altering energy metabolism in the cell [14].

Apart from metformin influence on immunocompetent cell number, this drug also can modulate their functional activity. As expected for an AMPK activator, metformin enhances cell mobility and phagocytosis, in particular in macrophages that show enhanced uptake of bacteria, synthetic beads, or apoptotic cells. The effects of AMPK activation may be due to its ability to increase availability of cell surface receptors, including αM integrin or Fc receptors or due to mechanisms that involve suppression of TLR4-associated signaling pathways. Metformin by activating AMPK regulates the process of inflammation resolution—efferocytosis and enhanced uptake of bacteria by phagocytic cells [12, 13].

Additionally, in patients with prediabetes, metformin treatment reduces the concentration of neutrophil extracellular trap (NET) components independently from glycemic control [14].

The normalization of phagocytosis processes and NETosis under metformin administration could suggest an effect of this drug on neutrophil activation. Indeed, metformin attenuates neutrophil activation via inhibition of mitochondrial respiratory complex I, potentially through intracellular H_2O_2-mediated inhibition of IκB-α degradation and thus prevention of NF-κB activation [18].

Immune system modulation by metformin can be realized not only by its direct influence on the immunocompetent cells but also by its ability to regulate chemokine level. Metformin causes a decrease in inflammatory markers in plasma, including soluble intercellular adhesion molecule, vascular cell adhesion molecule-1, macrophage migration inhibitory factor, C-reactive protein, IL-6, and IL-8. The anti-inflammatory action of metformin is realized by suppressing Akt, Erk1/2, and NF-B translocation. Such changes lead to blocking of pro-inflammatory signal transduction via the phosphoinositide 3 kinase pathway [19].

Immunosuppressive effect of metformin can be mediated by its ability to inhibit the expression of pro-inflammatory mediators (IFN-, TNF-, IL-1, IL-6, IL-17, iNOS, MMP9, and RANTES) and infiltration of immune cells, which was blocked by reducing the expression of CAMs (ICAM, VCAM, and E-selectin) on vascular cells [20, 21].

2.3 Effects of metformin on oxidative stress

Oxidative stress is the leading cause of microvascular and cardiovascular diabetes complications [22]. Disruption of glucose metabolism causes mitochondrial superoxide overproduction in cells. An increased amount of superoxide leads to overactivity of polyol and hexosamine pathways, increased formation of AGEs (advanced glycation end products) and its receptors, and activation of protein kinase C isoforms. Altogether, this leads to the development of complications of diabetes. Simultaneously endothelial nitric oxide synthase is inactivated. Changes in the activity of these signaling pathways result in increased intracellular ROS and activation of pro-inflammatory pathways [22].

Considering such intimate link between diabetes and oxidative stress, anti-diabetes treatments should not only reduce blood sugar but should also possess strong antioxidant properties. Metformin satisfies both criteria; as in addition to a hypoglycemic effect, it improves the immunological parameters of patients, presumably through its antioxidant properties [23]. In aortic endothelial cells, metformin has been shown to inhibit high glucose-dependent ROS overproduction, which was mediated by a reduction in NADPH oxidase activity and an inhibition of the respiratory chain complex 1. Another possible mechanism of metformin antioxidant properties is its ability to activate AMPK with the ensuing induction of manganese superoxide dismutase and expression of the antioxidant thioredoxin and endothelial NO synthase (eNOS). Additionally, metformin is able to reduce AGEs synthesis and the expression of their specific cell receptor called RAGE in endothelial cells [16, 23]. In addition to the abovementioned indirect mechanisms of modulation of superoxide anion intracellular production, it was found that metformin can directly scavenge ROS, in particular $^{\bullet}OH$ but not $O_2^{\bullet}$ [16].

While leukocytes actively participate in ROS generation, they are highly sensitive to ROS-mediated oxidative damage. Metformin was demonstrated to have a protective effect against oxidative stress in immunocompetent cells [24].

Furthermore, metformin modulates the function of fMLP-activated polymorphonuclear neutrophils that quench the products of oxidative burst. Researchers hypothesized that metformin may recognize specific cell membrane sites, thereby inducing intracellular signal transduction resulting in changes in NADPH oxidase activity or in other sources of intracellular ROS [25]. Furthermore, metformin-induced decrease in ROS levels led to a partial inhibition of lipid peroxidation in lymphocytes [26].

2.4 A protective role of metformin against apoptosis

Most chronic diseases, including diabetes mellitus, are accompanied by oxidative stress, which may result in apoptosis of different types of cells [27]. Metformin has been shown to have protective role on apoptosis. The inhibition of apoptosis by metformin has been described in many cell types and under various conditions. There may be several mechanisms of apoptosis prevention. Firstly, metformin possesses good radical scavenging activity. Secondly, metformin can regulate caspase levels and induce xenobiotic phase II enzymes [28].

A number of authors have concluded that metformin exerts a neuroprotective effect by decreasing mitochondria-dependent apoptosis. This is achieved through the inhibition of permeability transition pore opening, blocking the release of cytochrome c and preventing subsequent cell death [29]. A protective role of metformin against programmed cell death is likely mediated by maintaining mitochondria integrity and reducing Ca^{2+}. This drug also lowers the expression of caspase-3, cytochrome c, and cleaved caspase-9 and reduces fragmentation of PARP-1 while increasing the expression of Bcl-2 [29]. A similar protective effect of metformin has been described for primary rat hepatocytes. Metformin may protect against apoptosis by induction of menadione-induced heme oxygenase-1 and bcl-xl expression and the reduction of c-Jun N-terminal kinase activation [30, 31].

Given the ability of metformin to inhibit apoptosis of different cells in a variety of pathologies, it is possible to assume that it has a similar effect on immunocompetent blood cells. Indeed, it was shown that metformin markedly decreased the percentage of apoptotic cells in bone marrow cells of rats [32]. It also reduces the activation of macrophages and inhibits the expression of COX-2 and caspase-3, thereby attenuating inflammatory responses and apoptosis [33].

Treatment with metformin reduces the amount of oxidant-induced DNA damage in lymphocytes. It was shown that pharmacological concentration (50 μM) of metformin could protect against prooxidant stimulus-induced DNA damage at early but not late stages. Thus, metformin likely exerts an antiapoptotic effect by reducing caspase-3 and caspase-8 activities [28].

3. Effects of *Galega officinalis* L. on immunocompetent cells under diabetes mellitus

Galega officinalis (goat's rue) is a toxic leguminous plant originated in the Eastern Mediterranean and Black Sea regions but now has been spread in southeastern parts of Europe and the Middle East. In the medieval period, this plant was traditionally used for the treatment of diabetes [5, 34]. *G. officinalis* contains a large number of secondary metabolites with pronounced biological properties, among which are alkaloids, saponins, flavonoids, tannins, fatty acids, and phytoestrogens [35].

3.1 Component composition and hypoglycemic effect of non-alkaloid extract of *Galega officinalis*

The non-alkaloid extract of *G. officinalis* can be obtained by a two-step extraction [6, 7]. In the first stage, the biologically active substances are obtained by plant material infusion in 96 % ethanol. After alcohol evaporation, equal volumes of water and chloroform are added to the residue. The obtained chloroform fraction should be evaporated to obtain the solid residue, which is then dissolved in water to form an emulsion. The latter is not stable and eventually forms a precipitate. The stability of emulsions is very important; their stratification affects the accuracy of active substance content measurement. To solve this problem, the biocomplex PS (surface-active products of *Pseudomonas* sp. PS-17 biosynthesis) can be used [7]. Using gas chromatography/mass spectrometry method, it was established that the biocomplex PS consists of methyl ester of decenoic acid and dodecenoic acid. These surfactants were added to the initial mixture obtained by the addition of water to non-alkaloid fraction of *G. officinalis*. Such extraction and stabilization yield a stable water emulsion without toxic alkaloids [6, 36].

Crucially, such non-alkaloid fraction of *G. officinalis* extract exhibited a hypoglycemic effect in streptozotocin-induced diabetes mellitus if administered for 14 days at 600 mg/kg per day. Notably, blood glucose concentration decreased to physiological values [6, 7].

Blood glucose measurement evaluates current glucose concentration, which may depend on many factors (the intake and composition of food, physical activity and their intensity, the emotional state of the patient, and even the time of the day) [37]. Thus, blood glucose concentration may not reflect the actual degree of diabetes compensation, potentially resulting in medication under- or overdosing. Therefore, today, the key indicator for treatment quality and risk of diabetes complications is the level of glycosylated hemoglobin (HbA1c) [37]. Notably, the non-alkaloid fraction of *Galega officinalis* extract normalizes HbA1c content under diabetes [6].

Sugar-reducing effect of non-alkaloid extract may be due to its complex composition [6, 36, 38]. Gas chromatography/mass spectrometry detected phytol as a component of non-alkaloid fraction of *Galega officinalis* extract. Phytol might contribute to the extract's sugar-lowering effect, as it is known to lower insulin resistance and sensitivity of muscles to insulin and to reduce gluconeogenesis [39]. It has been shown that phytol can increase the expression of *GLUT2* and *glucokinase* genes through activation of RXR (retinoid X receptor) [39], which are otherwise downregulated under diabetes mellitus. Palmitic acid esters in the extract could also cause a dose-dependent decrease in blood plasma glucose in animals with experimental diabetes mellitus [40]. Furthermore, non-alkaloid fraction of *Galega officinalis* extract contains high levels of phytosterols (campesterol and stigmasterol) that, in addition to the ability to inhibit cholesterol adsorption, can reduce the level of glycosylated hemoglobin [41, 42].

Another notable biologically active substance from *Galega officinalis* is α-amyrin. It has a hypoglycemic action and can influence endocannabinoid system. Some ligands for cannabinoid CB1 receptors can directly bind and allosterically regulate Kir6.2/SUR1 K (ATP) channels, thereby controlling glucose-stimulated insulin release. In addition, α- and β-amyrin, due to their anti-inflammatory and antioxidant properties, have a positive effect on the state of animals with streptozotocin diabetes [43].

It has been shown that quinazoline derivatives are capable to lower blood glucose level and body weight in obese animals [44]. Notably, the non-alkaloid fraction of *Galega officinalis* contains such substances (2-methyl-1,2,3a,4,5-hexahydropyrrolo[1,2-a]quinazoline). These derivatives can increase the activity of AMPK, which results in increased glucose adsorption by muscle cells. It has been found that AMPK, in addition to regulating insulin release by pancreatic cells, inhibits the activity of acetyl-CoA-carboxylase and hydroxymethylglutaryl-CoA-reductase in fat cells, thereby inhibiting the biosynthesis of fatty acids and cholesterol [45].

High content of alpha-linolenic acid in *Galega* extract is also noteworthy. Omega-3 polyunsaturated fatty acids increase cell membrane fluidity, as well as the number of insulin receptors, the affinity of insulin to these receptors, and the number of type 4 glucose transporters; they also regulate the balance between pro- and antioxidants [46].

Based on the above statement, the sugar-lowering effect of the non-alkaloid fraction of *Galega officinalis* extract is likely due to the presence of phytol, ethyl ester of palmitic acid, phytosterols (campesterol and stigmasterol), and quinazoline derivatives, acting separately or synergistically [6].

3.2 Regulation of bone marrow cells proliferation by *Galega officinalis*

Many of diabetes complications are induced by the intensification of chronic inflammation and attenuation of the immune response. Leukocytes play major roles in inflammation and immune responses. Diabetes mellitus is accompanied by infectious and inflammatory processes, of which the most frequent are bacterial infections, which are accompanied by relapses and are difficult to treat. Changes in the proliferative activity and ratio of leukocytes and changes in their functional properties and activation of free radical oxidation are among probable causes of the propensity of patients with diabetes mellitus to infectious processes and their compromised immunological status [2].

Therefore, the measurement of the hypoglycemic effect is insufficient when testing the effectiveness of new antidiabetic agents. It is also necessary to evaluate the effect of potential hypoglycemic drugs on cells that are susceptible to metabolic changes in diabetes mellitus. Cells whose function is very significantly affected in the course of diabetes mellitus are white blood cells. High levels of glucose in the bloodstream cause inflammation, which primarily affects blood cells, in particular, leukocytes [47, 48].

In addition to a broad spectrum of substances with a hypoglycemic effect, the non-alkaloid fraction of *Galega officinalis* extract contains compounds with potential immunomodulatory effect. *Galega officinalis* normalizes differential count of leukocytes in conditions of diabetes mellitus. In particular, it leads to an increase in the number of segmented and band neutrophils while overall lowering the number of lymphocytes to almost control values [49]. This indicates a normalization of the cell-mediated immune response, as one of the most important factors determining the activity of the immune system of an organism [49]. The normalization of the content of immunocompetent cells in blood after treatment of diabetic rats with *Galega* extract may be due to the influence of its biologically active substances on the proliferation of these cells.

The non-alkaloid fraction of *Galega officinalis* extract, as a source of biologically active substances with wide range of actions, significantly affects the proliferative activity of bone marrow cells in conditions of diabetes. In particular, in rats with streptozotocin-induced diabetes mellitus, the administration of *Galega officinalis* extract caused a significant decrease in leukocyte proliferation, which is otherwise very high under diabetes. However, a more detailed analysis showed that despite the overall growth of leukocyte proliferation under diabetes mellitus, the abundance of not all leukocyte types increases in the bone marrow [38]. In particular, under diabetes a reduction in the number of myeloblasts was shown, with the following decrease of juvenile and staff neutrophils. By contrast, lymphoblast numbers increased. Interestingly, the number of lymphocytes in the bone marrow does not undergo significant changes, potentially because immature lymphocytes leave the bone marrow towards the bloodstream. Since the non-alkaloid fraction of *Galega officinalis* extract can regulate the proliferative activity of leukocyte precursors, it is able to influence on the content of different types of leukocytes. *Galega officinalis* extract administration causes a decline in lymphoblasts and segmented granulocytes number, as well as an increase in numbers of lymphocytes and juvenile and staff granulocytes in the bone marrow of animals with diabetes mellitus. It has been proposed that this effect is due to the extract's ability to regulate the tumor necrosis factor α (TNF-α) content, the amount of which significantly increases in diabetes mellitus [38].

Furthermore, the revealed influence of *Galega officinalis* extract on the proliferative activity of leukocytes may relate to the presence of inositol [50], fatty acids [51, 52], especially α-linolenic acid [53–55], flavonoids [56–59], phytol [60], squalene [61], campesterol, and stigmasterol [62] as well as α-amyrin [38, 63].

3.3 Influence of *Galega officinalis* on functional state of leukocytes and their antioxidant-prooxidant balance

In diabetes, abnormal immune response manifests itself not only in the imbalance in the process of leukocytes proliferation but also in the disruption of these cells' functional activity. The main effectors of the inflammatory process are phagocytes [64]. The effectiveness of phagocytic response is largely determined by the nature and intensity of its initial stage—chemotaxis. However, because of its complexity, chemotaxis is one of the most vulnerable forms of neutrophil reactivity [65]. Therefore, the impairment of the functional capacity of phagocytes and other immunocytes is associated with the pathology of movement of these cells. The main mechanism that allows cell motility is actin polymerization, as it underlies in the formation of stress fibrils, lamellipodia, and filopodia [66].

In animals with diabetes, the non-alkaloid fraction of *Galega officinalis* extract causes a decrease in filamentous actin (F-actin) content; this can testify about the reduction in the formation of short pseudopodia on the leukocytes surface. These data indicate that the use of this extract reduces the change in the structural and functional properties of leukocytes, as well as decrease of leukocyte pre-activated state [67]. It is possible that the extract-induced decrease in actin polymerization might regulate integrin-dependent interaction with vascular endothelium necessary for leukocytes penetration through the blood vessel wall during inflammatory processes [68].

F-actin is represented by two pools: (1) long microfilaments (the constitutive fraction of cytoskeleton) located near the cell membrane and reaching towards the center of the cell and (2) short microfilaments located in the submembrane cortical network. Short filaments form a very dynamic fraction, since they are the first ones to initiate polymerization of actin membrane filaments at the time of leukocytes activation [69]. Along with F-actin high content in blood leukocytes in diabetes mellitus condition, the process of its polymerization is intensified with the formation of fraction of short actin filaments. The source of monomers for this polymerization is, to a large extent, products of cytoskeleton filaments depolymerization and, to a lesser extent, the cellular pool of monomeric actin. The increase in actin polymerization may be due to an increase in the phosphatidylinositol amount observed in diabetes mellitus [70]. These cellular messengers may act as inhibitors of phosphorylation of actin regulatory proteins that affect the redistribution of actin filaments and reduce the content of cytoskeleton actin filaments and proportionally increase the level of actin in the short filaments and monomers fractions [71].

The administration of the non-alkaloid fraction of *Galega officinalis* extract in leukocytes of animals with diabetes causes a pronounced depolymerization of short actin filaments. It is accompanied by the formation of actin monomers and their polymerization to a fraction of cytoskeleton filaments. *Galega*-induced changes in actin cytoskeleton organization of leukocytes under prolonged hyperglycemia are probably due to a decrease in the pre-activated state of leukocytes. This effect is mainly achieved by a decrease in the intensity of activation and translocation of the phosphatidylinositol-3′-kinase regulatory subunit in the cytoskeleton sites [68, 72]. Reduced amount of phosphatidylinositol-3′-kinase reaction products (phosphatidylinositol-3,4-diphosphate and phosphatidylinositol-1,3,4-triphosphate) in the cell results in association of the CAP protein with actin filaments, resulting in inhibition of actin polymerization [71].

As mentioned above, diabetes mellitus type 1 is characterized by pre-activated state of leukocytes. This state is associated with the structural and functional rearrangement of the receptor apparatus of these cells. Often, such alterations are realized through changes in the structure of surface glycoproteins that contain sialic acid [73]. In diabetes, N-acetyl-β,D-glucosamine residues are exposed to a greater degree compared to healthy subjects, while the exposure of sialic acids linked by $\alpha2\rightarrow3$ and $\alpha2\rightarrow6$-glycoside bonds to subterminal residues (β, D-galactose, or N-acetylgalactosamine) decreases. Quantitative redistribution of glycoconjugates in leukocyte membranes leads to the modification of signaling networks involved in intercellular interactions, as well as, to the disruption of the aggregation and adhesiveness of these cells [67]. Activation of membrane-bound neuraminidases in diabetes mellitus leads to a decrease in the total level of sialic acids on the cell membrane. Desialylation is accompanied by increased content of subterminal monosaccharide—β, D-galactose. Galactose-containing glycoproteins regulate leukocyte migration during the inflammatory process, accompanied by a dynamic rearrangement of actin cytoskeleton [74].

The non-alkaloid fraction of *Galega officinalis* extract normalizes the content and structures of the glycoproteins' carbohydrate determinants that form leukocytes' glycocalyx.

Reduction in N-acetyl-β,D-glucosamine residue content upon *Galega officinalis* administration is important to restore normal leukocyte function. Normalized content of such receptors indicates completion of leukocytes pre-activation. It is known that N-acetyl-β,D-glucosamine-containing glycoproteins include a receptor for N-formyl-methionyl-leucyl-phenylalanine, which stimulates a respiratory burst in neutrophil granulocytes by activating NADPH oxidase [75]. Also, N-acetyl-β,D-glucosamine-containing glycoconjugates are involved in the adhesion of leukocytes to the endothelium during inflammation (through cell surface receptor macrophage-1 antigen or complement receptor 3, which mediates the interaction of neutrophil granulocytes with intercellular adhesion molecule-1) [75]. Thus, the normalization of the receptor content, which has N-acetyl-β,D-glucosamine in its structure, improves the cell's response to extracellular stimuli with a corresponding restoration of the functional state of leukocytes.

Under streptozotocin-induced diabetes, the administration of the non-alkaloid fraction of *Galega officinalis* extract increases the content of α(2→3)-bond sialic acids to physiological levels. It is possible that this effect is due to the influence of the extract's biologically active substances on the activity of enzymes involved in the cleavage or transfer of sialic acid residues (neuraminidase and trans-sialidase) [67, 76]. Glycoproteins that contain sialic acids are structural components of the leukocyte co-receptor complex CD3, which is present in all mature T-lymphocytes and is involved in their activation. It can be assumed that the use of *Galega officinalis* may lead to the restoration of the structure of carbohydrate determinants of the glycoprotein subunit CD3-γ or CD3-ε in the CD3 co-receptor. This in turn inhibits the attenuation of T cells maturation and, as a consequence, prevents the development of the immune deficiency [77–79].

Consequently, receptor apparatus restoration by *Galega officinalis* extract determines the normalization of the cells' response to extracellular signals, which ultimately leads to the reorganization of actin cytoskeleton elements. However, the leukocyte migration, and therefore the state of actin cytoskeleton, depends on the presence of adhesion molecules on leukocyte surface and on the presence of chemokines. One of these chemokines is TNF-α, a pleiotropic pro-inflammatory cytokine. Through the activation of various signaling cascades, it regulates cell proliferation, differentiation, migration, and apoptosis [80, 81]. An increase in cytokine concentrations under diabetes [38, 67] stimulates leukocyte actin polymerization. TNF-α induces a brief increase in polymerized actin content by activating the Rho/ROCK (Rho-related protein kinase) signaling pathway in neutrophils. The activation of the Rho/ROCK signaling pathway leads to the reorganization of the neutrophil cytoskeleton inducing the formation of stress fibers [82–84]. *Galega* extract decreases TNF-α content to physiological levels. This effect is believed to be related to the presence of anti-inflammatory compounds, including flavonoids, methyl ester of linolenic acid, and α-amyrin [67].

Thus, the non-alkaloid fraction of *Galega officinalis* extract reduces leukocyte pre-activation by acting both on cellular receptor apparatus and on chemokine content in the medium. Reducing diabetes-induced leukocytes pre-activated state by *Galega* extract can significantly improve these cells' functional state. One of the most important functional properties of neutrophils is their bactericidal action. It has been discovered that *Galega officinalis* greatly improved the microbe killing properties of cells. In particular, the non-alkaloid fraction of *Galega officinalis* extract causes a decrease in neutrophils myeloperoxidase content, whereas in conditions of diabetes, the content of this enzyme increases [38, 85]. Inhibition of myeloperoxidase production by neutrophils can play an important role in the prevention of vascular damage mediated by leukocytes. It is known that the excessive amount of myeloperoxidase can cause damage of the blood vessel walls by producing strong oxidants (HOCl and HOBr) or by nitration of the tyrosine residues in proteins. Altogether this can eventually result in cardiovascular diseases [86, 87]. It has been proposed that such inhibiting effect of *Galega officinalis* extract may be due to the synergistic action of phytol, flavonoids, squalene, phytosterols, and amyrin [38].

Along with the decrease in the content of myeloperoxidase, the non-alkaloid fraction of the *Galega officinalis* extract also reduces the content of cationic proteins [38] that mediate the killing of a variety of microorganisms through ion pore formation in their membranes [88]. The latter effect is associated with the presence of flavonoids in the extract [38], because these compounds are able to inhibit cationic protein secretion [89].

Thus, the use of alkaloid-free *Galega officinalis* extract for the treatment of diabetes leads to the restoration of functional properties of leukocytes, as indicated by the reconstitution of glycoconjugate receptors on leukocyte membranes, normalization of the ratio of polymerized and unpolymerized actin, as well as restoration of bactericidal properties of these cells.

Diabetes is accompanied by neutrophil malfunction caused, to a large extent, by the development of oxidative-nitrative stress [90]. Oxidative stress leads to the activation of immunocompetent blood cells and their aggregation and adhesion. Further, an increase in the synthesis of arachidonic acid and its metabolites, cytokines, oxygen radicals, and secretion of lysosomal enzymes take place in activated leukocytes. Altogether, it ultimately leads to the development of atherosclerosis [91].

Due to the presence of a large number of biologically active substances with a potential antioxidant effect in the non-alkaloid fraction of *Galega officinalis* extract, it is possible to use this extract as a potential source of antioxidants. Indeed, under diabetes mellitus, the non-alkaloid fraction of *Galega officinalis* extract causes a significant reduction in ROS content in leukocytes, which is otherwise elevated in the pathology [92]. Reduction of ROS generation by leukocytes may be due to the influence of *Galega* extract on the activity of the three main enzymatic systems responsible for generation ROS: membrane-bound NADPH oxidase, peroxidase—myeloperoxidase in neutrophils and eosinophil peroxidase in eosinophils, as well as NO synthase. Indeed, a decrease in the content of myeloperoxidase in polymorphonuclear leukocytes [38] and reduction of the total activity of NO synthase was confirmed [93]. In addition to decreasing the activity of ROS synthesis enzymatic systems, the non-alkaloid extract of *Galega officinalis* significantly reduces the processes of protein and lipid oxidative modification. This effect is due to a decrease in total ROS content and NO stable metabolites (nitrite and nitrate anions), with the corresponding termination of biosubstrate oxidation by free radicals. Reduction of oxidative modified proteins and lipids stops the chain reaction of oxidative-nitric stress in conditions of diabetes and confirms the antioxidant effect of the *Galega officinalis* extract [38, 93].

The negative action of ROS in the body is counterbalanced by an antioxidant system, whose functioning is aimed at neutralizing free radicals, as well as repairing damages caused by them [94]. However, in conditions of oxidative-nitrative stress, which is largely activated during diabetes, antioxidant system of blood cells cannot fully implement its protective and adaptive mechanisms. The abnormal functioning of the immune system is evident from a decrease in the superoxide dismutase, catalase, and glutathione peroxidase activity in leukocytes. Under diabetes, the non-alkaloid fraction *of Galega officinalis* extract has a protective effect on the key components of the antioxidant defense system, causing a significant increase in superoxide dismutase and catalase activities [92]. Restoration of antioxidant defense enzymes activity by biologically active substances may be caused by inhibition of the glycosylation of these enzymes, mediated by the hypoglycemic effect of the extract. The increased activity of the antioxidant enzymes is in line with the observed suppression of the formation of oxygen and nitrogen reactive forms, as well as protein and lipid oxidation [38, 93].

The protective effect of the non-alkaloid fraction of *Galega officinalis* extract on blood cells can be explained by its ability to regulate the prooxidant-antioxidant balance by means of scavenging free radicals and preventing the inhibition of key components of enzymatic antioxidant system. The main active ingredients of the extract that exhibit antioxidant properties are phytol, showing its properties due to its hydroxyl group [95] and, flavonoids, serving as a traps for electrons and free radicals and thus suppressing the chain reactions of free radical biosubstrate oxidation [38, 89, 93]. Also, α-amyrin [43] and α-linoleic acid [46] possess pronounced antioxidant activities.

3.4 *Galega officinalis* prevents leukocytes apoptosis induced by diabetes mellitus

The development of diabetes mellitus is accompanied by a significant intensification of oxidative-nitrative stress, resulting in the formation of substances with a strong proapoptotic effect. Especially sensitive to such substances are blood cells, including leukocytes. The response of immune cells to antigenic stimuli, as well as the nature, dynamics, and duration of the immune response and immunological tolerance formation are partially regulated through programmed cell death [96]. The non-alkaloid fraction of *Galega officinalis* extract causes inhibition of DNA fragmentation, which is a biochemical marker of apoptosis [97].

Other studies have shown that the use of the non-alkaloid fraction of *Galega officinalis* extract in animals with diabetes leads to a reduction of lymphocytes with features of apoptosis, in particular to reduction of phosphatidylserine (PS) residue translocation from the inner to the outer side of the membrane [38]. Changes in the intensity of lymphocyte apoptosis may be due to the effect of extract on the content of TNF-α. It is known that TNF-α reacts with the so-called death receptors and activates procaspases that trigger the apoptotic cascade [98]. Thus, a decrease in TNF-α content might suggest that one of the mechanisms by which *Galega officinalis* inhibits apoptosis in immunocompetent cells is by suppressing the extrinsic, or death receptor, apoptosis pathway [38].

Another evidence for the activation of the extrinsic apoptosis pathway under diabetes is exposure on leukocytes' immature membrane epitopes with modified sialic acid content. It takes place in response to the loss of surface membrane during cytoplasmic membrane blebbing [99]. The administration of *Galega officinalis* extract to diabetic animals causes an increase in the content of sialic acid residues linked by $\alpha(2\rightarrow3)$ and $\alpha(2\rightarrow6)$ glycosidic bonds with the subterminal surface glycoconjugate residues of rat leukocytes [75].

On the other hand, it has been found that *Galega officinalis* is able to regulate the processes of the intrinsic (mitochondrial) pathway of apoptosis. In particular, it reduces the levels of the apoptosis regulatory proteins p53 and Bcl-2 [75, 97]. It is known that cell damage results in p53 translocation from the cytoplasm into the mitochondria [100]. In the mitochondria this protein undergoes rapid enzymatic de-ubiquitination that yields an active form which interacts with BH4 domain of antiapoptotic proteins Bcl-XL and Bcl-2 [100]. Binding to antiapoptotic proteins induces the release and activation of proapoptotic proteins Bax and Bid. Such interactions lead to the release of cytochrome c and induction of apoptosis [101, 102]. At the same time, *Galega officinalis* in leukocytes regulates the content of Bcl-2, a protein that inhibits both p53-dependent and p53-independent pathways of apoptosis. Reduction of this protein content promotes the formation of ion channels in mitochondria membrane, thus stabilizing the mitochondrial cytochrome c oxidase and regulating the activation of proteins that are involved in apoptosis [75, 97].

Another significant confirmation of *Galega officinalis* antiapoptotic action is the reduction of the content of PARylated proteins in leukocytes under diabetes [75].

This indicates a decrease in DNA damage with the corresponding inhibition of DNA repair complex (base excision repair in response to single-stranded DNA breaks and nucleotide excision repair), which includes poly (ADP-ribose) polymerase enzyme [103]. Thus, *Galega*-induced decrease in protein PARylation could stem from inhibition of poly (ADP-ribose) polymerase activity, which can be assumed to prevent ribosylation of a number of proteins, including glyceraldehyde-3-phosphate dehydrogenase. In the presence of excess glucose, this results in inactivation of the polyol and hexosamine pathways, thereby preventing the accumulation of products and precursors of nonenzymatic glycosylation and activation of protein kinase C. As the final result, this leads to the inhibition of oxidative-nitric stress manifestations and prevents the occurrence of chronic diabetic lesions [75].

The established antiapoptotic effect of *Galega officinalis* extract is mediated by sugar-reducing, antioxidant, and anti-inflammatory properties of its components. In particular, the composition of the extract revealed a number of compounds that have potentially hypoglycemic (phytol, ethyl ester of palmitic acid, campesterol, stigmasterol, and quinazoline derivatives), antioxidant (phytol, flavonoids, vitamin E), and anti-inflammatory (flavonoids, methyl ester of linolenic acid, α-amyrin) effects [38].

4. Conclusions

Metformin has become widely used in the treatment of diabetes mellitus type 2 over the last period of time. This is due to the fact that metformin, along with its hypoglycemic effect, has the potential to modulate the functioning of immunocompetent blood cells. Metformin transiently inhibits NADH:ubiquinone oxidoreductase of the mitochondrial electron transport chain. This inhibition leads to the activation of the energy sensor 5′-AMP-activated protein kinase. The activation of this enzyme results in a whole range of metabolic changes in the immunocompetent cells. Metformin is able to regulate the processes of bone marrow cell proliferation, affect the functional activity, and regulate the apoptosis processes of immunocompetent cells.

To date, practically all mechanisms of therapeutic influence of metformin are well described. Instead, the plant from which this biguanide was first obtained somewhat become underestimated. Under diabetes mellitus type 1, the non-alkaloid fraction of *Galega officinalis* possesses pronounced hypoglycemic effect. The non-alkaloid fraction of *Galega officinalis* normalizes the leukocyte proliferation processes by restoring the neutrophils bone marrow pool and reducing the lymphoblasts number. This extract affects the functional state of immunocompetent cells in blood, leading to quantitative redistribution and structural alterations of carbohydrate determinants in leukocyte membranes, reorganization of actin cytoskeleton, as well as affecting the bactericidal function of neutrophils. Furthermore, non-alkaloid fraction of *Galega officinalis* predetermines the suppression of leukocyte to genetically programmed death. The multifactorial effect of *Galega officinalis* extract under diabetes may be, on the one hand, due to its potent hypoglycemic effect, and, on the other hand, due to its ability to regulate the prooxidant-antioxidant balance by scavenging free radicals and preventing the inhibition of key enzymatic components of the antioxidant defense system.

Conflict of interest

The authors declare no conflict of interest.

Author details

Mariia Nagalievska*, Halyna Hachkova and Nataliia Sybirna
Department of Biochemistry, Faculty of Biology, Ivan Franko National University of Lviv, Lviv, Ukraine

*Address all correspondence to: khmarija@gmail.com

References

[1] Bajpai A, Tilley DG. The role of leukocytes in diabetic cardiomyopathy. Frontiers in Physiology. 2018;**9**:1547. DOI: 10.3389/fphys.2018.01547

[2] Takeda Y, Asao H, Wakabayashi I. An analysis of the intracellular signal transduction of peripheral blood leukocytes in animal models of diabetes using flow cytometry. Methods in Molecular Biology. 1916;**2019**:177-193. DOI: 10.1007/978-1-4939-8994-2_17

[3] de Souza Prestes A, Dos Santos MM, Ecker A, de Macedo GT, Fachinetto R, Bressan GN, et al. Methylglyoxal disturbs the expression of antioxidant, apoptotic and glycation responsive genes and triggers programmed cell death in human leukocytes. Toxicology In Vitro. 2019;**55**:33-42. DOI: 10.1016/j.tiv.2018.11.001

[4] Pan S, Zhou S, Gao S, Yu Z, Zhang S, Tang M, et al. New perspectives on how to discover drugs from herbal medicines: CAM's outstanding contribution to modern therapeutics. Evidence-based Complementary and Alternative Medicine. 2013;**2013**:627375. DOI: 10.1155/2013/627375

[5] Shokri F, Shokoohi M, Niazkar HR, Abadi ARR, Kalarestaghi H, Ahin M. Investigation the spermatogenesis and testis structure in diabetic rats after treatment with *Galega officinalis* extract. Crescent Journal of Medical and Biological Sciences. 2019;**6**(1):31-36

[6] Lupak M, Khokhla M, Hachkova G, Shulga O, Sheglova N, Vildanova R, et al. Application of biogenic surfactants for stabilization of alkaloid-free fraction isolated from *Galega officinalis* extract. Biologica Studia. 2015;**9**(1):25-36. DOI: 10.30970/sbi.0901.397

[7] Khokhla M, Kleveta G, Kotyk A, Skybitska M, Chajka Y, Sybirna N. Sugar-lowering effects of *Galega officinalis* L. Annales Universitatis Mariae Curie-Sklodowska, Sectio DDD: Pharmacia. 2010;**23**(4):177-182

[8] Khodadadi S. Administration of *Galega officinalis* in experimental and clinical investigations; A narrative review. Annals of Research in Antioxidants. 2016;**1**(1):e03

[9] Ursini F, Russo E, Pellino G, D'Angelo S, Chiaravalloti A, De Sarro G, et al. Metformin and autoimmunity: A "new deal" of an old drug. Frontiers in Immunology. 2018;**9**:1236. DOI: 10.3389/fimmu.2018.01236

[10] Queiroz EAIF, Puukila S, Eichler R, Sampaio SC, Forsyth HL, Barbosa AM, et al. Metformin induces apoptosis and cell cycle arrest mediated by oxidative stress, AMPK and FOXO3a in MCF-7 breast cancer cells. PLoS One. 2014;**9**(5):e98207. DOI: 10.1371/journal.pone.0098207

[11] de Oliveira S, Houseright RA, Graves AL, Golenberg N, Korte BG, Miskolci V, et al. Metformin modulates innate immune-mediated inflammation and early progression of NAFLD-associated hepatocellular carcinoma in zebrafish. Journal of Hepatology. 2019;**70**:710-721. DOI: 10.1016/j.jhep.2018.11.034

[12] Bae H, Zmijewski JW, Deshane JS, Tadie J, Chaplin DD, Takashima S, et al. AMP-activated protein kinase enhances the phagocytic ability of macrophages and neutrophils. The FASEB Journal. 2011;**25**(12):4358-4368. DOI: 10.1096/fj.11-190587

[13] Park DW, Jiang S, Tadie J, Stigler WS, Gao Y, Deshane J, et al. Activation of AMPK enhances neutrophil chemotaxis and bacterial killing. Molecular Medicine.

2013;**19**:387-398. DOI: 10.2119/molmed.2013.00065

[14] Pollak M. The effects of metformin on gut microbiota and the immune system as research frontiers. Diabetologia. 2017;**60**:1662-1667. DOI: 10.1007/s00125-017-4352-x

[15] Zhang Q, Tang W, Deater M, Phan N, Marcogliese AN, Li H, et al. Metformin improves defective hematopoiesis and delays tumor formation in Fanconi anemia mice. Blood. 2016;**128**(24):2774-2784. DOI: 10.1182/blood2015-11-683490

[16] Xu G, Wu H, Zhang J, Li D, Wang Y, Wang Y, et al. Metformin ameliorates ionizing irradiation-induced long-term hematopoietic stem cell injury in mice. Free Radical Biology and Medicine. 2015;**87**:15-25. DOI: 10.1016/j.freeradbiomed.2015.05.045

[17] Orio F, Manguso F, Di Biase S, Falbo A, Giallauria F, Labella D, et al. Metformin administration improves leukocyte count in women with polycystic ovary syndrome: A 6-month prospective study. European Journal of Endocrinology. 2007;**157**:69-73. DOI: 10.1530/EJE-07-0133

[18] Kebir DE, Filep JG. Role of neutrophil apoptosis in the resolution of inflammation. The Scientific World Journal. 2010;**10**:1731-1748. DOI: 10.1100/tsw.2010.169

[19] Isoda K, Young JL, Zirlik A, MacFarlane LA, Tsuboi N, Gerdes N, et al. Metformin inhibits proinflammatory responses and nuclear factor-B in human vascular wall cells. Arteriosclerosis, Thrombosis, and Vascular Biology. 2006;**26**:611-617. DOI: 10.1161/01.ATV.0000201938.78044.75

[20] Nath N, Khan M, Paintlia MK, Hoda MN, Giri S. Metformin attenuated the autoimmune disease of the central nervous system in animal models of multiple sclerosis. The Journal of Immunology. 2009;**182**:8005-8014. DOI: 10.4049/jimmunol.0803563

[21] Han J, Li Y, Liu X, Zhou T, Sun H, Edwards P, et al. Metformin suppresses retinal angiogenesis and inflammation in vitro and in vivo. PLoS One. 2018;**13**(3):e0193031. DOI: 10.1371/journal.pone.0193031

[22] Giacco F, Brownlee M. Oxidative stress and diabetic complications. Circulation Research. 2010;**107**:1058-1070. DOI: 10.1161/CIRCRESAHA.110.223545

[23] Foretz M, Guigas B, Bertrand L, Pollak M, Viollet B. Metformin: From mechanisms of action to therapies. Cell Metabolism. 2014;**20**(6):953-966. DOI: 10.1016/j.cmet.2014.09.018

[24] Victor VM, Rovira-Llopis S, Banuls C, Diaz-Morales N, Castello´ R, Falcon1 R, et al. Effects of metformin on mitochondrial function of leukocytes from polycystic ovary syndrome patients with insulin resistance. European Journal of Endocrinology. 2015;**173**:683-691. DOI: 10.1530/EJE-15-0572

[25] Bonnefont-Rousselot D, Raji B, Walrand S, Garde's-Albert M, Jore D, Legrand A, et al. An intracellular modulation of free radical production could contribute to the beneficial effects of metformin towards oxidative stress. Metabolism. 2003;**52**(5):586-589. DOI: 10.1053/meta.2003.50093

[26] Onaran I, Guven GS, Ozdas SB, Kanigur G, Vehid S. Metformin does not prevent DNA damage in lymphocytes despite its antioxidant properties against cumene hydroperoxide-induced oxidative stress. Mutation Research. 2006;**611**:1-8. DOI: 10.1016/j.mrgentox.2006.06.036

[27] Lee SC, Pervaiz S. Apoptosis in the pathophysiology of diabetes

mellitus. The International Journal of Biochemistry & Cell Biology. 2007;**39**(3):497-504. DOI: 10.1016/j.biocel.2006.09.007

[28] Kanigür-Sultuybek G, Ozdas ŞB, Curgunlu A, Tezcan V, Onaran I. Does metformin prevent short term oxidant-induced DNA damage? In vitro study on lymphocytes from aged subjects. Journal of Basic and Clinical Physiology and Pharmacology. 2007;**18**(2):129-140. DOI: 10.1515/jbcpp.2007.18.2.129

[29] Ullah I, Ullah N, Naseer MI, Lee HY, Kim MOK. Neuroprotection with metformin and thymoquinone against ethanol-induced apoptotic neurodegeneration in prenatal rat cortical neurons. BMC Neuroscience. 2012;**13**:11. DOI: 10.1186/1471-2202-13-11

[30] de la Rosa LC, Vrenken TE, Buist-Homan M, Faber KN, Moshage H. Metformin protects primary rat hepatocytes against oxidative stress-induced apoptosis. Pharmaceutical Research & Perspectives. 2015;**3**(2):e00125. DOI: 10.1002/prp2.125

[31] Wiernsperger N. Metformin as a cellular protector; a synoptic view of modern evidences. Journal of Nephropharmacology. 2015;**4**(1):31-36

[32] Cheki M, Ghasemi MS, Rashnoudi AMR, Majd NE. Metformin attenuates cisplatin-induced genotoxicity and apoptosis in rat bone marrow cells. Drug and Chemical Toxicology. 2019;**9**:1-8. DOI: 10.1080/01480545.2019.1609024

[33] Wang Z, Liu X, Wang M, Jiang G, Qiu T, Chen Z, et al. Metformin attenuated the inflammation after renal ischemia/reperfusion and suppressed apoptosis of renal tubular epithelial cell in rats. Acta Cirúrgica Brasileira. 2015;**30**(9):617-623. DOI: 10.1590/S0102-865020150090000006

[34] Bromfield ESP, Cloutier S, Robidas C, Thi TVT, Darbyshire SJ. Invasive *Galega officinalis* (Goat's rue) plants in Canada form a symbiotic association with strains of *Neorhizobium galegae* sv. officinalis originating from the Old World. Ecology and Evolution. 2019;**00**:1-6. DOI: 10.1002/ece3.5266

[35] Karakas FP, Turker AU, Karakas A, Mshvildadze V. Cytotoxic, anti-inflammatory and antioxidant activities of four different extracts of *Galega officinalis* L (Goat's rue). Tropical Journal of Pharmaceutical Research. 2016;**15**(4):751-757. DOI: 10.4314/tjpr.v15i4.12

[36] Khokhla M, Kleveta H, Lupak M, Kaniuka O, Chaika IA, Skybitska M, et al. The research of *Galega officinalis* extract components. Visnyk of L'viv University. Biological Series. 2013;**62**: 55-60 (in Ukrainian)

[37] Alqahtani N, Khan WA, Alhumaidi MH, Ahmed YA. Use of glycated hemoglobin in the diagnosis of diabetes mellitus and pre-diabetes and role of fasting plasma glucose, oral glucose tolerance test. International Journal of Preventive Medicine. 2013;**4**(9):1025-1029

[38] Nagalievska M, Sabadashka M, Hachkova H, Sybirna N. *Galega officinalis* extract regulate the diabetes mellitus related violations of proliferation, functions and apoptosis of leukocytes. BMC Complementary and Alternative Medicine. 2018;**18**(1):4. DOI: 10.1186/s12906-017-2079-3

[39] Elmazar M, El-Abhar HS, Schaalan MF, Schaalan MF, Farag NA. *P*hytol/phytanic acid and insulin resistance: Potential role of phytanic acid proven by docking simulation and modulation of biochemical alterations. PLoS One. 2013;**8**(1):1-10. DOI: 10.1371/journal.pone.0045638

[40] Sarkodie J, Fleischer T, Edoh DA, Dickson RA, Mensah MLK, Annan K, et al. Antihyperglycaemic activity of ethanolic extract of the stem of *Adenia lobata* Engl (Passifloraceae). International Journal of Pharmaceutical Sciences and Research. 2013;**4**(4):1370-1377

[41] Lee YM, Haastert B, Scherbaum W, Hauner H. A phytosterol-enriched spread improves the lipid profile of subjects with type 2 diabetes mellitus. A randomized controlled trial under free-living conditions. European Journal of Nutrition. 2003;**42**:111-117. DOI: 10.1007/s00394-003-0401-y

[42] Tanaka M, Misawa E, Ito Y, Habara N, Nomaguchi K, Yamada M, et al. Identification of five phytosterols from Aloe vera gel as antidiabetic compounds. Biological & Pharmaceutical Bulletin. 2006;**29**(7):1418-1422. DOI: 10.1248/bpb.29.1418

[43] Santos FA, Frota JT, Arruda BR, de Melo TS, da Silva AA, Brito GA, et al. Antihyperglycemic and hypolipidemic effects of α,β-amyrin, a triterpenoid mixture from *Protium heptaphyllum* in mice. Lipids in Health and Disease. 2012;**11**:98. DOI: 10.1186/1476-511X-11-98

[44] Nam Kyu Lee (SuwonSi, KR), Jun Won Lee (Gunpo-Si, KR), Sukho Lee (Suwon-Si, KR), Guang-Jin Im (Ansan-Si, KR), Hye Young Han (Seoul, KR), Tae Kon Kim (Suwon-Si, KR), Yong Hyuk Kim (Suwon-Si, KR), Wie-Jong Kwak (Seoul, KR), Wie-Jong Kwak (Seoul, KR), Sang Woong Kim (Daejeon, KR), Joohun Ha (Seoul, KR), Eon Kyum Kim (Daejeon, KR), Jung Kyu Lee (Daejeon, KR), Choong Yeul Yoo (Daejeon, KR), Dae Yeon Lee (Daegu, KR). Quinazoline derivatives for the treatment and prevention of diabetes and obesity. Patent application number: 20080207614

[45] Leclerc I, Woltersdorf WW, da Silva Xavier G, Rowe RL, Cross SE, Korbutt GS, et al. Metformin, but not leptin, regulates AMP-activated protein kinase in pancreatic islets: Impact on glucose-stimulated insulin secretion. American Journal of Physiology-Endocrinology and Metabolism. 2004;**286**(6):E1023-E1031. DOI: 10.1152/ajpendo.00532.2003

[46] Rodriguez-Leyva D, Dupasquier CM, McCullough R, Pierce GN. The cardiovascular effects of flaxseed and its omega-3 fatty acid, alphalinolenic acid. The Canadian Journal of Cardiology. 2010;**26**(9):489-496. DOI: 10.1016/s0828-282x(10)70455-4

[47] Lontchi-Yimagou E, Sobngwi E, Matsha TE, Kengne AP. Diabetes mellitus and inflammation. Current Diabetes Reports. 2013;**13**(3):435-444. DOI: 10.1007/s11892-013-0375-y

[48] Erbağcia AB, Tarakçioğlua M, Coşkunb Y, Sivaslib E, Namidurua ES. Mediators of inflammation in children with type I diabetes mellitus: Cytokines in type I diabetic children. Clinical Biochemistry. 2001 Nov;**34**(8):645-650. DOI: 10.1016/S0009-9120(01)00275-2

[49] Khokhla MR, Kleveta GY, Chajka YP, Skybitska MI, Sybirna NO. Cytological and biochemical characteristics of rats' peripheral blood under the condition of experimental diabetes mellitus type 1 and *Galega officinalis* admission. Biological Studies. 2012;**6**(1):37-46. DOI: 10.30970/sbi.0601.189

[50] Deliliers GL, Servida F, Fracchiolla NS, Ricci C, Borsotti C, Colombo G, et al. Effect of inositol hexaphosphate (IP6) on human normal and leukaemic haematopoietic cells. British Journal of Haematology. 2002;**117**(3):577-587. DOI: 10.1046/j.1365-2141.2002.03453.x

[51] Thies F, Nebe-von-Caron G, Powell JR, Yaqoob P, Newsholme EA, Calder PC. Dietary supplementation

with g-linolenic acid or fish oil decreases T lymphocyte proliferation in healthy older humans. The Journal of Nutrition. 2001;**131**(7):1918-1927. DOI: 10.1093/jn/131.7.1918

[52] Yaqoob P, Newsholme EA, Calder PC. The effect of fatty acids on leucocyte subsets and proliferation in rat whole blood. Nutrition Research. 1995;**15**(2):279-287. DOI: 10.1016/0271-5317(95)92592-8

[53] Sravan Kumar G, Das UN, Vijay Kumar K, Madhavi N, Das NP, Tan BKH. Effect of n-6 and n-3 fatty acids on the proliferation of human lymphocytes and their secretion of TNF-α and IL-2 in vitro. Nutrition Research. 1992;**12**(7):815-823

[54] Calder PC, Yaqoob P, Thies F, Wallace FA, Miles EA. Fatty acids and lymphocyte functions. British Journal of Nutrition. 2002;**87**(1):S31-S48. DOI: 10.1079/BJN2001455

[55] Caughey GE, Mantzioris E, Gibson RA, Cleland LG, James MJ. The effect on human tumor necrosis factor A and interleukin 1 production of diets enriched in n-3 fatty acids from vegetable oil or fish oil. American Journal of Clinical Nutrition. 1996;**63**(1):16-22. DOI: 10.1093/ajcn/63.1.116

[56] Hirano T, Oka K, Kawashima E, Akiba M. Effects of synthetic and naturally occurring flavonoids of mitogen-induced proliferation of human peripheral-blood lymphocytes. Life Sciences. 1989;**45**(15):1407-1411. DOI: 10.1016/0024-3205(89)90028-3

[57] Nijveldt RJ, van Nood E, van Hoorn DEC, Boelens PG, van Norren K, van Leeuwen PAM. Flavonoids: A review of probable mechanisms of action and potential applications. The American Journal of Clinical Nutrition. 2001;**74**:418-425. DOI: 10.1093/ajcn/74.4.418

[58] Saraf S, Singh MA, Saraf A. Flavonoids: A nutritional protection against oxidative and UV induced cellular damages. Pharmacognosy Reviews. 2007;**1**:30-40

[59] Kim HP, Son KH, Chang HW, Kang SS. Anti-inflammatory plant flavonoids and cellular action mechanisms. Journal of Pharmacological Sciences. 2004;**96**: 229-245. DOI: 10.1254/jphs.CRJ04003X

[60] Silva RO, Sousa FBM, Damasceno SRB, Carvalho NS, Silva VG, Oliveira FRMA, et al. Phytol, a diterpene alcohol, inhibits the inflammatory response by reducing cytokine production and oxidative stress. Fundamental & Clinical Pharmacology. 2014;**28**(4):455-464. DOI: 10.1111/fcp.12049

[61] Cárdeno A, Aparicio-Soto M, Montserrat-de la Paz S, Bermudez B, Muriana FJG, Alarcón-de-la-Lastra C. Squalene targets pro- and anti-inflammatory mediators and pathways to modulate over-activation of neutrophils, monocytes and macrophages. Journal of Functional Foods. 2015;**14**:779-790. DOI: 10.1016/j.jff.2015.03.009

[62] Brüll F, Mensink RP, Plat J. Plant sterols: Functional lipids in immune function and inflammation? Clinical Lipidology. 2009;**4**(3):355-365. DOI: 10.2217/clp.09.26

[63] Silva KA, Paszcuk AF, Passos GF, Silva ES, Bento AF, Meotti FC, et al. Activation of cannabinoid receptors by the pentacyclic triterpene α,β-amyrin inhibits inflammatory and neuropathic persistent pain in mice. Pain. 2011;**152**(8):1872-1887. DOI: 10.1016/j.pain.2011.04.005

[64] Rosales C, Juliano RL. Signal transduction by cell adhesion receptors in leukocytes. Journal of Leukocyte

Biology. 1995;**57**(2):189-198. DOI: 10.1002/jlb.57.2.189

[65] Koval'chuk LV, Saĭgitov RT. Chemokines—A new family of cytokines regulating leukocyte migration. Journal of Microbiology, Epidemiology and Immunobiology. 2000;**1**:69-70

[66] Carlier M, editor. Actin-based Motility: Cellular, Molecular and Physical Aspects. Springer; 2010. 435 p

[67] Lupak M, Hachkova H, Khokhla M, Chajka Y, Skybitska M, Sybirna N. Leukocyte actin cytoskeleton reorganization and redistribution of sialylated membrane glycoconjugates under experimental diabetes mellitus and against the administration of the *Galega officinalis* L. extract. Cytology and Genetics. 2017;**51**(3):162-172. DOI: 10.3103/S0095452717030070

[68] Advani A, Marshall S, Thomas T. Increasing neutrophil F-actin corrects CD11b exposure in type 2 diabetes. European Journal of Clinical Investigation. 2004;**34**(5):358-364. DOI: 10.1111/j.1365-2362.2004.01346.x

[69] Hannigan M, Zhan L, Ai Y, Huang CK. Leukocyte-specific gene 1 protein (LSP1) is involved in chemokine KC-activated cytoskeletal reorganization in murine neutrophils in vitro. Journal of Leukocyte Biology. 2001;**69**(3):497-504. DOI: 10.1189/jlb.69.3.497

[70] Sybirna N, Zdioruk M, Brodyak I, Bars'ka M, Vovk O. Activation of the phosphatidylinositol-3′-kinase pathway with lectin induced signal through sialocontaining glycoproteins of leukocyte membranes under type 1 diabetes mellitus. Ukrainskiĭ Biokhimicheskiĭ Zhurnal. 2011;**83**(5):22-31

[71] Kleveta G, Borzęcka K, Zdioruk M, Czerkies M, Kuberczyk H, Sybirna N, et al. LPS induces phosphorylation of actin-regulatory proteins leading to actin reassembly and macrophage motility. Journal of Cellular Biochemistry. 2012;**113**(1):80-92. DOI: 10.1002/jcb.23330

[72] Samstag Y, Eibert SM, Klemke M, Wabnitz G. Actin cytoskeletal dynamics inT-lymphocyte activation and migration. Journal of Leukocyte Biology. 2003;**73**(1):30-48. DOI: 10.1189/jlb.0602272

[73] Sybirna NO, Brodyak IV, Bars'ka ML, Vovk OI. Participation of phosphatidylinositol-3′-kinase in signal transduction through galactosyl-containing glycoprotein receptors of segmentonuclear leukocytes under type 1 diabetes mellitus. Fiziologicheskiĭ Zhurnal. 2012;**58**(6):9-22

[74] Fernández-Rodríguez J, Feijoo-Carnero C, Merino-Trigo A, Páez de la Cadena M, Rodríguez-Berrocal FJ, de Carlos A, et al. Immunohistochemical analysis of sialic acid and fucose composition inhuman colorectal adenocarcinoma. Tumour Biology. 2000;**21**(3):153-164. DOI: 10.1159/000030122

[75] Karlsson A. Wheat gernagglutinin induced NADPH-oxidase in human neutrophils by interaction with mobilizable receptors. Infection and Immunity. 1999;**67**(7):3461-3468

[76] Khokhla M, Kleveta G, Lupak M, Skybitska M, Chajka Y, Sybirna N. The inhibition of rat leukocytes apoptosis under the condition of experimental diabetes mellitus type 1 by *Galega officinalis* L. extract. Current Issues in Pharmacy and Medical Sciences. 2013;**26**(4):393-397. DOI: 10.12923/j.2084-980X/26.4/a.09

[77] Soudais C, de Villartay JP, Le Deist F, Fischer A, Lisowska-Grospierre B. Independent mutations of the human CD3-έ gene resulting in a T cell receptor/CD3 complex

immunodeficiency. Nature Genetics. 1993;**3**(1):77-81. DOI: 10.1038/ng0193-77

[78] Eash S, Tavares R, Stopa EG, Robbins SH, Brossay L, Atwood WJ. Differential distribution of the JC virus receptor-type sialic acid in normal human tissues. The American Journal of Pathology. 2004;**164**(2):419-428. DOI: 10.1016/S0002-9440(10)63132-X

[79] Aiba Y, Kameyama M, Yamazaki T, Tedder TF, Kurosaki T. Regulation of B-cell development by BCAP and CD19 through their binding to phosphoinositide 3-kinase. Blood. 2008;**111**(3):1497-1503. DOI: 10.1182/blood-2007-08-109769

[80] Baud V, Karin M. Signal transduction by tumor necrosis factor and its relatives. Trends in Cell Biology. 2001;**11**(9):372-377. DOI: 10.1016/S0962-8924(01)02064-5

[81] Nakao S, Kuwano T, Ishibashi T, Kuwano M, Ono M. Synergistic effect of TNF-alpha in soluble VCAM-1-induced angiogenesis through alpha 4 integrins. Journal of Immunology. 2003;**170**(11):5704-5711. DOI: 10.4049/jimmunol.170.11.5704

[82] Hahmann C, Schroeter T. Rho-kinase inhibitors as therapeutics: From pan inhibition to isoform selectivity. Cellular and Molecular Life Sciences. 2010;**67**(2):171-177. DOI: 10.1007/s00018-009-0189-x

[83] Riento K, Ridley AJROCKS. Multifunctional kinases in cell behaviours. Nature Reviews. Molecular Cell Biology. 2003;**4**(6):446-456. DOI: 10.1038/nrm1128.

[84] Arita R, Nakao S, Kita T, Kawahara S, Asato R, Yoshida S, et al. A key role for ROCK in TNF-a–mediated diabetic microvascular damage. Investigative Ophthalmology & Visual Science. 2013;**54**(3):2373-2383. DOI: 10.1167/iovs.12-10757

[85] Allen RC, Stephens JT. Myeloperoxidase selectively binds and selectively kills microbes. Infection and Immunity. 2011;**79**(1):474-485. DOI: 10.1128/IAI.00910-09

[86] Gorudko V, Kostevich VA, Sokolov AV, Shamova EV, Buko IV, Konstantinova EE, et al. Functional activity of neutrophils in diabetes mellitus and coronary heart disease: Role of myeloperoxidase in the development of oxidative stress general pathology and pathophysiology. Bulletin of Experimental Biology and Medicine. 2012;**154**(1):23-26. DOI: 10.1007/s10517-012-1865-7

[87] Nicholls SJ, Hazen SL. Myeloperoxidase and cardiovascular disease. Arteriosclerosis, Thrombosis, and Vascular Biology. 2005;**25**:1102-1111. DOI: 10.1161/01.ATV.0000163262.83456.6d

[88] Cruse JM, Lewis RE. Atlas of Immunology. 2nd ed. CRC Press LLC; 2004. 958 p

[89] Middleton E. Biological properties of plant flavonoids: An overview. International Journal of Pharmacognosy. 1996;**34**(5):344-348. DOI: 10.1076/phbi.34.5.344.13245

[90] Lee HB, Ha H, King GL. Reactive oxygen species and diabetic nephropathy. Journal of the American Society of Nephrology. 2003;**14**(3):209-210. DOI: 10.1097/01.ASN.0000077403.06195.D2

[91] Morel O, Pereira B, Averous G, Faure A, Jesel L, Germain P, et al. Increased levels of procoagulant tissue factor-bearing microparticles within the occluded coronary artery of patients with ST-segment elevation myocardial infarction:

Role of endothelial damage and leukocyte activation. Atherosclerosis. 2009;**204**(2):636-641. DOI: 10.1016/j.atherosclerosis.2008.10.039

[92] Lupak MI, Khokhla MR, Hachkova GY, Kanyuka OP, Klymyshyn NI, Chajka YP, et al. The alkaloid-free fraction from *Galega officinalis* extract prevents oxidative stress under experimental diabetes mellitus. Ukranian Biochemical Journal. 2015;**87**(4):78-86. DOI: 10.15407/ubj87.04.078

[93] Lupak MI, Kanyuka OP, Hachkova GY, Chajka YP, Skybitska MI, Sybirna NO. Influence of alkaloid-free fraction of *Galega officinalis* extract on L-arginin/NO system of rats leukocytes under the experimental diabetes mellitus type 1. Medical and Clinical Chemistry. 2014;**16**(3):108-110

[94] Atalay V, Laaksonen DE, Niskanen L. Altered antioxidant enzyme defenses in insulin-dependent diabetic men with increased resting and exercise-induced oxidative stress. Acta Physiologica Scandinavica. 1997;**161**:195-201. DOI: 10.1046/j.1365-201X.1997.00200.x

[95] De Menezes Patrício Santos CC, Salvadori MS, Mota VG, Costa LM, De Almeida AAC, Lopes De Oliveira GA, et al. Antinociceptive and antioxidant activities of phytol in vivo and in vitro models. Neuroscience Journal. 2013;**2013**:1-9. DOI: 10.1155/2013/949452

[96] Hetts SW. To die or not to die: An overview of apoptosis and its role in disease. Journal of the American Medical Association. 1998;**279**(4):300-307. DOI: 10.1001/jama.279.4.300

[97] Khokhla M, Kleveta G, Chajka YA, Skybitska M, Sybirna N. The influence of *Galega officinalis* on rats leukocytes apoptosis under the experimental diabetes mellitus type 1. Visnyk of Lviv University. Biological Series. 2012;**60**:117-125

[98] Deng Y, Ren X, Yang L, Lin Y, Wu X. A JNK-dependent pathway is required for TNFalpha-induced apoptosis. Cell. 2003;**115**(1):61-70. DOI: 10.1016/S0092-8674(03)00757-8

[99] Meesmann HM, Fehr EM, Kierschke S, Herrmann M, Bilyy R, Heyder P, et al. Decrease of sialic acid residues as an eat-me signal on the surface of apoptotic lymphocytes. Journal of Cell Science. 2010;**123**(Pt19):3347-3356. DOI: 10.1242/jcs.066696

[100] Braithwaite A, Royds J, Jackson P. The p53 story: Layers of complexity. Carcinogenesis. 2005 Jul;**26**(7):1161-1169. DOI: 10.1093/carcin/bgi091

[101] Erster S, Mihara M, Kim R. In vivo mitochondrial p53 translocation triggers a rapid first wave of cell death in response to DNA damage that can precede p53 target gene activation. Molecular and Cellular Biology. 2004;**24**(15):6728-6741. DOI: 10.1128/MCB.24.15.6728-6741.2004

[102] Janicke RU, Sohn D, Schulze-Osthoff K. The dark side of a tumor suppressor: Anti-apoptotic p53. Cell Death and Differentiation. 2008 Jun;**15**(6):959-976. DOI: 10.1038/cdd.2008.33

[103] Schmitz H. Reversible nuclear translocation of glyceraldehyde-3-phosphate dehydrogenase upon serum depletion. European Journal of Cell Biology. 2001;**80**(6):419-427. DOI: 10.1078/0171-9335-00174

Section 2

Metformin and Reproductive System

Chapter 6

Metformin in Health Issues and Reproductive System

Elham Pourmatroud

Abstract

Metformin is one of oldest drug in reproductive medicine era; but most of times it is equal to polycystic ovary (PCO) syndrome especially obese patients. If it is still valuable or not, could have another health benefit or new fertility roles, and could be effective as well in male reproductive system will be discussed. According to increased rate of metabolic disorders and cardiovascular problems and cancers, there are several investigations on this old used drug. Those studies had been magnified its role as "the aspirin of current century," which might have a promising role in longevity of the life. So, the chapter will be interesting.

Keywords: metformin, reproductive, health, fertility, metabolic

1. Introduction

Metformin is a component of many herbal therapeutic substances, which has been known since 1500 BCE in Egyptian medicine [1]. In Europe, a herbal remedy was used for ameliorating polyuria and polydipsia; from the Middle Ages, its name was *Galega officinalis* (or the French lilac) [2]. However, just in the early 1900s, the effective element "guanidine" was extracted [3].

Everybody knows that the incidence and prevalence of diabetes mellitus (DM) is increasing constantly. Diabetes is one of the most common noncommunicable diseases and is considered as one of the top five universal causes of precocious death in both developed and non-developed countries. So the immense numbers of studies about metformin, which is the most prevalent and popular remedy for it, could be predictable. As a result, it is no wonder that there is a scanty paper about other worthful aspects of metformin.

Metformin has been called "the aspirin of the twenty-first century [4]." This old-fashioned drug was famous only as antidiabetic drug until recent years. So, what makes this drug so hear saying and impressive for life longevity [5], prevention from cancers [6] and useful in patients with chronic kidney disease, congestive heart failure or chronic liver disease [7]. At the present time, evidence suggests that metformin's wide-spectrum advantages are mediated by at least two relevant pathways: first, by inhibition of intracellular metabolic activity of mitochondria and second, the cellular nutrition-sensing system mediated by mTOR [4]. ("The mammalian target of rapamycin" is one kind of the kinase family that mediates metabolism and cell growth as a reaction to growth factors, nutrients, and stress [8].)

IntechOpen

In this chapter we are going to talk about three different fields of metformin action in detail.

2. Health issues

In accordance with aging, there are some significant changes in the body and elevation in prevalence of some specific disease and abnormality [9].

- Endocrine system: type 2 diabetes, thyroid disease, osteoporosis, and orthostatic hypotension
- Cardiovascular: hearth failure, hypertension, and CVD
- Neurological: delirium, cognitive impairment, and dementia
- Optical: macular degeneration, cataract, and presbyopia
- Muscular: impaired mobility, muscular strength, and sarcopenia
- Auditory: presbycusis and conductive hearing loss
- Skeletal: osteoporosis, kyphosis, and scoliosis
- Gastrointestinal: dysphagia, constipation, and malabsorption
- Renal: chronic kidney disease
- Immune: increased risk of infections
- Dermal: dryness and lower elasticity and pressure ulcer

The life span has been regulated by pharmacologic, genetic, and dietary interferences in several sample systems. The most considerable mechanism in aging phenomenon is DNA damage; the endogenous, potent factors are reactive oxygen species (ROS), alkylation, and hydrolysis [10]. Thus, most studies in this subject are focusing on it.

Through the metformin role in aging, it leads to decreased insulin levels, inhibition of mTOR, decreased IGF-1 signaling, endogenous production of reactive oxygen species, inhibition of mitochondrial complex 1, activation of AMP-activated protein kinase (AMPK), and reduction in DNA damage.

Nuclear factor kappa-light-chain-enhancer of activated B cells (NF-kB) is a protein complex that governs transcription of DNA. Metformin inhibits NF-kB, a key point in inflammatory process [11]. Also, by lowering the reactive oxygen species and improving the endothelial function [12], reduction in coronary heart diseases and cerebrovascular accidents after metformin administration could be expected. With those mechanisms, the effectiveness in blood hemostasis is considerable; reduction in systemic production of the tissue type plasminogen activator, Von Willibrand factor, and plasminogen activator inhibitor [13], furthermore modulation the fibrin threads formation in both diabetic and non-diabetic patients [14].

According to one recent meta-analysis, metformin is operative in reducing body weight of simple obesity (in nondiabetic, non-polycystic ovary syndrome (PCOS) patients), by reducing the absorption of glucose in the intestine, decreasing production of glucose in the liver, and ameliorating insulin sensitivity via increasing muscle glucose uptake and use [15].

The role of metformin in the nervous system is proposed excitingly. Alzheimer is a disease with an advanced insulin resistance of the brain cell which leads to formation of the amyloid cells [16]. Undesirable oxidative damages and inactivation of AMPK pathway [17] and making delay in mitochondria programmed cell death could be mediated by metformin [18]. Besides Alzheimer, other neurological diseases like Parkinson and amyotrophic lateral sclerosis have the same mechanism.

As a result of conversion in the insulin resistance, depletion in intestinal absorption of carbohydrate and leptin secretion, and enhancing effects of glucagon-like peptide-1 on fat cells, metformin could be applied for weight reduction [19].

Additionally, prescription of metformin with antiretroviral agents (especially in HIV treatment) has been showed a reduction in their side effects like the risk of insulin insensitivity, weight obtain, dyslipidemia, and hyperglycemia [20].

In cancerous issue, there are several studies that depict the effectiveness of metformin.

One meta-analysis has concluded that metformin plays a role in the decline of liver cancer risk in type 2 diabetes patients [21]. The anti-tumorigenic sequel of metformin in pancreatic cancer [22], colorectal cancer [23], prostate cancer [24], and lung cancer [25] and its role in lowering the risk of cancer-related mortality have been proposed. From another aspect, in colorectal cancers' cell, metformin inhibits an essential energy source: adenosine A1 receptor (ADORA1) [26].

As we mentioned before, lowering the insulin levels by metformin ends in reduction in the levels of P13K pathway. (The PI3K/AKT/mTOR pathway is an intracellular signaling pathway with significant regulating function in all of the cellular stages: quiescence, proliferation, cancer, and longevity.) Moreover metformin by forcing effect on AMPK lowers the ATP ratio in cells causing switch-off of cell growth and proliferation in breast cell [27]. In breast cancer, metformin has an inhibitory effect at early stages of cell differentiation [28]; indeed, the antineoplastic effects need higher-dose consumption and more clinical evidences [29]. With those outstanding impressive mechanisms of metformin, a smaller size and slower progression of thyroid cancer [30] and advantageous effect on endometrium cancer including progesterone-resistant cancer cells [31] have been pointed.

Metformin could have an adjuvant task in treating cervical cancer, particularly in types with liver kinase B1 (LKB1) positive (a gen with tumor suppression efficacy) [32]. Eventually, there is an update study about metformin's anti-metastatic effects on aggressive malignancies like melanomas [33].

From another aspect, metformin decreases the frequency of preeclampsia, by reduction in the production of anti-angiogenic factors (soluble vascular endothelial growth factor receptor-1 and soluble endoglin) and the modification in endothelial dysfunction [34].

It must be highlighted that all of mentioned witnesses are extra glycemic effects of metformin in health jeopardies in nondiabetic patients.

3. Fertility issues

Metformin as a hydrophilic biguanide is present in many tissues like the hypothalamus, pituitary, and gonads moreover than famous places (liver, pancreas, and adipose tissues). It could be accumulating in specific tissues more than plasma level by particular transportation system, in which one of those places is the reproductive system [35]. Metformin activates the cytoplasmic protein kinase, which is a well-known enzyme: AMPK.

AMPK is a sensitive and important sensor of cellular energy homeostasis.

Hypothalamic neurons secrete gonadotropin-releasing hormone (GnRH) that stimulates follicle-stimulating hormone (FSH) and luteinizing hormone (LH) production from the pituitary gland. GnRH function in the brain has an AMPK-dependent pathway. Metformin as an AMPK activator decreases the amplitude of FSH and LH secretion.

3.1 Male reproductive system

Spermatogenesis is under noticeable hormonal regulation, especially by pituitary hormones (FSH and LH). LH stimulates the Leydig cells (LCs) to secrete testosterone and dihydrotestosterone, although FSH arouses Sertoli cells (SCs) of seminiferous tubules to maintain the cycle of spermatogenesis and inhibin secretion. Respectively, testosterone and inhibin secretion from the testis cause a negative feedback with inhibitory effects on FSH and LH. This regular system is necessary for normal spermatogenesis [36].

During spermatogenesis, the evolution process of germ cells into mature and motile spermatozoa needs specific nutrient sources which are obtained mainly from sugars (particularly glucose and fructose) and other metabolites such as lactate and citrate. Those metabolites are the most principal fuels for ATP production in germ cells and spermatozoa [37].

Moreover, production of lactate by glycolytic pathway in the SCs [38] and secretion into intratubular fluid is a necessary step for germ cell spermatogenesis. This is another energy-making way, important for motility enhancement. This process is controlled directly by glucose metabolism [39]. After primary spermatozoa production, they will store in the epididymis. Here final maturation occurs by advancement in motility function and fertilization capacity. All of those processes demand high energy and depend on glucose transporter (GLUT) proteins for carrying glucose through sperm's lipidic membrane inside the sperm cell [40]. In effect, regular and correct male fertility through this long journey is closely related to glucose metabolism.

Metformin's effect on human male reproductive function still is obscure. Extensively, current data are extracted from normal animal model studies, particularly rodents and diabetic men.

In healthy male animals, exposure to metformin displays adverse reproductive outcomes like:

1. Decrease in testosterone production [41].

2. Reduction in seminiferous tubules diameter and testis size.

3. Reduction in Sertoli cell numbers [42].

4. Decrease in sperm quality parameters [43].

In diabetic men, according to hyperglycemic state and excessive ROS production, metformin improves antioxidant environment of the testis and enhances steroidogenesis. This favorable amelioration in the testis leads to increase in concentration of motile sperm and normal morphological sperm [44]. Furthermore, metformin increases endothelial nitric oxide synthase phosphorylation [45] and the contractility in the corpora cavernosa [46], so sexual disorders like retrograde ejaculation or erectile dysfunction could be mended.

Recently, evidences of metformin efficacy in nondiabetic men are increasing. As remarked above, lactate synthesis by SCs is a crucial step in testicular metabolic cycle, which produces more desirable energy substrate for springing up germ cells and has a prominent anti-apoptotic effect [47]. Also, some studies showed that metformin plays a role as a suppressor of complex I of the mitochondrial electron transport chain that directly decreases oxidative metabolism and accordingly increases anaerobic respiration and lactate secretion [48].

Surprisingly, adding metformin in cryopreservation media during sperm freezing practice (for fertility preservation) reduces sperm permanent damage and improves the rate of success in fertilization process and decreases the number of abnormal zygotes after in vitro fertilization [49].

3.2 Female reproductive system

As it is well-known, metformin has a crucial role in PCOS pathogenesis amelioration and not surprising the large number of studies about its efficacy and widespread utilization. But, when we are looking for its usage in non-PCOS infertile or subfertile woman, unexpectedly, there is scanty study about it.

Insulin resistance could have significant negative role in various conditions such as stress [50], aging [51], obesity [52], depression [53], and inactive lifestyle [54]. Infertile women often have one of those conditions. Moreover, ovarian dysfunction induces "stress response mechanism" owing to abnormal cortisol secretion and increased level of catecholamines [55]. Besides that, by enhancing in insulin-like growth factor-binding protein-1 and glycodelin level, uterine vascularity and blood flow could be increased [56].

Those beneficial effects had been demonstrated in a study on about 200 patients (non-PCOS) with repeated IVF failure. In this study in a period of 8–12 weeks, low-dose (500 mg/day) metformin administration before IVF cycle significantly increases the pregnancy rate by improving in oocyte quality and endometrium, receptivity [57].

In another bovine study, it was shown that IGF-1 has a dual positive role in follicle regulation which increases FSH effectiveness as an autocrine regulator of granulosa cell growth that could illustrate metformin worth in infertility treatment procedures [58]. Moreover, in vitro experiment studies show that metformin could decrease the progesterone [59] and estradiol [60] secretion from granulosa cells and androstenedione [61] from theca cells.

4. Conclusion

As we reviewed in this chapter, metformin did not equal to NIDDM and PCOS, anymore. In all of the mentioned fields, researches are increasing more and more.

Conflict of interest

The author declares no conflict of interest.

Author details

Elham Pourmatroud
Payam IVF Center, Tehran, Iran

*Address all correspondence to: e.pourmatroud@yahoo.com

References

[1] Witters LA. The blooming of the French lilac. The Journal of Clinical Investigation. 2001;**108**(8):1105-1107. DOI: 10.1172/JCI14178

[2] Thomas I, Gregg B. Metformin; a review of its history and future: From lilac to longevity. Pediatric Diabetes. 2017;**18**(1):10-16. DOI: 10.1111/pedi.12473

[3] Watanabe C. Studies in the metabolic changes induced by the administration of guanidine bases. The Journal of Biological Chemistry. 1918;**33**:253-265

[4] Romero R, Erez O, Hüttemann M, Maymon E, et al. Metformin, the aspirin of the 21st century: Its role in gestational diabetes mellitus, prevention of preeclampsia and cancer, and the promotion of longevity. American Journal of Obstetrics and Gynecology. 2017;**217**(3):282-302. DOI: 10.1016/j.ajog.2017.06.003

[5] Onkan B, Driscoll M. Metformin induces a dietary restriction-like state and the oxidative stress response to extend *C. elegans* healthspan via AMPK, LKB1, and SKN-1. PLoS One. 2010;**5**(1):e8758. DOI: 10.1371/journal.pone.0008758

[6] Wu L, Zhu J, Prokop LJ, Murad MH. Pharmacologic therapy of diabetes and overall cancer risk and mortality: A meta-analysis of 265 studies. Scientific Reports. 2015;**5**:10147. DOI: 10.1038/srep10147

[7] Crowley MJ, Diamantidis CJ, McDuffie JR, Cameron CB, Stanifer JW, Mock CK, et al. Clinical outcomes of metformin use in populations with chronic kidney disease, congestive heart failure, or chronic liver disease: A systematic review. Annals of Internal Medicine. 2017;**166**(3):191-200. DOI: 10.7326/M16-1901

[8] Hall MN. mTOR-what does it do? Transplantation Proceedings. 2008;**40**(10 Suppl):S5-S8. DOI: 10.1016/j.transproceed.2008.10.009

[9] Barzilai N, Crandall JP, Kritchevsky SB, Espeland MA. Metformin as a tool to target aging. Cell Metabolism. 2016;**23**(6):1060-1065. DOI: 10.1016/j.cmet.2016.05.011

[10] Hoeijmakers JHJ. DNA damage, aging, and cancer. The New England Journal of Medicine. 2009;**361**:1475-1485. DOI: 10.1056/NEJMra0804615

[11] Isoda K, Young JL, Zirlik A, MacFarlane LA, Tsuboi N, Gerdes N, et al. Metformin inhibits proinflammatory responses and nuclear factor-kappaB in human vascular wall cells. Arteriosclerosis, Thrombosis, and Vascular Biology. 2006;**26**(3):611-617. DOI: 10.1161/01.ATV.0000201938.78044.75

[12] De Jager J, Kooy A, Lehert P, Bets D, Wulffele MG, Teerlink T, et al. Effects of short-term treatment with metformin on markers of endothelial function and inflammatory activity in type 2 diabetes mellitus: A randomized, placebo-controlled trial. Journal of Internal Medicine. 2005;**257**(1):100-109. DOI: 10.1111/j.1365-2796.2004.01420.x

[13] Grant PJ. Beneficial effects of metformin on haemostasis and vascular function in man. Diabetes & Metabolism. 2003;**29**(4 Pt 2):6S44-6S52. DOI: 10.1016/S1262-3636(03)72787-6

[14] Charles MA, Morange P, Eschwege E, Andre P, Vague P, Juhan-Vague I. Effect of weight change and metformin on fibrinolysis and the von Willebrand factor in obese nondiabetic subjects: The BIGPRO1 study. Biguanides and the prevention of the risk of obesity. Diabetes Care.

1998;**21**(11):1967-1972. DOI: 10.2337/diacare.21.11.1967

[15] Ning HH, Le J, Wang Q, et al. The effects of metformin on simple obesity: A meta-analysis. Endocrine. 2018;**62**(3):528-534. DOI: 10.1007/s12020-018-1717-y

[16] Culmsee C, Monnig J, Kemp BE, Mattson MP. AMP-activated protein kinase is highly expressed in neurons in the developing rat brain and promotes neuronal survival following glucose deprivation. Journal of Molecular Neuroscience. 2001;**17**(1):45-58. DOI: 10.1385/JMN:17:1:45

[17] Santomauro Junior AC, Ugolini MR, Santomauro AT, Souto RP. Metformin and AMPK: An old drug and a new enzyme in the context of metabolic syndrome. Arquivos Brasileiros de Endocrinologia e Metabologia. 2008;**52**(1):120-125. DOI: 10.1590/S0004-27302008000100017

[18] Kroemer G, Reed JC. Mitochondrial control of cell death. Nature Medicine. 2000;**6**(5):513-519. DOI: 10.1038/74994

[19] Glueck CJ, Fontaine RN, Wang P, Subbiah MT, Weber K, Illig E, et al. Metformin reduces weight, centripetal obesity, insulin, leptin, and low-density lipoprotein cholesterol in nondiabetic, morbidly obese subjects with body mass index greater than 30. Metabolism. 2001;**50**(7):856-861. DOI: 10.1053/meta.2001.24192

[20] Sheth SH, Larson RJ. The efficacy and safety of insulin-sensitizing drugs in HIV-associated lipodystrophy syndrome: A meta-analysis of randomized trials. BMC Infectious Diseases. 2010;**10**:183. DOI: 10.1186/1471-2334-10-183

[21] Zhang ZJ, Zheng ZJ, Shi R, Su Q, Jiang Q, Kip KE. Metformin for liver cancer prevention in patients with type 2 diabetes: A systematic review and meta-analysis. The Journal of Clinical Endocrinology and Metabolism. 2012;**97**(7):2347-2353. DOI: 10.1210/jc.2012-1267

[22] Cerullo M, Gani F, Chen SY, Canner J, Pawlik TM. Metformin use is associated with improved survival in patients undergoing resection for pancreatic cancer. Journal of Gastrointestinal Surgery. 2016;**20**(9):1572-1580. DOI: 10.1007/s11605-016-3173-4

[23] Zhang ZJ, Zheng ZJ, Kan H, Song Y, Cui W, Zhao G, et al. Reduced risk of colorectal cancer with metformin therapy in patients with type 2 diabetes: A meta-analysis. Diabetes Care. 2011;**34**(10):2323-2328. DOI: 10.2337/dc11-0512

[24] Yu H, Yin L, Jiang X, Sun X, Wu J, Tian H, et al. Effect of metformin on cancer risk and treatment outcome of prostate cancer: A meta-analysis of epidemiological observational studies. PLoS One. 2014;**9**(12):e116327. DOI: 10.1371/journal.pone.0116327

[25] Sakoda LC, Ferrara A, Achacoso NS, Peng T, Ehrlich SF, Quesenberry CP, et al. Metformin use and lung cancer risk in patients with diabetes. Cancer Prevention Research (Philadelphia, Pa.). 2015;**8**(2):174-179. DOI: 10.1158/1940-6207.CAPR-14-0291

[26] Lan B, Zhang J, Zhang P, Zhang W, Yang S, Lu D, et al. Metformin suppresses CRC growth by inducing apoptosis via ADORA1. Frontiers in Biosciences (Landmark Ed). 2017;**22**:248-257. DOI: 10.2741/4484

[27] Camacho L, Dasgupta A, Jiralerspong S. Metformin in breast cancer—An evolving mystery. Breast Cancer Research. 2015;**17**:88. DOI: 10.1186/s13058-015-0598-8

[28] Hadad SM, Hardie DG, Appleyard V, Thompson AM. Effects

of metformin on breast cancer cell proliferation, the AMPK pathway and the cell cycle. Clinical & Translational Oncology. 2014;**16**(8):746-752. DOI: 10.1007/s12094-013-1144-8

[29] Iliopoulos D, Hirsch HA, Struhl K. Metformin decreases the dose of chemotherapy for prolonging tumor remission in mouse xenografts involving multiple cancer cell types. Cancer Research. 2011;**71**(9):3196-3201. DOI: 10.1158/0008-5472.CAN-10-3471

[30] Klubo-Gwiezdzinska J, Jensen K, Costello J, Patel A, Hoperia V, Bauer A, et al. Metformin inhibits growth and decreases resistance to anoikis in medullary thyroid cancer cells. Endocrine-Related Cancer. 2012;**19**(3):447-456. DOI: 10.1530/ERC-12-0046

[31] Zhuo Z, Wang A, Yu H. Metformin targeting autophagy overcomes progesterone resistance in endometrial carcinoma. Archives of Gynecology and Obstetrics. 2016;**294**(5):1055-1061. DOI: 10.1007/s00404-016-4148-0

[32] Xiao X, He Q, Lu C, Werle KD, Zhao RX, Chen J, et al. Metformin impairs the growth of liver kinase B1-intact cervical cancer cells. Gynecologic Oncology. 2012;**127**(1):249-255. DOI: 10.1016/j.ygyno.2012.06.032

[33] Cerezo M, Tichet M, Abbe P, Ohanna M, Lehraiki A, Rouaud F, et al. Metformin blocks melanoma invasion and metastasis development in AMPK/p53-dependent manner. Molecular Cancer Therapeutics. 2013;**12**(8):1605-1615. DOI: 10.1158/1535-7163.mct-12-1226-t

[34] Kalafat E, Sukur YE, Abdi A, Thilaganathan B, Khalil A. Metformin for prevention of hypertensive disorders of pregnancy in women with gestational diabetes or obesity: Systematic review and meta-analysis of randomized trials. Ultrasound in Obstetrics & Gynecology. 2018 Dec;**52**(6):706-714. DOI: 10.1002/uog

[35] Viollet B, Guigas B, Garcia NS, Leclerc J, Foretz M. Cellular and molecular mechanisms of metformin: An overview. Clinical Science (London, England). 2012;**122**(6):253-270. DOI: 10.1042/CS20110386

[36] Cheng CY, Mruk DD. A local autocrine axis in the testes that regulates spermatogenesis. Nature Reviews. Endocrinology. 2010;**6**:380-395. DOI: 10.1038/nrendo.2010.71

[37] Grootegoed JA, Oonk RB, Jansen R, et al. Metabolism of radiolabelled energy-yielding substrates by rat Sertoli cells. Journal of Reproduction and Fertility. 1986;**77**:109-118. DOI: 10.1530/jrf.0.0770109

[38] Coonrod S, Vitale A, Duan C, et al. Testis-specific lactate dehydrogenase (LDH-C4; Ldh3) in murine oocytes and pre-implantation embryos. Journal of Andrology. 2006;**27**:502-509. DOI: 10.2164/jandrol.05185

[39] Mita M, Hall PF. Metabolism of round spermatids from rats: Lactate as the preferred substrate. Biology of Reproduction. 1982;**26**:445-455. DOI: 10.1095/biolreprod26.3.445

[40] Scheepers A, Joost HG, Schurmann A. The glucose transporter families SGLT and GLUT: Molecular basis of normal and aberrant function. JPEN Journal of Parenteral and Enteral Nutrition. 2004;**28**:364-371. DOI: 10.1177/0148607104028005364

[41] Tartarin P, Moison D, Guibert E, Dupont J, Habert R, et al. Metformin exposure affects human and mouse fetal testicular cells. Human Reproduction. 2012;**27**(11):3304-3314. DOI: 10.1093/humrep/des264

[42] Riera MF, Regueira M, Galardo MN, et al. Signal transduction pathways

in FSH regulation of rat Sertoli cell proliferation. American Journal of Physiology. Endocrinology and Metabolism. 2012;**302**:E914-E923

[43] Adaramoye O, Akanni O, Adesanoye O, Labo-Popoola O, Olaremi O. Evaluation of toxic effects of metformin hydrochloride and glibenclamide on some organs of male rats. Nigerian Journal of Physiological Sciences. 2012;**27**(2):137-144. DOI: 10.3389/fendo.2018.00675

[44] Rabbani SI, Devi K, Khanam S. Role of pioglitazone with metformin or glimepiride on oxidative stress-induced nuclear damage and reproductive toxicity in diabetic rats. Malaysian Journal of Medical Sciences. 2010;**17**(1):3-11

[45] Labazi H, Wynne BM, Tostes R, Webb RC. Metformin treatment improves erectile function in an angiotensin II model of erectile dysfunction. The Journal of Sexual Medicine. 2013;**10**(9):2154-2164. DOI: 10.1111/jsm.12245

[46] Phé V, Rouprêt M. Erectile dysfunction and diabetes: A review of the current evidence-based medicine and a synthesis of the main available therapies. Diabetes & Metabolism. 2012;**38**(1):1-13. DOI: 10.1016/j.diabet.2011.09.003

[47] Owen M, Doran E, Halestrap A. Evidence that metformin exerts its anti-diabetic effects through inhibition of complex 1 of the mitochondrial respiratory chain. Biochemical Journal. 2000;**348**(3):607-614. DOI: 10.1042/bj3480607

[48] Dias TR, Martins AD, Reis VP, Socorro S, Silva BM, et al. Glucose transport and metabolism in Sertoli cell: Relevance for male fertility. Current Chemical Biology. 2013;7(3):282-293

[49] Bertoldo MJ, Guibert E, Tartarin P, Guillory V, Froment P. Effect of metformin on the fertilizing ability of mouse spermatozoa. Cryobiology. 2014;**68**(2):262-268. DOI: 10.1016/j.cryobiol.2014.02.006

[50] Vanltallie TB. Stress: A risk factor for serious illness. Metabolism. 2002;**51**:40-45. DOI: 10.1053/meta.2002.33191

[51] Paolisso G, Tagliamonte MR, Rizzo MR, Giugliano D. Advancing age and insulin resistance: New facts about an ancient history. European Journal of Clinical Investigation. 1999;**29**:758-769. DOI: 10.1046/j.1365-2362.1999.00522.x

[52] Bjorntorp P, Rosmond R. The metabolic syndrome—A neuroendocrine disorder? The British Journal of Nutrition. 2000;**83**:S49-S57. DOI: 10.1017/s0007114500000957

[53] Wolkowitz OM, Epel ES, Reus VI. Stress hormone-related psychopathology: Pathophysiological and treatment implications. The World Journal of Biological Psychiatry. 2001;**2**:115-143. DOI: 10.3109/15622970109026799

[54] Rosenthal M, Haskell WL, Solomon R, Widstrom A, Reaven GM. Demonstration of a relationship between levels of physical training and insulin-stimulated glucose utilisation in normal humans. Diabetes. 1983;**32**:408-411. DOI: 10.2337/diab.32.5.408

[55] Jinno M, Watanabe A, Takahashi S, Urakami C. A novel method to detect dysfunction of stress-response-mechanism in women with ovarian dysfunction: Implications of circadian rhythm in salivary cortisol for diagnosis and treatment. Fertility and Sterility. 2007;**88**(Suppl 1):S171. DOI: 10.1016/j.fertnstert.2007.07.594

[56] Jakubowicz DJ, Seppala M, Jakubowicz S, et al. Insulin reduction with metformin increases luteal phase serum glycodelin and insulin-like

growth factor-binding protein 1 concentrations and enhances uterine vascularity and blood flow in the polycystic ovary syndrome. Journal of Clinical Endocrinology and Metabolism. 2001;**86**:1126-1133. DOI: 10.1210/jcem.86.3.7295

[57] Fogle RH, Minkhorst OR, Reagan M, Denis AL, Toner TP, Hasty LA. Metformin may improve embryo quality and pregnancy rates in ovulatory (non-PCOS) patients undergoing *in vitro* fertilization (IVF). Fertility and Sterility. 2009;**92**(3):S167. DOI: 10.14310/horm.2002.1266

[58] Armstrong DT, Xia P, de Gannes G, Tekpetey FR, Khamsi F. Differential effects of insulin-like growth factor-I and follicle-stimulating hormone on proliferation and differentiation of bovine cumulus cells and granulosa cells. Biology of Reproduction. 1996;**54**(2):331-338. DOI: 10.1095/biolreprod54.2.331

[59] Tosca L, Solnais P, Ferre P, et al. Metformin-induced stimulation of adenosine 5′ monophosphate-activated protein kinase (PRKA) impairs progesterone secretion in rat granulosa cells. Biology of Reproduction. 2006;**75**:342-351

[60] Tosca L, Chabrolle C, Uzbekova S, et al. Effects of metformin on bovine granulosa cells steroidogenesis: Possible involvement of adenosine 5′ monophosphate-activated protein kinase (AMPK). Biology of Reproduction. 2007;**76**:368-378

[61] Attia GR, Rainey WE, Carr BR. Metformin directly inhibits androgen production in human thecal cells. Fertility and Sterility. 2001;**76**:517-524

Section 3

Metformin and Cancer

Chapter 7

Metformin and Its Implication in Cancer Therapy

Laura Mazilu, Dana Stanculeanu, Andreea Gheorghe, Adrian-Paul Suceveanu, Irinel Parepa, Felix Voinea, Doina Catrinoiu and Andra-Iulia Suceveanu

Abstract

Metformin has been used for almost half a century as the first line of treatment for type 2 diabetes. Mechanisms of action are still incompletely known, recent studies have shown that metformin exerts its effects through several mechanisms, including the stimulation of AMP-activated protein kinase, decreasing production of cyclic AMP, inhibition of mitochondrial complex I of the electron transport chain, targeting glycerophosphate dehydrogenase and altering gut microbiota. In recent years, studies have shown that patients with type 2 diabetes mellitus have a lower risk of developing cancer, and patients with cancer and type 2 diabetes have a lower mortality. Experimental studies have demonstrated that metformin has anti-tumor activity by inhibiting mTORC1 signaling pathway and mitochondrial complex, inhibiting tumor growth and proliferation, and inducing cellular apoptosis. There are multiple studies showing that combination of metformin with different types of anti-cancer therapies may reduce toxicities and tumor resistance. This chapter is focused on the progress made in understanding the anti-tumor effect of metformin and its association with cancer therapy.

Keywords: metformin, cancer, chemotherapy, targeted therapy

1. Introduction

Guanidine derivatives, metformin, buformin and phenoformin, were discovered in the 1920s, extracted from the isoamylene plant [1]. Metformin it is a biguanide extracted from herb *Galega officinalis*, and it was first proposed by Emile Werner and James Bell in 1922, when they found that metformin is reducing the amount of glucose in rabbits and does not affect heart and blood pressure [2, 3]. Due to the increased risk of lactic acidosis and of cardiac death, buformin and phenoformin were withdrawn from the market in 1970 [4]. Due to the good safety profile of metformin, the use of this drug was extended beyond type 2 diabetes to ovarian polycystic disease, gestational diabetes, diabetic nephropathy and cardiovascular complications associated with type 2 diabetes [5].

The association between cancer and diabetes was first proven in 1930 by Marble [6]. Over the past 20 years, numerous studies have shown that diabetic patients have a higher incidence of cancers, increased mortality [7, 8], and the fact that patients with diabetes and cancer are less sensitive to chemotherapy [9–11].

Regarding the anti-tumor effect of metformin, numerous studies have shown that metformin-treated diabetes patients have a low incidence of cancers and low mortality compared with patients treated with other types of anti-diabetics such as sulfonylureas or insulin [9, 12, 13].

In vivo and in vitro studies have demonstrated that metformin has an anti-tumoral effect both directly and indirectly, which translates into inhibition of tumor cell proliferation, induction of apoptosis, and cell cycle arrest [14–16].

Taking all these into consideration, metformin appears to be useful as an adjuvant to cancer treatment.

2. Anti-tumor mechanism of action of metformin

Metformin's mechanisms of action and its anti-tumor effects are multiple and have been described over the years in numerous studies, both in vivo and in vitro, but they are not yet completely understood. The main mechanisms of actions are activation of liver kinase B1 (LKB1) and AMP-activated kinase (AMPK), and inhibition of mammalian target of rapamycin (mTOR). Other mechanisms described in literature are inhibition of protein synthesis, activation of apoptosis by p21 and p53, inhibition of unfolded protein response (UPR), activation of immune system, prevention of angiogenesis, reduction of blood insulin levels and reduction of hyperlipidemia [17, 18].

Metformin is entering the cells with the help of organic cation transporter 1 and 3, and as a result is blocking the complex I of electron transfer chain (ETC) and an enzyme named mitochondrial glycerophosphate 3 dehydrogenase (mGDP). Introduction of Metformin into the cell results in reduced activity of adenosine triphosphate (ATP) and reduced oxygen consumption, which further increase the levels of adenosine monophosphate within the cells and activate AMPK, and in the end this will put the cells under stressful conditions [19, 20].

Metformin inhibits mTOR pathway by activating LKB1 and AMPK, resulting in reduction of protein synthesis and inhibition of angiogenesis. AKPK inhibits mTOR pathway by activation of tuberculous sclerosis complex (TSC2) and by direct phosphorylation of co-signaling molecules that will attached to mTOR molecules [21, 22]. Metformin is also inhibiting mTOR by reducing phosphorylation of ribosomal protein S6 kinase (S6Ks) [23].

Ataxia teleangectasia mutated (ATM) and LKB1 are proteins with an important role in cell cycle. Both ATM and LKB1 are tumor suppressors. The response of ATM to metformin is phosphorylation of LKB and in the end the activation of AMPK [24].

Inhibition of unfolded protein response (UPR) is another mechanism by which metformin exerts its anti-tumor effect. UPR activity is vital for cell survival of under stress conditions. Metformin inhibits the activity of UPR and determine cells to undergo apoptosis [25].

Insulin and insulin growth-like factor (IGF) promote mitosis and cell growth and inhibit apoptosis. All this processes are very important in carcinogenesis and the relation between hyperinsulinemia, insulin resistance and cancer promotion are well known [26]. Metformin inactivates I/IGF pathway by reducing blood insulin levels and by inhibiting glucose absorption by intestinal cells [27, 28].

3. Metformin: epidemiologic evidence of its anti-tumor effect

Metformin was approved by Food and Drug Administration (FDA) in 1957 for type 2 diabetes and became the first line treatment due to its superior safety profile and hypoglycemic and cardiovascular protective effect [29].

The effect of metformin on cancer risk reduction was first observed in a study published in 2005 by Evans et al., which included 11,776 patients with type 2 diabetes; this observation was reiterated in another trial in 2009, involving more than 4,000 patients with diabetes treated with metformin, the risk of developing cancer being 7.3% for patients receiving metformin vs. 11.6% in the control group [30, 31].

In 2009, a study conducted at the MD Anderson Cancer Center by Li et al., showed that metformin use is associated with a low risk of pancreatic cancer in patients with type 2 diabetes [32].

A very large retrospective study that evaluated more than 62.000 patients with diabetes showed that metformin treatment reduces the risk of cancer compared to other antidiabetic therapies (insulin, sulfonylureas), and also showed that the combination of metformin with insulin or sulfonylureas reduces the risk of cancer associated with these therapies. This study showed that the risk of developing colorectal and pancreatic cancer is higher in patients with diabetes treated with insulin, compared to patients treated with metformin, and that metformin does not reduce the risk of breast or prostate cancer [33].

In terms of mortality, in 2006 a study conducted by Bowker el al, retrospectively reported that mortality is higher in patients with type 2 diabetes using insulin and sulfonylurea, comparing with those using metformin [34].

In 2010, a prospective study, ZODIAC-16, evaluating the influence of metformin on cancer mortality in 1353 patients with type 2 diabetes showed that metformin-treated patients had a lower mortality rate (with a median of 9.6 years) compared to the control group [35].

3.1 Metformin in hepatocellular carcinoma and pancreatic cancer

Hepatocellular carcinoma is one of the leading causes of death in cancer patients. Well known risk factors implicated in etiology of hepatocellular carcinoma are chronic hepatitis B and C and hepatic cirrhosis. In the last years, due to the rising incidence of obesity and diabetes worldwide, non-alcoholic steatosis, non-alcoholic fatty liver disease and type 2 diabetes are newly described risk factors.

Donadon has focused his studies on patients with hepatocarcinoma and has shown that metformin significantly reduces the risk of hepatocarcinoma in diabetic patients, compared to patients treated with sulfonylureas or insulin, and also reduces the risk of hepatocarcinoma in patients with diabetes and chronic liver disease [36–39].

There are several meta-analyses supporting this data, for example a 31% incidence reduction of pancreatic and hepatocellular carcinoma for patients using metformin was reported by a meta-analyses of 11 trials [40]. Another meta-analysis evaluating 37 trials of patients with colorectal, pancreatic, breast and hepatic cancer, reported a reduced incidence of cancer in patients using metformin, comparing with non-users [41].

One meta-analysis stated that metformin does not significantly reduce the risk of hepatocellular carcinoma. This meta-analysis excluded all the studies with time-related biases [42, 43].

3.2 Metformin in colorectal cancer

Colorectal cancer is increasing in incidence and mortality worldwide, especially in countries with low and middle income, but also in high developed countries mainly due to life style.

The first data that reported the relationship between metformin and colorectal cancer risk emerged in 2004 and since then numerous studies have evaluated this association and had different outcomes, reporting a decrease risk, an increased risk or no association [43, 44].

The first clinical trial that examine the chemopreventive effect of low-dose metformin on metachronous colorectal adenoma/polyp formation, was conducted in 2016, and the observation was that Metformin suppress the formation of metachronous colorectal adenoma/polyp [45].

Another study investigating the use of Metformin as chemopreventive therapy was performed in 2018 on a small number of patients without diabetes, and showed that metformin is reducing the risk of developing polyps. The adverse events were mild and with no differences between groups [46].

3.3 Metformin in breast cancer

A meta-analysis that included 11 clinical trials of patients with breast cancer, reported a 65% improvement in overall survival for patients with breast cancer and diabetes that are treated with metformin [47].

There are also studies suggesting that the use of metformin is changing the type of cancers diagnosed in patients with diabetes. For example, a study conducted by Berstein reported that in patients using metformin, breast cancer is much more frequent, especially the progesterone receptor positive-type [46], and another study reported that triple negative-type is less common [47]. Other data suggests that response rate is higher in diabetic patients with breast cancer receiving neo-adjuvant chemotherapy and metformin, comparing with those not receiving metformin [48].

3.4 Metformin in renal cancer

Kidney cancers incidence is increasing mainly due to the increasing rates of hypertension and due to the improvement of imaging techniques, because kidney cancers are most often asymptomatic. Renal cell carcinoma is the most common type of kidney cancer.

There are several studies reporting that patients with renal cancer and diabetes have a poor prognosis, and that diabetes has a negative impact on survival of these patients [49]. Also some articles suggest that type 2 diabetes may be an independent risk factor for renal cancers [50].

A meta-analysis performed in 2017 which included 8 publications on kidney cancer showed that metformin could improve the survival of renal cancer patients, especially for patients with localized renal cell carcinoma, and concluded that further investigation is needed regarding the effect of metformin on patients with localized and metastatic renal carcinoma in order to exclude disease heterogeneity [51].

3.5 Metformin in lung cancer

Lung cancer is the leading cause of death all over the world in both sexes and despite the recent advances in therapy, the prognosis of these patients is still no satisfactory.

Regarding lung cancer, Mazzone et al. and Tan et al. reported that in patients receiving metformin the incidence of adenocarcinomas is higher comparing with other histopathological types, and that patients receiving metformin had a better response to chemotherapy [52, 53].

A meta-analysis conducted in 2017 reported that metformin demonstrates a significant improvement of overall survival and progression free survival of patients with lung cancer [54].

Although, numerous trials reported a reduction in cancer incidence in patients receiving metformin, there are recent studies on diabetic patients with breast, endometrial, prostate and renal cancer receiving metformin that suggests no association between the use of metformin and cancer incidence [55].

For prostate cancer, studies and meta-analysis showed that diabetes may reduce the risk of prostate cancer [56], but also showed that patients with diabetes and prostate cancer have higher rates of mortality and relapse after prostatectomy [57, 58]. All these results are in conflict with other studies that reported that metformin may reduce the risk for prostate cancer and may improve survival [59, 60].

4. Metformin: combination with antineoplastic drugs

Taking in consideration all the information available stating that metformin has a positive effect on cancer incidence and mortality, over the years numerous trial have evaluated or are underway to evaluate the combination of metformin with different antineoplastic drugs in breast, endometrial, prostate, lung, pancreatic and colorectal cancers.

4.1 Metformin: combination with chemotherapy

There are numerous chemotherapeutic drugs evaluated in combination with metformin. For example doxorubicin, cyclophosphamide, docetaxel, trastuzumab, exemestane, letrozole, carboplatin, 5-flurouracyl.

Combination of 5-fluorouracyl and metformin showed a modest activity in patients with colorectal cancer [61], but when used as chemopreventive treatment in monotherapy, metformin showed a reduced incidence of colorectal metachronous adenoma or polyp [45].

Metformin in combination with medroxyprogesterone acetate in endometrial cancer and atypical endometrial hyperplasia, showed a complete response rate of 14% in endometrial cancer and 81% in atypical endometrial hyperplasia and a good clinical profile with no severe adverse events [62].

For patients with diabetes and breast cancer receiving neo-adjuvant chemotherapy and metformin, Jiralerspong et al. reported a superior rate of complete pathological response [63].

In patients with prostate cancer the combination of bicalutamide and metformin may reduce cancer cells growth rate; in androgen receptor positive cells (AR) the reduction of cell growth appear to be mediated by anti-proliferative effect, and in androgen receptor negative cells by pro-apoptotic effect [64].

4.2 Metformin: combination with targeted therapies

Targeted therapies are used with success in the treatment of many cancer types, but usually the disease becomes unresponsive to treatment and shows acquired resistance, and this is a challenge for clinicians. Preclinical and clinical data showed that the combination of metformin with targeted therapies have good results. Targeted therapies comprise mostly of kinase inhibitors. At present more than 35 different types of kinase inhibitors are approved by FDA [65].

First targeted therapy approved by the FDA, was Gefitinib, a molecule targeting epidermal growth factor receptor (EGFR) in 2003 for the treatment of patients with locally advanced and metastatic non-small cell lung cancer (NSCLC) after failure of platinum and docetaxel chemotherapy [66]. A high percent of patients receiving gefitinib have high response rate, but despite this, patients rapidly develop resistance. Mechanisms involved in resistance to Gefitinib are activation of mTOR pathway and upregulation of insulin-like growth factor-1 receptor (IGF-1R), and taking into consideration the effect of metformin on mTOR pathway inhibition and IGF-1R pathway suppression, multiple studies started to evaluate this relationship. The result were that the addition to metformin to Gefitinib reduce proliferation and can revert resistance to gefitinib [67, 68]. Combination of metformin and Gefitinib also improve prognosis of patients with NSCLC, by increasing survival and by delaying resistance to targeted therapy [69]. At this moment, a phase II multicenter double blind trial evaluating gefitinib in combination with metformin as first-line treatment for patients with locally advanced NSCLC, is ongoing [70].

Sorafenib was approved in 2007 for treatment of advanced hepatocellular carcinoma, but showed low response rate and serious adverse events [71]. Combination of Sorafenib and other drugs was necessary in order to improve treatment efficacy. So far, data showed that metformin has the capability to increase sorafenib efficacy by reducing lung metastasis in patients with hepatocellular carcinoma. The mechanism of action of this combination is targeting the mTOR pathway [72].

Trastuzumab was approved in 1998 for the treatment of HER2-positive breast cancer. Combination of Trastuzumab and metformin in clinical trials conducted over the years, showed that metformin suppresses the proliferation of trastuzumab-resistant breast cancer cells and also have a cardio-protective effect, against cardiac events related to trastuzumab [73, 74].

Bevacizumab, inhibits VEGF-A, the result being inhibition of angiogenesis and regression of tumor vascularization, thereby inhibiting cancer growth. It was approved in 2004 in combination with chemotherapy for metastatic colorectal cancer and now it is used in the treatment of numerous cancer types-metastatic breast cancer, renal cell carcinoma, advanced epithelial ovarian cancer, non-squamous NSCLC [75]. Combination of metformin with bevacizumab was found to be effective in the treatment of ovarian cancer and metastatic non-squamous NSCLC in combination with chemotherapy [76, 77].

4.3 Metformin: combination with radiotherapy

Metformin in combination with radiotherapy may increase cancer response to treatment. As already mentioned, one of the mechanism of action of metformin is affecting complex I in the electron transfer chain, reducing the oxygen consumption and increasing the reactive oxygen species (ROS) within the cells, resulting in DNA damage [78]. Another proposed mechanism is activation of p53 by activating AMPK, and as a result cell cycle arrest. Both, metformin and radiotherapy can activate p53 and stop cell proliferation [79]. There are several articles and case reports, showing a better response for patients receiving radiotherapy and metformin, comparing with those without metformin in: esophageal cancer, rectal cancer and head and neck carcinomas [80].

5. Conclusions

Many studies reported a reduced incidence of cancer in patients receiving metformin in standard dose, but also these trials have limitations: most of the trials were retrospective, others included both patients with invasive and non-invasive neoplasms, others trials did not exclude patients exposed to other antidiabetic treatments, all these findings being responsible for potential biases.

In general, chemopreventive agents are used as long term therapies. Metformin meets all necessary criteria as a long term chemopreventive agent, because it is safe, has a well-known mechanism of action, it is well tolerated with few adverse effects and it is cost effective.

Based on the available information, we can conclude that metformin is reducing cancer incidence and mortality, is increasing tumor response when used in combination with different types of cancer therapies, either chemotherapy, targeted therapies or radiotherapy, is improving the outcome of cancer patients, and can be used in cancer prevention.

Clinical trials which evaluated the effect of metformin in combination with different types of antineoplastic treatment included only patients with diabetes, therefore clinical trials evaluating the effect of metformin in non-diabetic population are needed in order to explore the benefit of metformin and also to evaluate the adverse events of combinations compared with monotherapy in this particular population.

Conflict of interest

Authors report no conflicts of interest.

Author details

Laura Mazilu[1*], Dana Stanculeanu[2], Andreea Gheorghe[1], Adrian-Paul Suceveanu[1], Irinel Parepa[1], Felix Voinea[1], Doina Catrinoiu[2] and Andra-Iulia Suceveanu[1]

1 Ovidius University of Constanta, Faculty of Medicine, Constanta, Romania

2 Carol Davila University of Medicine and Pharmacy, Bucharest, Romania

*Address all correspondence to: lauragrigorov@gmail.com

References

[1] Bailey CJ, Day C. Traditional plant medicines as treatments for diabetes. Diabetes Care. 1989;**12**:553-564. DOI: 10.2337/diacare.12.8.553

[2] Gul W. Metformin: Methods of analysis and its role in lowering the risk of cancer. Journal of Bioequivalence & Bioavailability. 2016;**8**:254-259

[3] Suissa S, Azoulay L. Metformin and cancer: Mounting evidence against an association. Diabetes Care. 2014;**37**(7):1786-1788. DOI: 10.2337/dc14-0500

[4] Luft D, Schmülling RM, Eggstein M. Lactic acidosis in biguanide-treated diabetics: A review of 330 cases. Diabetologia. 1978;**14**:75-87. DOI: 10.1007/BF01263444

[5] Viollet B, Guigas B, Sanz Garcia N, Leclerc J, Foretz M, Andreelli F. Cellular and molecular mechanisms of metformin: An overview. Clinical Science. 2012;**122**:253-270. DOI: 10.1042/CS20110386

[6] Marble A. Diabetes and cancer. The New England Journal of Medicine. 1934;**211**:339-349. DOI: 10.1056/NEJM193408232110801

[7] Pandey A, Forte V, Abdallah M, Alickaj A, Mahmud S, Asad S, et al. Diabetes mellitus and the risk of cancer. Minerva Endocrinologica. 2011;**36**:187-209

[8] Simon D. I.15 diabetes and cancer. Diabetes Research and Clinical Practice. 2014;**103**:S5. DOI: 10.1016/S0168-8227(14)70016-6

[9] Currie CJ, Poole CD, Jenkins-Jones S, Gale EA, Johnson JA, Morgan CL. Mortality after incident cancer in people with and without type 2 diabetes: Impact of metformin on survival. Diabetes Care. 2012;**35**:299-304. DOI: 10.2337/dc11-1313

[10] Coughlin SS, Calle EE, Teras LR, Petrelli J, Thun MJ. Diabetes mellitus as a predictor of cancer mortality in a large cohort of US adults. American Journal of Epidemiology. 2004;**159**:1160-1167. DOI: 10.1093/aje/kwh161

[11] Barone BB, Yeh HC, Snyder CF, Peairs KS, Stein KB, Derr RL, et al. Long-term all-cause mortality in cancer patients with preexisting diabetes mellitus: A systematic review and meta-analysis. Journal of the American Medical Association. 2008;**300**:2754-2764. DOI: 10.1001/jama.2008.824

[12] Lee MS, Hsu CC, Wahlqvist ML, Tsai HN, Chang YH, Huang YC. Type 2 diabetes increases and metformin reduces total, colorectal, liver and pancreatic cancer incidences in Taiwanese: A representative population prospective cohort study of 800,000 individuals. BMC Cancer. 2011;**11**:20. DOI: 10.1186/1471-2407-11-20

[13] Kumar S, Meuter A, Thapa P, Langstraat C, Giri S, Chien J, et al. Metformin intake is associated with better survival in ovarian cancer: A case-control study. Cancer. 2013;**119**:555-562. DOI: 10.1002/cncr.27706

[14] Zi F, Zi H, Li Y, He J, Shi Q, Cai Z. Metformin and cancer: An existing drug for cancer prevention and therapy. Oncology Letters. 2018;**15**(1):683-690. DOI: 10.3892/ol.2017.7412

[15] Rizos CV, Elisaf MS. Metformin and cancer. European Journal of Pharmacology. 2013;**705**:96-108. DOI: 10.1016/j.ejphar.2013.02.038

[16] Bost F, Sahra IB, Le Marchand-Brustel Y, Tanti JF. Metformin and cancer therapy. Current Opinion in Oncology. 2012;**24**:103-108. DOI: 10.1097/CCO.0b013e32834d8155

[17] Foretz M, Guigas B, Bertrand L, Pollak M, Viollet B. Metformin: From mechanisms of action to therapies. Cell Metabolism. 2014;**20**(6):953-966. DOI: 10.1016/j.cmet.2014.09.018

[18] Muaddi H, Chowdhury S, Vellanki R, Zamiara P, Koritzinsky M. Contributions of AMPK and p53 dependent signaling to radiation response in the presence of metformin. Radiotherapy and Oncology. 2013;**108**(3):446-450. DOI: 10.1016/j.radonc.2013.06.014

[19] Wheaton WW, Weinberg SE, Hamanaka RB, et al. Metformin inhibits mitochondrial complex I of cancer cells to reduce tumorigenesis. eLife. 2014;**3**:e02242. DOI: 10.7554/eLife.02242

[20] Madiraju AK, Erion DM, Rahimi Y, et al. Metformin suppresses gluconeogenesis by inhibiting mitochondrial glycerophosphate dehydrogenase. Nature. 2014;**510**(7506):542. DOI: 10.1038/nature13270

[21] Kourelis TV, Siegel RD. Metformin and cancer: New applications for an old drug. Medical Oncology. 2012;**29**(2):1314-1327. DOI: 10.1007/s12032-011-9846-7

[22] Gwinn DM, Shackelford DB, Egan DF, et al. AMPK phosphorylation of raptor mediates a metabolic checkpoint. Molecular Cell. 2008;**30**(2):214-226. DOI: 10.1016/j.molcel.2008.03.003

[23] Anisimov VN, Berstein LM, Egormin PA, et al. Effect of metformin on life span and on the development of spontaneous mammary tumors in HER-2/neu transgenic mice. Experimental Gerontology. 2005;**40**(8):685-693. DOI: 10.1016/j.exger.2005.07.007

[24] Huang X, Wullschleger S, Shpiro N, et al. Important role of the LKB1–AMPK pathway in suppressing tumorigenesis in PTEN-deficient mice. The Biochemical Journal. 2008;**412**(2):211-221. DOI: 10.1042/BJ20080557

[25] Saito S, Furuno A, Sakurai J, et al. Chemical genomics identifies the unfolded protein response as a target for selective cancer cell killing during glucose deprivation. Cancer Research. 2009;**69**(10):4225-4234. DOI: 10.1158/0008-5472.CAN-08-2689

[26] Pollak M. The insulin and insulin-like growth factor receptor family in neoplasia: An update. Nature Reviews. Cancer. 2012;**12**:159-169

[27] Pollak M. Insulin and insulin-like growth factor signalling in neoplasia. Nature Reviews. Cancer. 2008;**8**:915-928. DOI: 10.1038/nrc2536

[28] Goodwin PJ, Pritchard KI, Ennis M, Clemons M, Graham M, Fantus IG. Insulin-lowering effects of metformin in women with early breast cancer. Clinical Breast Cancer. 2008;**8**:501-505. DOI: 10.3816/CBC.2008.n.060

[29] American Diabetes Association. Standards of medical care in diabetes-2014. Diabetes Care. 2014;**37**(Suppl. 1):S14-S80. DOI: 10.2337/dc14-S014

[30] Evans JM, Donnelly LA, Emslie-Smith AM, Alessi DR, Morris AD. Metformin and reduced risk of cancer in diabetic patients. BMJ. 2005;**330**:1304-1305. DOI: 10.1136/bmj.38415.708634.F7

[31] Libby G, Donnelly LA, Donnan PT, Alessi DR, Morris AD, Evans JM. New users of metformin are at low risk of incident cancer: A cohort study among people with type 2 diabetes. Diabetes Care. 2009;**32**:1620-1625. DOI: 10.2337/dc08-2175

[32] Li D, Yeung SC, Hassan MM, KonoplevaM,AbbruzzeseJL.Antidiabetic

therapies affect risk of pancreatic cancer. Gastroenterology. 2009;**137**:482-488. DOI: 10.1053/j.gastro.2009.04.013

[33] Currie CJ, Poole CD, Gale EA. The influence of glucose-lowering therapies on cancer risk in type 2 diabetes. Diabetologia. 2009;**52**:1766-1777. DOI: 10.1007/s00125-009-1440-6

[34] Bowker SL, Majumdar SR, Veugelers P, Johnson JA. Increased cancer-related mortality for patients with type 2 diabetes who use sulfonylureas or insulin. Diabetes Care. 2006;**29**:254-258. DOI: 10.2337/dc06-0997

[35] Landman GW, Kleefstra N, van Hateren KJ, Groenier KH, Gans RO, Bilo HJ. Metformin associated with lower cancer mortality in type 2 diabetes: ZODIAC-16. Diabetes Care. 2010;**33**:322-326. DOI: 10.2337/dc09-1380

[36] Donadon V, Balbi M, Valent F, Avogaro A. Glycated hemoglobin and antidiabetic strategies as risk factors for hepatocellular carcinoma. World Journal of Gastroenterology. 2010;**16**:3025-3032. DOI: 10.3748/wjg.v16.i24.3025

[37] Donadon V, Balbi M, Mas MD, Casarin P, Zanette G. Metformin and reduced risk of hepatocellular carcinoma in diabetic patients with chronic liver disease. Liver International. 2010;**30**:750-758. DOI: 10.1111/j.1478-3231.2010.02223.x

[38] Donadon V, Balbi M, Casarin P, Vario A, Alberti A. Association between hepatocellular carcinoma and type 2 diabetes mellitus in Italy: Potential role of insulin. World Journal of Gastroenterology. 2008;**14**:5695-5700

[39] Donadon V, Balbi M, Zanette G. Hyperinsulinemia and risk for hepatocellular carcinoma in patients with chronic liver diseases and type 2 diabetes mellitus. Expert Review of Gastroenterology & Hepatology. 2009;**3**:465-467

[40] Decensi A, Puntoni M, Goodwin P, Cazzaniga M, Gennari A, et al. Metformin and cancer risk in diabetic patients: A systematic review and meta-analysis. Cancer Prevention Research (Philadelphia, Pa.). 2010;**3**:1451-1461. DOI: 10.1158/1940-6207.CAPR-10-0157

[41] Zhang P, Li H, Tan X, Chen L, Wang S. Association of metformin use with cancer incidence and mortality: a meta-analysis. Cancer Epidemiology. 2013;**37**:207-218. DOI: 10.1016/j.canep.2012.12.009

[42] Fujita K, Iwama H, Miyoshi H, et al. Diabetes mellitus and metformin in hepatocellular carcinoma. World Journal of Gastroenterology. 2016;**22**(27):6100-6113. DOI: 10.3748/wjg.v22.i27.6100

[43] Gandini S, Puntoni M, Heckman-Stoddard BM, et al. Metformin and cancer risk and mortality: A systematic review and meta-analysis taking into account biases and confounders. Cancer Prevention Research (Philadelphia, Pa.). 2014;**7**(9):867-885. DOI: 10.1158/1940-6207.CAPR-13-0424

[44] Yang YX, Hennessy S, Lewis JD. Insulin therapy and colorectal cancer risk among type 2 diabetes mellitus patients. Gastroenterology. 2004;**127**:1044-1050. DOI: 10.1053/j.gastro.2004.07.011

[45] Higurashi T, Hosono K, Takahashi H, Komiya Y, Umezawa S, Sakai E, et al. Metformin for chemoprevention of metachronous colorectal adenoma or polyps in post-polypectomy patients without diabetes: A multicentre double-blind, placebo-controlled, randomised phase 3 trial. The Lancet Oncology. 2016;**17**:475-483. DOI: 10.1016/S1470-2045(15)00565-3

[46] Higurashi T, Nakajima A. Metformin and colorectal cancer. Frontiers in Endocrinology (Lausanne). 2018;**9**:622. DOI: 10.3389/fendo.2018.00622

[47] Calip GS, Yu O, Elmore JG, Boudreau DM. Comparative safety of diabetes medications and risk of incident invasive breast cancer: A population-based cohort study. Cancer Causes & Control. 2016;**27**(5):709-720. DOI: 10.1007/s10552-016-0744-3

[48] Berstein LM, Boyarkina MPT, syrlina EVT, urkevich EA, Semiglazov VF. More favorable progesterone receptor phenotype of breast cancer in diabetics treated with metformin. Medical Oncology. 2010;**28**:1260-1263. DOI: 10.1007/s12032-010-9572-6

[49] Chen L, Li H, Gu L, Ma X, Li X, et al. The impact of diabetes mellitus on renal cell carcinoma prognosis: A meta-analysis of cohort studies. Medicine (Baltimore). 2015;**94**:e1055. DOI: 10.1097/MD.0000000000001055

[50] Otunctemur A, Ozbek E, Sahin S, Dursun M, Besiroglu H, et al. Diabetes mellitus as a risk factor for high grade renal cell carcinoma. Asian Pacific Journal of Cancer Prevention. 2014;**15**:3993-3996. DOI: 10.7314/APJCP.2014.15.9.3993

[51] Li Y, Hu L, Xia Q, Yuan Y, Mi Y. The impact of metformin use on survival in kidney cancer patients with diabetes: A meta-analysis. International Urology and Nephrology. 2017;**49**(6):975-981. DOI: 10.1007/s11255-017-1548-4

[52] Mazzone PJ, Rai H, Beukemann M, Xu M, Jain A, Sasidhar M. The effect of metformin and thiazolidinedione use on lung cancer in diabetics. BMC Cancer. 2012;**12**:410. DOI: 10.1186/1471-2407-12-410

[53] Tan BX et al. Prognostic influence of metformin as first-line chemotherapy for advanced nonsmall cell lung cancer in patients with type 2 diabetes. Cancer. 2011;**117**:5103-5111. DOI: 10.1002/cncr.26151

[54] Cao X, Wen ZS, Wang XD, Li Y, Liu KY, Wang X. The clinical effect of metformin on the survival of lung cancer patients with diabetes: A comprehensive systematic review and meta-analysis of retrospective studies. Journal of Cancer. 2017;**8**(13):2532-2541. DOI: 10.7150/jca.19750

[55] Coperchini F, Leporati P, Rotondi M, et al. Expanding the therapeutic spectrum of metformin: From diabetes to cancer. Journal of Endocrinological Investigation. 2015;**38**:1047. DOI: 10.1007/s40618-015-0370-z

[56] Kasper JS, Giovannucci E. A meta-analysis of diabetes mellitus and the risk of prostate cancer. Cancer Epidemiology, Biomarkers & Prevention. 2006;**15**:2056-2062. DOI: 10.1158/1055-9965.EPI-06-0410

[57] Snyder CF, Stein KB, Barone BB, Peairs KS, Yeh HC, Derr RL, et al. Does pre-existing diabetes affect prostate cancer prognosis? A systematic review. Prostate Cancer and Prostatic Diseases. 2010;**13**:58-64. DOI: 10.1038/pcan.2009.39

[58] Patel T, Hruby G, Badani K, Abate-Shen C, McKiernan JM. Clinical outcomes after radical prostatectomy in diabetic patients treated with metformin. Urology. 2010;**76**:1240-1244. DOI: 10.1016/j.urology.2010.03.059

[59] Wright JL, Stanford JL. Metformin use and prostate cancer in Caucasian men: Results from a population-based case-control study. Cancer Causes & Control. 2009;**20**:1617-1622. DOI: 10.1007/s10552-009-9407-y

[60] He XX, Tu SM, Lee MH, Yeung SC. Thiazolidinediones and metformin associated with improved survival of diabetic prostate cancer patients. Annals of Oncology. 2011;**22**:2640-2645. DOI: 10.1093/annonc/mdr020

[61] Miranda VC, Braghiroli MI, Faria LD, et al. Phase 2 trial of metformin combined with 5-fluorouracil in patients with refractory metastatic colorectal cancer. Clinical Colorectal Cancer. 2016;**15**(4):321-328. DOI: 10.1016/j.clcc.2016.04.011

[62] Mitsuhashi A, Sato Y, Kiyokawa T, Koshizaka M, Hanaoka H, Shozu M. Phase II study of medroxyprogesterone acetate plus metformin as a fertility-sparing treatment for atypical endometrial hyperplasia and endometrial cancer. Annals of Oncology. 2016;**27**(2):262-266. DOI: 10.1093/annonc/mdv539

[63] Jiralerspong S, Palla SL, Giordano SH, et al. Metformin and pathologic complete responses to neoadjuvant chemotherapy in diabetic patients with breast cancer. Journal of Clinical Oncology. 2009;**27**(20):3297-3302. DOI: 10.1200/JCO.2009.19.6410

[64] Colquhoun AJ, Venier NA, Vandersluis AD, Besla R, Sugar LM, Kiss A, et al. Metformin enhances the antiproliferative and apoptotic effect of bicalutamide in prostate cancer. Prostate Cancer and Prostatic Diseases. 2012;**15**:346-352. DOI: 10.1038/pcan.2012.16

[65] Ferguson FM, Gray NS. Kinase inhibitors: The road ahead. Nature Reviews. Drug Discovery. 2018;**17**(5):353-377. DOI: 10.1038/nrd.2018.21

[66] Cohen MH, Williams GA, Sridhara R, et al. FDA drug approval summary: Gefitinib (ZD1839) (Iressa) tablets. The Oncologist. 2003;**8**(4):303-306. DOI: 10.1634/theoncologist.8-4-303

[67] Wheeler DL, Dunn EF, Harari PM. Understanding resistance to EGFR inhibitors-impact on future treatment strategies. Nature Reviews. Clinical Oncology. 2010;**7**(9):493-507. DOI: 10.1038/nrclinonc.2010.97

[68] Pan YH, Jiao L, Lin CY, et al. Combined treatment with metformin and gefitinib overcomes primary resistance to EGFR-TKIs with EGFR mutation via targeting IGF-1R signaling pathway. Biologics. 2018;**12**:75-86. DOI: 10.2147/BTT.S166867

[69] Chen H, Yao W, Chu Q, et al. Synergistic effects of metformin in combination with EGFR-TKI in the treatment of patients with advanced non-small cell lung cancer and type 2 diabetes. Cancer Letters. 2015;**369**(1):97-102. DOI: 10.1016/j.canlet.2015.08.024

[70] Li KL, Li L, Zhang P, et al. A multicenter double-blind phase II study of metformin with gefitinib as first-line therapy of locally advanced non-small-cell lung cancer. Clinical Lung Cancer. 2017;**18**(3):340-343. DOI: 10.1016/j.cllc.2016.12.003

[71] Guan YS, He Q. Sorafenib: Activity and clinical application in patients with hepatocellular carcinoma. Expert Opinion on Pharmacotherapy. 2011;**12**(2):303-313. DOI: 10.1517/14656566.2011.546346

[72] Ling S, Song L, Fan N, et al. Combination of metformin and sorafenib suppresses proliferation and induces autophagy of hepatocellular carcinoma via targeting the mTOR pathway. International Journal of Oncology. 2017;**50**(1):297-309. DOI: 10.3892/ijo.2016.3799

[73] Vazquez-Martin A, Oliveras-Ferraros C, Del Barco S, et al.

The anti-diabetic drug metformin suppresses self-renewal and proliferation of trastuzumab-resistant tumor-initiating breast cancer stem cells. Breast Cancer Research and Treatment. 2011;**126**(2):355-364. DOI: 10.1007/s10549-010-0924-x

[74] Smith TA, Phyu SM, Akabuogu EU. Effects of administered cardioprotective drugs on treatment response of breast cancer cells. Anticancer Research. 2016;**36**(1):87-93

[75] Yamazaki K, Nagase M, Tamagawa H, et al. Randomized phase III study of bevacizumab plus FOLFIRI and bevacizumab plus mFOLFOX6 as first-line treatment for patients with metastatic colorectal cancer (WJOG4407G). Annals of Oncology. 2016;**27**(8):1539-1546. DOI: 10.1093/annonc/mdw206

[76] Markowska A, Sajdak S, Markowska J, et al. Angiogenesis and cancer stem cells: New perspectives on therapy of ovarian cancer. European Journal of Medicinal Chemistry. 2017;**142**:87-94. DOI: 10.1016/j.ejmech.2017.06.030

[77] Marrone KA, Zhou X, Forde PM, et al. A randomized phase II study of metformin plus paclitaxel/carboplatin/bevacizumab in patients with chemotherapy-naïve advanced or metastatic nonsquamous non-small cell lung cancer. The Oncologist. 2018;**23**(7):859-865. DOI: 10.1634/theoncologist.2017-0465

[78] Samsuri NAB, Leech M, Marignol L. Metformin and improved treatment outcomes in radiation therapy–A review. Cancer Treatment Reviews. 2017;**55**:150-162. DOI: 10.1016/j.ctrv.2017.03.005

[79] Baskar R, Dai J, Wenlong N, Yeo R, Yeoh K-W. Biological response of cancer cells to radiation treatment. Frontiers in Molecular Biosciences. 2014;**1**:24. DOI: 10.3389/fmolb.2014.00024

[80] Rao M, Gao C, Guo M, Law BYK, Xu Y. Effects of metformin treatment on radiotherapy efficacy in patients with cancer and diabetes: A systematic review and meta-analysis. Cancer Management and Research. 2018;**10**:4881-4890. DOI: 10.2147/CMAR.S174535

Chapter 8

Preventive and (Neo)Adjuvant Therapeutic Effects of Metformin on Cancer

Yile Jiao, Xiaochen Wang and Zhijun Luo

Abstract

Metformin, the first-line antidiabetic drug, has become an attractive candidate in cancer therapy since retrospective clinical investigations reported that patients with type 2 diabetes receiving metformin had lower incidence of cancer than those with other glucose lowering drugs. In line with this, preclinical studies have demonstrated that the antitumor activity of metformin could proceed through several mechanisms. Thus far, metformin has been used in cancer prevention with reduced risk as consequence and treatment of various cancers as an adjuvant or neoadjuvant drug. Thus, existing data support the beneficial effects of metformin on many types of cancers such as reducing metastasis and mortality and improving pathological responses and survival rates. However, some reports do not support this and even show adverse effects. The discrepancy may be attributed to expression levels of its transporters or genetic background. Hence, this chapter briefly reviews information on the mechanism of metformin action and summarizes both completed and ongoing clinical trials in an attempt to evaluate the value of metformin in prevention and treatment of various cancer types.

Keywords: metformin, AMPK, mTORC1, diabetes, lipogenesis, cancer prevention and therapy, clinical trials

1. Introduction

Metformin is derived from *Galega officinalis*, a natural herbal medicine. The herb was first used to relieve polyuria, a symptom of diabetes in ancient Egypt and medieval Europe [1]. Metformin is a widely used frontline drug for type 2 diabetes mellitus (T2DM). The major function of metformin is to decrease hepatic gluconeogenesis and enhance insulin sensitivity by increasing glucose uptake in muscle and adipose [2]. In addition to antidiabetes, metformin has proved to be beneficial to metabolic syndrome and nonalcoholic fatty liver disease [3, 4]. Cancer is characteristic of a metabolic disorder, inasmuch as metabolism is reprogrammed by switching oxidative phosphorylation into aerobic glycolysis, and thus, many of key molecules in these two routes are altered in their expression or posttranslational modification [5]. The incidence of cancer is higher in patients with T2DM than those without diabetes, indicating that diabetes is a risk factor of cancer [6]. Since Evan et al. reported in 2005 lower cancer incidence in patients with T2DM taking metformin than those with other antidiabetic drugs, great efforts have been made to elucidate the antitumor activity of metformin [7]. A considerable number of preclinical and clinical investigations support the beneficial effects of metformin on both prevention and treatment of various cancers. At the same time, some of mechanisms underlying metformin action on cancer cells have been unraveled, although much of them is still incomplete. Thus far, more than 300 clinical trials using metformin as a single or adjuvant agent in combination with other chemotherapies have been initiated in the treatment of various types of cancer in the world (www.clinicaltrials.gov).

2. Targets of metformin

Many functions of metformin are mediated by adenosine monophosphate-activated protein kinase (AMPK). Metformin at high doses leads to elevation of AMP, which binds to and allosterically activates AMPK, while at low doses, it engages lysosomes in the absence of AMP [8, 9]. The upstream kinases that phosphorylate AMPK α subunits at Thr172 include liver kinase B1 (LKB1), calmodulin-dependent kinase beta, and TGF-β-activated protein kinase [10–12].

AMPK plays important roles in regulating lipid and protein metabolisms by phosphorylating a series of target proteins. Thus, LKB1-AMPK pathway is critically important for metabolic adaption under stress condition, which aims to protect cells in the beginning [13]. However, persistent activation of AMPK by metformin can also cause cytostatic and even cytotoxic effects. Mounting evidence shows that metabolic syndrome and diabetes increase the risk of cancer, and correction of metabolic abnormalities alleviates cancer burdens and improves survival [14–16]. Drugs that target AMPK or downstream molecules are research focus nowadays for cancer prevention and treatment. Some of pathways downstream of AMPK essential for tumorigenesis and cancer progression are depicted in **Figure 1**.

PI3K-protein kinase B (AKT)-mammalian target of rapamycin (mTOR) pathway is well received as the target of AMPK. Mammalian target of rapamycin complex 1 (mTORC1) consists of mTOR, regulatory-associated protein of mTOR (Raptor), mammalian lethal with SEC13 protein 8, proline-rich AKT substrate 40 kDa, and DEP domain-containing mTOR-interacting protein [17]. Tuberous sclerosis complex 2 (TSC2) is a GTPase-activating protein that forms a complex with TSC1 to stimulate GTPase activity of Ras homolog enriched in brain (Rheb) and thus inhibits mammalian target of rapamycin complex 1 (mTORC1) activation. TSC2 is subjected to inhibition by AKT and activation by AMPK via phosphorylation at different sites. In addition, AMPK phosphorylates and inhibits Raptor, a scaffold of mTORC1. A plethora of cellular events, such as protein translation, lipogenesis, cell cycle progression, and autophagy, are regulated by the activated mTOR pathway, which are counteracted by AMPK [18]. Thus, control of mTORC1 activity is crucial for prevention and treatment of cancer.

Cancer cells always require large amount of building blocks for dividing progenitor cells. Thus, synthesis of fatty acid and cholesterol is very active [19]. Acutely, AMPK inhibits acetyl CoA carboxylase (ACC) and HMG-CoA reductase (HMGCR), which are rate-limiting enzymes for de novo synthesis of fatty acid and cholesterol, respectively [20]. In addition, AMPK activates malonyl-CoA decarboxylase (MAD) that converts malonyl-CoA to acetyl CoA. As cytosolic malonyl-CoA decreases, fatty acid synthesis is attenuated [17, 21]. AMPK also influences de novo synthesis of glycerolipid by inhibiting the rate-limiting enzyme glycerol phosphate acyltransferase (PAT) [17, 22]. Chronically, AMPK phosphorylates sterol regulatory element-binding protein-1c (SREBP-1c) and its related protein carbohydrate-response-element-binding protein (ChREBP), restricting the nuclear localization of

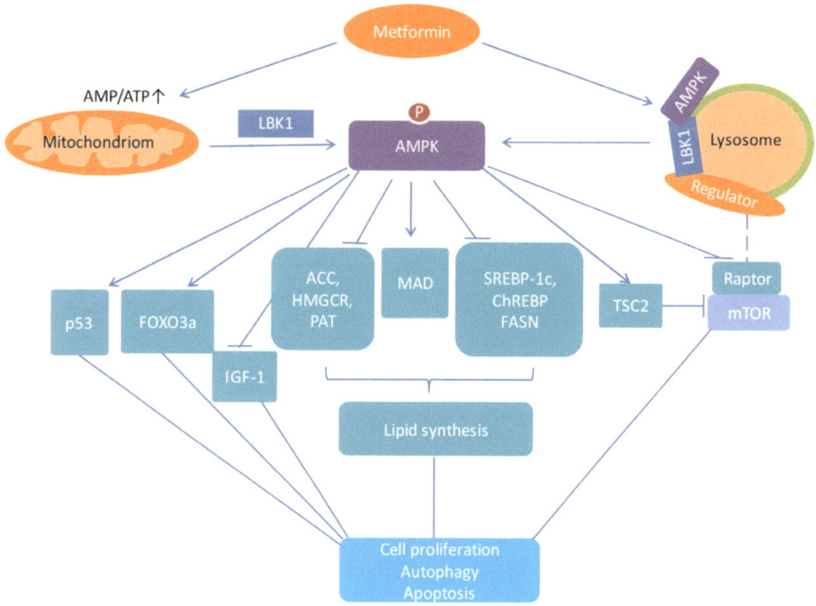

Figure 1.
AMPK activation and its biological functions. AMPK is activated by increased AMP:ATP ratio induced by metabolic stress and metformin. In addition, metformin can activate AMPK through lysosomal pathway, where v-ATPase-regulator-AXIN/LKB1-AMPK complex is formed. After activation, AMPK acts on multiple molecules/pathways, including inhibition of mTORC1, lipogenesis and IGF-1 expression, and activation of p53 and FOXO3a [17, 22, 87–89]. As such, AMPK regulates cell proliferation, autophagy, and apoptosis of cancer cells.

these transcription factors, so as to inhibit transcription of target genes for lipogenesis, including those encoding ACC and fatty acid synthase (FASN) [23].

3. Clinical investigations

Decreases from 20 to 94% in cancer risk among patients with T2DM after the use of metformin have been reported since 2005 [24]. A large population study conducted by Taiwan National Health Insurance Data Survey evaluated 16,602 individuals treated with metformin or other antidiabetic drug between 2000 and 2007 and concluded a 88% reduction in the risk of various cancer types after metformin treatment [25, 26]. In line with this, numerous investigations provided supporting data that metformin reduced incidence of various cancers. For example, DeCenci et al. have found a 30% decrease in cancer incidence in patients with T2DM treated with metformin compared to those with other drugs [27, 28]. Currie et al. conducted a large cohort study with around 60,000 patients from the UK database and revealed that metformin alone decreased the incidence of colorectal and pancreatic cancer compared with insulin and sulfonylureas monotherapy after the adjustment of confound bias, but this was not seen in breast cancer (BC) and prostate cancer [29]. It is noteworthy that metformin plus insulin could alleviate the progression of cancer [hazard ratio (HR) = 0.54, 95% confidence interval (CI) 0.43–0.66] [29]. With respect to mortality, ZODIAC trial with a 10-year follow up has indicated a lower death rate of cancer among metformin users with T2DM [30]. According to Noto et al. meta-analysis, diabetic patients taking metformin showed significant reduction of incidence of multiple types of cancer [risk ratio (RR) = 0.67, 0.53–0.85], including colorectal cancer (CRC) (RR = 0.68, 0.53–0.88) and cancer mortality (RR = 0.66, 95% CI = 0.49–0.88) [31]. A study of Bowker et al. reported that metformin decreased cancer mortality in T2DM, as compared with insulin and/or sulfonylurea groups [32]. After 1-year observation, the cancer death rate of metformin, insulin, and sulfonylurea users is 3.5, 8.8, and 4.9 per 1000 patients, respectively.

Regarding tumor types, dosage of metformin, study setting, and period of intervention associated with the treatment outcomes, examples are listed in **Table 1**.

Cancer type	Intervention	Outcome
Breast cancer		
Bodmer et al. [39]	Metformin or other antidiabetic drugs	Diabetic patients treated with metformin ≧ 5 years had a lower incidence of cancer, compared with nonusers or short-term (<5 years treatment) metformin users
Jiralerspong et al. [45]	Metformin + chemotherapy	The pCR rate in 68 diabetic patients treated with metformin, 87 diabetic patients without metformin, and 2374 nondiabetic patients was 24, 8, and 16% (P = 0.02)
Niraula et al. [46]	Metformin	Reduction of cancer cell proliferation (Ki67) by 3% (P = 0.016) and increases in apoptosis by 0.49% (P = 0.004) was compared between pre- and post-surgery, despite minor change of fasting insulin level
Hou et al. [51]	Metformin + chemotherapy	1013 BC patients with diabetes and 4621 BC patients without diabetes were analyzed. Nondiabetic group had higher 5-year survival rate than diabetic group (82 vs. 79%, P < 0.001). In diabetic subgroup, metformin-treated group had significant higher 5-year survival rates than nonmetformin-treated group (88 vs. 73%, P< 0.001)
El-Haggar et al. [42]	Metformin + chemotherapy or +hormone therapy, tamoxifen	Non-diabetic women with newly diagnosed BC (68/129) were prescribed with metformin (860 mg b.i.d.) along with chemotherapy or hormone therapy compared to nonmetformin-treated control arm over 6 or 12 months. A 3.27-fold decrease (P = 0.023, 95% CI 1.17–9.06) at the time of developing metastasis and an increase in average DFS by 2.137 (P = 0.044) in the metformin-treated group. Also, the levels of IGF-1, the ratio of IGF-1 to IGFBP-3, insulin, fasting blood glucose, HOMA-IR index notably decease, while IGFBP-3 levels significantly increase after using of metformin
He et al. [53]	Metformin or other antidiabetic drugs	A cohort study evaluated a total of 1983 women with stage ≧ 2 Her2 positive BC. Among 154/1983 diabetic patients who had already responded to previous chemotherapy. Metformin users had prolonged OS (HR = 0.52, 95% CI 0.28–0.97, P = 0.041) and reduced cancer-specific mortality of BC (HR = 0.47, 95% CI 0.24–0.90, P = 0.023), compared with nonusers
Colon cancer		
Coyle et al. [33]	Metformin	Significant benefit of RFS (n = 623 patients in two studies), OS (n = 1936 patients in five studies), and CSS (n = 535 patients in two studies) was observed in metformin-treated patients from 3094 patients with early stage CRC in nine studies, compared with that in nonmetformin using group

Cancer type	Intervention	Outcome
Rokkas and Portincasa [55]	Metformin	A significant decrease in the risk of developing colon neoplasia [RRs (95% CI) = 0.75 (0.65–0.87), $Z = -3.95$, $P < 0.001$], including the reduction of colon cancer [0.79 (0.69–0.91), $Z = -3.34$, $P < 0.001$] and colon polyps [0.58 (0.42–0.80), $Z = -3.30$, $P < 0.001$] among patients with T2DB after metformin treatment
Garrett et al. [58]	Metformin or other antidiabetic drugs	After adjustment of cofound variates, a 30% increase in OS was demonstrated among 424/4758 patients who were diagnosed of T2DM and CRC and administrated to metformin as compared with that in other antidiabetics users
Higurashi et al. [59]	Metformin	A total of 151 nondiabetic patients with CRC after polypectomy was randomized to metformin-treated arm (250 mg daily over 1 year) or placebo control arm with 1-year endoscopy reports. The incidence of total polyps and adenomas decreased in metformin-treated group by 18.5% [RR = 0.67, 95% CI (0.47–0.97), $P = 0.034$] and 21% [RR = 0.60, 95% CI (0.39–0.92), $P = 0.16$], compared with that in control group
Endometrial cancer		
Sivalingam et al. [60]	Metformin	A total of 40 women with atypical endometrial hyperplasia (AEH) or EC was assigned to receive metformin 850 mg b.i.d. over average 20 day, or no treatment before hysterectomy. Ki67 was reduced by 17.2% (95% CI 27.4–7.0, $P < 0.002$) in metformin-treated group
Schuler et al. [61]	Metformin	20 nondiabetic women with EC and obesity (BMI ≥ 30) were administrated with metformin 850 mg daily for 1–4 weeks before surgery. The levels of Ki67 and p-S6 were reduced between pretreatment and postsurgery by 11.75% ($P = 0.008$) and 51.2% ($P = 0.0002$), respectively. Besides, the levels of p-AMPK ($P = 0.00001$), p-Akt ($P = 0.0002$), p-4EBP1 ($P = 0.001$), and ER ($P = 0.0002$) also decreased after surgery
Mitsuhashi et al. [63]	Metformin + MPA	17 AEH and 19 noninvasive EC patients received metformin (escalating from 750 to 2250 mg daily) after complete response treated by MPA and other drugs. Relapse rate among patients was 10%, and estimated 3-year RFS rate was 89%
Nevadunsky et al. [66]	Adjuvant metformin	Metformin significantly improved OS (HR = 0.54, 95% CI 0.30–0.97, $P < 0.04$) in diabetic patients with nonendometrioid EC when compared with that in nonusers with EC
Acute lymphoblastic leukemia		
Ramos-Peñafiel et al. [67]	Metformin + prednisone	A total of 102 nondiabetic patients with ALL was enrolled, 26 received metformin (850 mg t.i.d.) for 6 days during preinduction stage, and 76 were treated with traditional chemotherapy without metformin. The use of metformin prevented therapy failure and early relapse ($P = 0.025$) in patients bearing relative to high levels of ABCB1
Esophageal Cancer		
Skinner et al. [68]	Neoadjunvant metformin + CRT	Metformin users along with CRT resulted in higher pCR (34.5%) than nonmetformin cohort (4.8%,

Cancer type	Intervention	Outcome
		P = 0.01) and nondiabetic patients (19.6%, P = 0.05). Higher pCR rate was found to be associated with higher metformin dose (≥1500 mg/d). Post-CRT maximum SUV decreased significantly in patients taking metformin (P = 0.05)
Lee et al. [25]	Adjuvant metformin	Reduction of total CID and incidence of some gastroenterological cancers including CRC, HCC, and so on, among which the CID of esophageal cancer decreased in diabetic groups taking adjuvant metformin in comparison to non-DM groups. Metformin dosage giving rise to a significant decrease in cancer incidence was ≤500 mg/day
Leamm et al. [69]	Metformin + neoadjuvant chemo(radio)therapy	No statistically significant difference between metformin users and nonmetformin users for median overall survival (43.6 vs. 42.8 months, P = 0.66) or for median DFS (31.1 vs.47.0 months, P = 0.68)
Prostate cancer		
Wright et al. [70]	Metformin	A reduced risk of prostate cancer was showed among white men at age of 35–74 after the use of metformin, as reported by a case-control study
Rothermundt et al. [74]	Metformin	A total of 44 men with castration-resistant prostate cancer was assigned to receive metformin 500 mg b.i. d. until progression. After initial metformin treatment, changes in IGF and IGBP3 and improvement of insulin sensitivity from baseline were observed but without correlation with progression. At week 4, only four patients did not have progression (95% CI, 3–22). Average PFS was 2.8 months (95% CI, 2.8–3.2) and PSA double time declined in 23 patients but not significant
Joshua et al. [75]	Metformin	Metformin 500 mg t.i.d. was prescribed to 24 men with operable prostate cancer before prostatectomy. In a per patient and per tumor analyses, Ki67 was reduced by 29.5% (P = 0.0064) and 28.6% (P = 0.0042) in comparison with the initial biopsy and postprostatectomy sections
Rieken et al. [77]	Metformin	Metformin users with prostate cancer exhibited a minor improvement of RFS after prostatectomy
Spratt et al. [78]	Metformin	A retrospective study examined 2901 noninvasive prostate cancer patients through radiation therapy. In 157 patients treated with metformin, PSA-RFS and DMFS were improved and the castration-resistant prostate cancer progression was alleviated

Table 1.
Examples of clinical investigations of metformin used as a neoadjuvant and adjuvant agent in cancer therapy.

3.1 The role of metformin in radiotherapy and chemotherapy

Metformin has been reported to be a useful adjuvant drug to radiotherapy or chemotherapy for different cancers, especially prostate and colon cancers [33]. The effects of metformin on overall survival (OS), relapse-free survival (RFS), and cancer-specific survival (CSS) after concurrent chemotherapy and/or radiotherapy vary on cancer types.

A previous study has shown that metformin increases radiosensitivity of luminal BC by influencing expression of thioredoxin and intracellular redox homeostasis [34]. A high level of AMPKα expression correlates with the increased radiosensitivity and better prognosis. A systemic review and meta-analysis conducted in 2018 summarized the impact of metformin on the efficacy of radiotherapy in 17 studies, including prostate cancer, head and neck cancer, rectal cancer, lung cancer, esophageal cancer, and liver cancer [35]. The study compared diabetic patients with metformin (D + M) and diabetic or nondiabetic cohort without metformin (D − M or N − M) after radiotherapy. An improved pathologic complete response (pCR), 2y-OS, and 5y-OS vary in different cancer types when analyzing D + M and D − M groups, supporting that metformin is beneficial to OS of diabetic patients while distant metastasis-free survival (DMFS) and 5-year OS were not significantly different between D + M and N − M groups. With respect to the possible mechanisms by which metformin enhances radiosensitivity, studies have indicated that p53 and AMPKα are involved [36, 37]. Despite the increased sensitivity to radiotherapy and chemotherapy, cumulative side effects and toxicity concur with the use of metformin. For example, a study has shown that combination of metformin with radiochemotherapy can lead to less tolerance to cisplatin and radiotherapy and exacerbate gastrointestinal adverse effects such as grade ≥ 3 nausea/vomiting [38].

3.2 Breast cancer

Several lines of clinical investigations have been conducted to assess the beneficial effects of metformin on BC [39–52]. Two retrospective studies revealed that long-term use of metformin (>5 years) reduced the risk of BC in T2DM women as compared with other antidiabetic drugs [39, 40]. However, Currie et al. reported that metformin use did not affect risk of breast and prostate cancer, but the reduced risk was found in colon and pancreas cancer [29].

He et al. have shown improvement of disease-free survival (DFS), DMFS, and OS in diabetic women who well-responded to previous hormone therapy and then received metformin treatment. The results demonstrated that metformin synergizes with hormone therapy [53, 54].

Metformin was used as neoadjuvant chemotherapy of BC to improve pathological conditions prior to surgery [45–48]. The increased pCR in 2529 women with BC has been demonstrated in metformin-treated diabetic patients, compared to nonmetformin-treated patients with or without diabetes [45]. Another study by Niraula et al. evaluated the effect of metformin on serum biomarkers in nondiabetic BC patients before surgery [46]. The patients were treated with metformin for 2 weeks, and serum biomarkers were assessed. A notably reduction of Ki67 and elevation of apoptosis were observed in invasive tumor after the use of metformin. The significant decrease of homeostatic model assessment of insulin resistance (-HOMA-IR) was also observed, while insulin and leptin displayed a modest change. However, a study showed that metformin increased phospho-AMPK (p-AMPK) and decreased p-Akt and Ki67 without induction of apoptosis, suggesting a cytostatic effect [47].

The long-term use of metformin has been shown to reduce risk of distant metastasis and mortality of BC patients with type 2 diabetes [49–51]. Furthermore, metformin use as adjuvant therapy can also improve outcomes of BC in nondiabetic patients [41, 42, 52]. For example, a single-arm phase II trial enrolled nondiabetic women with M0 stage BC. After receiving metformin of 500 mg t.i.d. for 6 months, the result showed that fasting insulin level and HOMA-IR were significantly reduced. Total cholesterol, low density lipoprotein, and leptin also similarly declined [52]. Another study focused on the optimal dose of metformin that achieves favorable effects on BC by comparing dose between 1500 and 1000 mg daily [41]. For postmenopausal women with basal testosterone levels≥0.28 ng/mL, it seemed that metformin of 1500 mg/d was better than 1000 mg/d in reduction of insulin and testosterone levels, which were associated with cancer incidence and prognosis. Combination of metformin with other chemotherapy usually generates better outcomes in nondiabetic BC patients with the higher HOMA-IR (>2.8), and HOMA-IR can be improved by metformin [42–44, 48].

In summary, studies showing beneficial effects of metformin are more than those without effects. Metformin as an adjuvant agent can suppress BC at various doses ranging from 500 to 1500 mg. The outcomes mainly include reduced risk of BC, decreases in cancer-promoting markers and metastatic events, increases in apoptotic markers, and improvement of progression-free survival (PFS) and OS.

3.3 Colon cancer

The role of metformin in preventing colon cancer has been documented in the following studies conducted in both diabetic and nondiabetic patients. A meta-analysis was carried out in 709,980 individuals with T2DM from 17 studies showing a significant decrease in the risk of colon neoplasia among metformin-treated patients compared to those without metformin, with respective reduction for either cancer or polys [55]. A randomized study enrolled a total of 26 nondiabetic individuals with aberrant crypt foci (ACF) (biomarker of CRC development) and assigned them to either receive metformin 250 mg daily for 1 month or control group [56]. Significant decreases in the average number of ACF by a 3.67-fold (P = 0.007) and in proliferating cell nuclear antigen index were discovered in metformin arm. This indicates that metformin prevents CRC by attenuating cell proliferation and ACF development.

Metformin has been used as an adjuvant agent in the treatment of CRC. First, a single-arm study has demonstrated a median PFS of 1.8 months and an OS of 7.9 months in metastatic CRC with combination of metformin (850 mg b.i.d.) and 5-fluorouracil treatment. Surprisingly, the improvement in median survival was more obvious in obese patients [57]. Second, Coyle et al. have evaluated 3092 patients with early stage of CRC [33]. It was found that the use of metformin significantly improved RFS (HR = 0.63, 95% CI 0.47–0.85), OS (0.69, 95% CI 0.58–0.83), and CSS (0.58, 95% CI 0.39–0.86) in patients with T2DM, compared with other antidiabetic drugs. Likewise, progression of CRC is also inhibited by metformin. A similar study showed prolonged OS in patients with T2DM with CRC receiving metformin, as compared with nonmetformin users (79.6 vs. 56.9 months, P = 0.048) [58]. The last randomized trial used metformin (250 mg daily) for a year in nondiabetic patients with high-risk adenoma recurrence and no colorectal polyps after polypectomy [59]. The results showed that polyps and adenomas are noticeably fewer in the metformin arm than in the control arm. The study also showed that average HOMA-IR status was significantly reduced in nonrecurrent patients by metformin, while the value remained stable in recurrent patients, indicating that insulin resistance is associated with chemoprevention outcome.

3.4 Endometrial cancer

Clinical investigations support that metformin could serve as a potential drug for protection against endometrial cancer (EC) [60–65]. Several studies have evaluated the effects of short-term use of metformin as a neoadjuvant therapy between initial recruitment and hysterectomy surgery in nondiabetic women with EC [60–62]. The first nonrandomized trial has examined the change of Ki67 and shown a remarkable reduction after metformin use at 850 mg b.i.d. for average 20 days [60]. A significant reduction in phospho-4E-binding protein 1 (p-4EFBP1) downstream of mTOR was also observed by immunohistochemistry, while indirect serum markers of insulin resistance (fasting glucose, insulin, and HOMA-IR) and leptin only showed a decrease trend but not significant after adjusting difference. Another preoperative clinical trial was done in nondiabetic women with body mass index (BMI) ≧ 30 [61]. After taking metformin 850 mg daily for 1–4 weeks prior to surgery, Ki67, p-AMPK, p-Akt, phospho-S6 Ribosomal Protein (p-S6), and p-4EBP were significantly lower in resected specimens than in pretreatment. The reduction of p-AMPK is inconsistent with purported positive effect of metformin. This study also showed a decrease in estrogen receptor (ER) but not progesterone receptor.

According to a study evaluating the effect of metformin on EC of diabetic patients (n = 114) as compared with diabetic (n = 136) and nondiabetic (n = 735) patients without metformin from 1999 to 2009, metformin-treated group exhibits prolonged OS than nonusers before and after the adjustment of confound bias [66]. A phase II study has examined the effects of long-term metformin (2250 mg daily until recurrence) on RFS after a complete response to medroxyprogesterone acetate (MPA) in 17 individuals with atypical endometrial hyperplasia and 19 with EC [63]. The 3-year estimated RFS was 89%, and the 3-year recurrence rate showed a 4.7-fold decrease in this study compared with a previous study [64]. In contrast to short-term treatment, the other randomized factorial study does not have a significant change in PFS/OS after metformin treatment (1700 mg/d for 16 weeks and 1-year follow up) [65].

3.5 Acute lymphoid leukemia

A single study randomized to assign 102 patients with nondiabetic acute lymphoid leukemia (ALL) into a group of 26 with metformin at 850 mg t.i.d. for 10 days and the rest to the group without metformin before remission therapy [67]. Metformin displayed a beneficial effect on OS in the patients with high levels of ABCB1 expression, the gene encoding multidrug resistant protein-1. The failure rate of therapy was significantly reduced and early relapse after remission prevented by metformin, as compared with nonusers.

3.6 Oesophagal cancer

Oesophagal cancer is deadly cancer with poor prognosis, and patients usually do survive or die no longer than 30 months after chemoradiation and surgery [68]. A prospective cohort study by Taiwan National Health Insurance revealed a positive effect of metformin as an adjunct to standard chemotherapies on the cancer incidence density (CID) of gastroenterological cancers [25]. In this study, a decrease in total CID including esophageal cancer was found in diabetic groups taking adjuvant metformin in comparison to nondiabetic groups. Another study reported that metformin enhanced the efficacy of radiochemotherapy in patients with T2DM resulting in superior pCR and low postconcurrent chemoradiation (CRT) maximum SUV compared to patients with T2DM without metformin and non-DM patients [68]. Additionally, higher pCR rate was correlated with higher metformin dose (≥1500 mg/d). However, a report in 2015 demonstrated inconsistent results, in which no difference in pCR was found between metformin users and nonmetformin users [69]. Furthermore, it was shown that together with neoadjunvant chemoradiation, metformin did not improve the median OS or median DFS in diabetic patients with esophageal cancer.

3.7 Prostate cancer

The effect of metformin on prostate cancer is ambiguous. Studies of Wright and Stanford have provided a 44% decrease in the risk of prostate cancer among Caucasian men with diabetes [70]. However, investigations by others could not obtain the same conclusion on the incidence of prostate cancer in diabetic patients treated with metformin, but the mortality might be reduced [71–73]. A single-arm clinical trial has revealed a decrease in insulin-like growth factor-1 (IGF-1) and an increase in insulin-like growth factor-binding protein-3 (IGFBP-3), alongside lowering prostate-specific antigen (PSA), after giving metformin 500 mg b.i.d. over 12 weeks to patients with castration-resistant prostate cancer [74]. In a single-arm study on men with biopsy-proven localized prostate cancer, 22 patients were selected to receive metformin at 500 mg/d or b.i.d., followed by t.i.d. for 28–84 days preceding their prostatectomy. The results revealed that Ki67 index was reduced by comparing the initial biopsy with postprostatectomy sections [75]. However, the changes were not recapitulated by another study, although metformin in the prostate tissue was detected after a median of 34 days prior to prostatectomy [76]. In a retrospective study, metformin-treated diabetic individuals gained the improvement of RFS among 6863 patients after radical prostatectomy [77]. Study of Spratt et al. also demonstrated the significantly elevated PSA-RFS, DFS, and lower cancer mortality in localized prostate cancer with metformin treatment compared with that of nonusers [78].

4. Ongoing clinical trials

Previous studies of metformin use as neoadjuvant or adjuvant therapy for various types of cancer provide strong rationale of clinical trials in more vigorous settings. Thus far, more than 300 clinical trials have initiated in the world despite some are somehow either terminated or withdrawn. **Table 2** lists some of them. For example, NCT02065687 is a randomized, metformin-placebo, phase II/III study that enrolls a total of 540 participants and examines the effect of adjuvant metformin together with paclitaxel and carboplatin in treatment of stages III–IV or recurrent EC. Patients receive metformin twice a day in a 5-year follow up until disease progression or undesirable adverse effects appear. According to this trial, prolonged PFS and OS will be observed after the use of metformin together with other chemotherapeutic drugs. One of the ongoing phase II trials carrying out in 151 premenopausal BC patients with BMI $\geqq 25$ kg/m^2 evaluates treatment effect with 850 mg metformin b.i.d. vs. placebo for a year, by examining the primary outcome changes of breast density at time points of 6 and 12 months. This study spanning from March 7, 2014 to June 30, 2020 also identifies biomarkers associated with metabolic effects of metformin and attempts to find prediction factors of BC risk (NCT02028221). Also, a trial (NCT02614339) is undergoing to follow-up 3-year DFS and 5-year OS in nondiabetic patients with stage II high-risk/III CRC treated with metformin (1000 mg/day) for 48 months. This study has enrolled 593 participants and is still recruiting and expected to complete in July 2021.

The trial of double-blinded 2 × 2 factorial (aspirin × metformin) design registers 160 patients with stages I–III colon cancer who undertake a completed polypectomy within recent 24 months (NCT03047837). After randomized allocation, patients will receive metformin at 850 mg b.i.d. or aspirin at 100 mg daily or two drugs together vs. placebo over 1 year. Immunohistochemistry for NF-κB, glucose metabolism, pS6K, and other biomarker will be compared pre- and postintervention (ClinicalTrials.gov Identifier: NCT03047837).

NCT number	Status	Participants	Period	Intervention	Cancer type
NCT02581137 https://ClinicalTrials.gov/show/NCT02581137	Active	(a) 26, (b)18 years and older (adult, older adult), (c) all sex	June 10, 2016 to not indicated	Drug: metformin hydrochloride	Oral cancer
NCT02028221 https://ClinicalTrials.gov/show/NCT02028221	Active	(a) 151, (b) 21 years to 54 years (adult), (c) female	March 7, 2014 to June 30, 2020	Drug: metformin & placebo	BC
NCT02431676 https://ClinicalTrials.gov/show/NCT02431676	Active	(a) 100, (b) 50 years to 65 years (adult, older adult), (c) female	May 1, 2013 to September 1, 2022	Drug: metformin & placebo	EC
NCT01697566 https://ClinicalTrials.gov/show/NCT01697566	Active	(a) 100, (b) 50 years to 65 years (adult, older adult), (c) female	May 1, 2013 to September 1, 2022	Drug: metformin & placebo	EC
NCT01797523 https://ClinicalTrials.gov/show/NCT01797523	Active	(a) 62, (b) 18 years and older (adult, older adult), (c) all sex	May 1, 2013 to October 1, 2020	Drug: metformin, letrozole, & everolimus	EC
NCT02065687 https://ClinicalTrials.gov/show/NCT02065687	Active	(a) 540, (b) 18 years to older (adult, older adult), (c) female	Match 17, 2014 to	Drug: carboplatin, metformin hydrochloride, paclitaxel, & placebo	EC
NCT03047837 https://ClinicalTrials.gov/show/NCT03047837	Recruiting	(a) 160, (b) 18 years to 80 years (adult, older adult), (c) all sex	March 15, 2017 to March 15, 2020	Drug: aspirin (ASA) + metformin (MET)|Drug: ASA|Drug: MET|Drug: placebos	Tertiary prevention in colon cancer
NCT01905046 https://ClinicalTrials.gov/show/NCT01905046	Recruiting	(a) 128, (b) 25 years to 55 years (adult), (c) female	August 2013 to	Drug: metformin hydrochloride & placebo	BC
NCT02614339 https://ClinicalTrials.gov/show/NCT02614339	Recruiting	(a) 593, (b) 20 years to 80 years (adult, older adult), (c) all sex	December 2015 to July 2021	Drug: metformin & placebo	CRC
NCT03378297 https://ClinicalTrials.gov/show/NCT03378297	Recruiting	(a) 143, (b) 18 years and older (adult, older adult), (c) female	May 4, 2018 to June 1, 2020	Drug: metformin & acetylsalicylic acid & drug: olaparib & drug: letrozole	Ovarian cancer
NCT03685409 https://ClinicalTrials.gov/show/NCT03685409	Recruiting	(a) 62, (b)20 years to 70 years (adult, older adult), (c) all sex	October 1, 2018 to September 30, 2020	Drug: metformin hydrochloride & placebo	Oral cancer

NCT number	Status	Participants	Period	Intervention	Cancer type
NCT01864096 https://ClinicalTrials.gov/show/NCT01864096	Recruiting	(a) 408, (b) 18 years to 79 years (adult, older adult), (c) male	October 1, 2013 to August 1, 2024	Drug: metformin & placebo	Prostate cancer

Table 2.
Summary of ongoing clinical trials approved by FDA.

5. Cautions to be considered

5.1 Cancer type-specific effects

Whether a cancer type is sensitive to metformin depends on expression level of OCT1 in the cell membrane. Thus far, majority of previous studies have demonstrated that metformin exerts beneficial effects on different types of cancer, while some do not respond. On contrary, in some cases, for example, in glioma and leukemia cancer cells, metformin reduces cisplatin-induced apoptosis, suggesting that metformin exerts a protective effect on cytotoxic agents in some cells [79]. Hence, before going to clinical trials, preclinical tests should be undertaken to ascertain if metformin enhances the inhibitory effect of other drugs. This is feasible when PDX animal models or organoid culture techniques are available.

5.2 Genetic background of cancer

Responses of cancer cells with and without LKB1 to metformin are different. Metformin exerts cytostatic effect on cancer cells with wild-type LKB1, while it causes cytotoxicity in cells lacking LKB1. If metformin is used together with most of chemotherapeutic drugs that are cytotoxic in cancer containing wild-type LKB1, the cooperative effects might not be achieved. The reason is that more rapidly dividing cells are more sensitive to cytotoxic drugs, while cytostatic drugs slow down speed of cell growth, which might compromise the efficacy of cytotoxic chemotherapy. In this scenario, it might be a good idea to take metformin and cytotoxic drug alternately. For example, patients take a couple of cycles of cytotoxic chemotherapy and then have rest for period of time during which metformin is alternately used. The purpose is to restrain cancer in dormancy and allow the patients to restore healthy condition. In addition, Birsoy et al. have delineated that the most metformin-sensitive cells contain mutations of genes responsible for upregulation of mitochondrial oxidative phosphorylation, for example, complex I components, or glucose utilization [80]. Thus, these genes may serve as biomarkers for metformin use. Altogether, these studies point to importance of personalized medicine to determine the efficacy of metformin in cancer therapy.

5.3 Sensitivity of cancer stem cells

Cancer stem cells (CSCs) are refractory to chemotherapy, leading to the relapse of cancer. These cells metastasize to distant organs after flowing in circulation, resulting in poor prognosis. Thus, CSCs have become an important target for anticancer therapies. Hirsch et al. have reported that the CSCs derived from BC are preferentially sensitive to metformin that is used from 10 to 100 times less dosage than nonstem cancer cells [81]. This finding suggests that metformin could effectively prevent metastasis. It is especially meaningful in the case of surgically resected cancer when local metastasis in lymph nodes is cytologically tested negative, but a few CSCs may escape to circulation. At this time, metformin can be used as preventive measure.

Previous studies have demonstrated that metformin selectively targets CSCs via regulation of different pathways in various cancer types including breast, pancreatic, prostate, and colon cancer [82, 83]. For example, Zhu et al. have shown that metformin inhibits $CD61^{high}/CD49f^{high}$ subpopulation, markers of tumor initiating cells, by inactivating epidermal growth factor receptor/ErbB2 signaling. Similarly, CD133+, aldehyde dehydrogenases 1+, and other molecules are inhibited in pancreatic and colon cancer through inhibition of the Akt/mTOR pathway [84, 85]. However, a recent study using head and neck squamous cell carcinoma has shown that metformin protects CSCs against the cisplatin-induced cell death when combining these two, which discord with previous studies [86]. Thus, it should be cautious to ascertain if metformin exerts inhibitory or protective effects on specifically originated CSCs.

6. Conclusion

Metformin is a cheap and nontoxic first-line antidiabetic medicine. It is an attractive drug that is being repurposed for multiple usages in treatment of other diseases in addition to diabetes. Metformin implements its function through AMPK-dependent and independent mechanisms. Preclinical and retrospective clinical investigations have inspired clinical trials of metformin use in various cancer therapies. It is a promising drug in neoadjuvant and adjuvant therapies. We hope these trials will come to end with positive or negative results in the next few years. In considering genetic heterogeneity of cancer, responses of different cancer types and subpopulations in the same cancer might be different. Therefore, we still have long way to go and loads of questions to be addressed.

Acknowledgements

ZL is supported by the National Natural Science Foundation of China (81572753, 31660332) and the Innovation and Entrepreneurship grant from Jiangxi Provincial Bureau of Foreign Experts, China.

Conflict of interest

The authors declare no conflict of interest.

Author details

Yile Jiao†, Xiaochen Wang† and Zhijun Luo*
Queen Mary School, Nanchang University, Nanchang, China

*Address all correspondence to: zluo559914@ncu.edu.cn

† Equal contribution to this work.

References

[1] Rena G, Hardie DG, Pearson ER. The mechanisms of action of metformin. Diabetologia. 2017;**60**(9):1577-1585. Available from: http://www.ncbi.nlm.nih.gov/pubmed/28776086

[2] Zhou M, Xia L, Wang J. Metformin transport by a newly cloned proton-stimulated organic cation transporter (plasma membrane monoamine transporter) expressed in human intestine. Drug Metabolism & Disposition. 2007;**35**(10):1956-1962. Available from: http://www.ncbi.nlm.nih.gov/pubmed/27011019

[3] Mazza A, Fruci B, Garinis GA, Giuliano S, Malaguarnera R, Belfiore A. The role of metformin in the management of NAFLD. Experimental Diabetes Research. 2012;**2012**:1-13. Available from: http://www.hindawi.com/journals/jdr/2012/716404/

[4] Ghatak SB, Dhamecha PS, Bhadada SV, Panchal SJ. Investigation of the potential effects of metformin on atherothrombotic risk factors in hyperlipidemic rats. European Journal of Pharmacology. 2011;**659**(2–3):213-223. Available from: https://linkinghub.elsevier.com/retrieve/pii/S0014299911003414

[5] Seyfried TN, Shelton LM. Cancer as a metabolic disease. Nutrition & Metabolism. 2010;**7**(1):7. Available from: http://nutritionandmetabolism.biomedcentral.com/articles/10.1186/1743-7075-7-7

[6] Kasznicki J, Sliwinska A, Drzewoski J. Metformin in cancer prevention and therapy. Annals of Translational Medicine. 2014;**2**(6):1-11

[7] Ikhlas S, Ahmad M. Metformin: Insights into its anticancer potential with special reference to AMPK dependent and independent pathways. Life Sciences. 2017;**185**:53-62. Available from: https://linkinghub.elsevier.com/retrieve/pii/S0024320517303685

[8] Zhang C-S, Hawley SA, Zong Y, Li M, Wang Z, Gray A, et al. Fructose-1,6-bisphosphate and aldolase mediate glucose sensing by AMPK. Nature. 2017;**548**(7665):112-116. Available from: http://www.nature.com/articles/nature23275

[9] Zhang C-S, Li M, Ma T, Zong Y, Cui J, Feng J-W, et al. Metformin activates AMPK through the lysosomal pathway. Cell Metabolism. 2016;**24**(4):521-522. Available from: https://linkinghub.elsevier.com/retrieve/pii/S1550413116304818

[10] Foretz M, Guigas B, Bertrand L, Pollak M, Viollet B. Metformin: From mechanisms of action to therapies. Cell Metabolism. 2014;**20**(6):953-966. Available from: https://linkinghub.elsevier.com/retrieve/pii/S1550413114004410

[11] Muaddi H, Chowdhury S, Vellanki R, Zamiara P, Koritzinsky M. Contributions of AMPK and p53 dependent signaling to radiation response in the presence of metformin. Radiotherapy and Oncology. 2013;**108**(3):446-450. Available from: https://linkinghub.elsevier.com/retrieve/pii/S0167814013002922

[12] Pollak MN. Investigating metformin for cancer prevention and treatment: The end of the beginning. Cancer Discovery. 2012;**2**(9):778-790. Available from: http://cancerdiscovery.aacrjournals.org/lookup/doi/10.1158/2159-8290.CD-12-0263

[13] Jeon S-M, Chandel NS, Hay N. AMPK regulates NADPH homeostasis to promote tumour cell survival during energy stress. Nature. 2012;**485**(7400):661-665. Available from: http://www.nature.com/articles/nature11066

[14] LeRoith D, Novosyadlyy R, Gallagher E, Lann D, Vijayakumar A, Yakar S. Obesity and type 2 diabetes are associated with an increased risk of developing cancer and a worse prognosis; epidemiological and mechanistic evidence. Experimental and Clinical Endocrinology and Diabetes. 2008;**116**(S 01):S4-S6. Available from: http://www.thieme-connect.de/DOI/DOI?10.1055/s-2008-1081488

[15] Nawroth P. Diabetes, obesity, insulin resistance: Different pathways to cancer? Experimental and Clinical Endocrinology & Diabetes. 2009; **117**(10):561-562. Available from: http://www.thieme-connect.de/DOI/DOI?10.1055/s-0029-1241797

[16] Percik R, Stumvoll M. Obesity and cancer. Experimental and Clinical Endocrinology & Diabetes. 2009; **117**(10):563-566. Available from: http://www.thieme-connect.de/DOI/DOI?10.1055/s-0029-1241870

[17] Beauchamp EM, Platanias LC. The evolution of the TOR pathway and its role in cancer. Oncogene. 2013;**32**(34): 3923-3932. Available from: http://www.nature.com/articles/onc2012567

[18] Saxton RA, Sabatini DM. mTOR signaling in growth, metabolism, and disease. Cell. 2017;**168**(6):960-976. Available from: https://linkinghub.elsevier.com/retrieve/pii/S0092867417301824

[19] Roux PP, Blenis J. ERK and p38 MAPK-activated protein kinases: A family of protein kinases with diverse biological functions. Microbiology and Molecular Biology Reviews. 2004;**68**(2): 320-344. Available from: http://mmbr.asm.org/cgi/doi/10.1128/MMBR.68.2.320-344.2004

[20] Luo Z, Saha AK, Xiang X, Ruderman NB. AMPK, the metabolic syndrome and cancer. Trends in Pharmacology Sciences. 2005; **26**(2):69-76. Available from: https://www.sciencedirect.com/science/article/abs/pii/S0165614704003402

[21] Li X, Wu C, Chen N, Gu H, Yen A, Cao L, et al. PI3K/Akt/mTOR signaling pathway and targeted therapy for glioblastoma. Oncotarget. 2016;**7**(22): 33440-33450. Available from: http://www.oncotarget.com/fulltext/7961

[22] Hay N. Upstream and downstream of mTOR. Genes & Development. 2004; **18**(16):1926-1945. Available from: http://www.genesdev.org/cgi/doi/10.1101/gad.1212704

[23] Dowling RJO, Topisirovic I, Fonseca BD, Sonenberg N. Dissecting the role of mTOR: Lessons from mTOR inhibitors. Biochimica et Biophysica Acta, Proteins and Proteomics. 2010; **1804**(3):433-439. Available from: https://linkinghub.elsevier.com/retrieve/pii/S1570963909003598

[24] Suissa S, Azoulay L. Metformin and cancer: Mounting evidence against an association. Diabetes Care. 2014;**37**(7): 1786-1788. Available from: http://www.ncbi.nlm.nih.gov/pubmed/24963109

[25] Lee M-S, Hsu C-C, Wahlqvist ML, Tsai H-N, Chang Y-H, Huang Y-C. Type 2 diabetes increases and metformin reduces total, colorectal, liver and pancreatic cancer incidences in Taiwanese: A representative population prospective cohort study of 800,000 individuals. BMC Cancer. 2011;**11**(1):20. Available from: http://bmccancer.biomedcentral.com/articles/10.1186/1471-2407-11-20

[26] Suissa S, Azoulay L. Metformin and cancer: Mounting evidence against an association: Figure 1. Diabetes Care. 2014;**37**(7):1786-1788. Available from: http://care.diabetesjournals.org/lookup/doi/10.2337/dc14-0500

[27] Rêgo DF, Pavan LMC, Elias ST, De Luca Canto G, Guerra ENS. Effects of metformin on head and neck cancer: A systematic review. Oral Oncology. 2015; **51**(5):416-422

[28] DeCensi A, Puntoni M, Goodwin P, Cazzaniga M, Gennari A, Bonanni B, et al. Metformin and cancer risk in diabetic patients: A systematic review and meta-analysis. Cancer Prevention Research. 2010;**3**(11):1451-1461

[29] Currie CJ, Poole CD, Gale EAM. The influence of glucose-lowering therapies on cancer risk in type 2 diabetes. Diabetologia. 2009;**52**(9):1766-1777. Available from: http://link.springer.com/10.1007/s00125-009-1440-6

[30] Landman GWD, Kleefstra N, van Hateren KJJ, Groenier KH, Gans ROB, Bilo HJG. Metformin associated with lower cancer mortality in type 2 diabetes: ZODIAC-16. Diabetes Care. 2010;**33**(2):322-326. Available from: http://care.diabetesjournals.org/cgi/doi/10.2337/dc09-1380

[31] Noto H, Goto A, Tsujimoto T, Noda M. Cancer risk in diabetic patients treated with metformin: A systematic review and meta-analysis. PLoS One. 2012;**7**(3):e33411. Available from: http://dx.plos.org/10.1371/journal.pone.0033411

[32] Bowker SL, Yasui Y, Veugelers P, Johnson JA. Glucose-lowering agents and cancer mortality rates in type 2 diabetes: Assessing effects of time-varying exposure. Diabetologia. 2010; **53**(8):1631-1637. Available from: http://link.springer.com/10.1007/s00125-010-1750-8

[33] Coyle C, Cafferty FH, Vale C, Langley RE. Metformin as an adjuvant treatment for cancer: A systematic review and meta-analysis. Annals of Oncology. 2016;**27**(12):2184-2195. Available from: https://linkinghub.elsevier.com/retrieve/pii/S0923753419365354

[34] Zhang Y, Storr SJ, Johnson K, Green AR, Rakha EA, Ellis IO, et al. Involvement of metformin and AMPK in the radioresponse and prognosis of luminal versus basal-like breast cancer treated with radiotherapy. Oncotarget. 2014;**5**(24):12936-12949. Available from: http://www.oncotarget.com/fulltext/2683

[35] Rao M, Gao C, Guo M, Law BYK, Xu Y. Effects of metformin treatment on radiotherapy efficacy in patients with cancer and diabetes: A systematic review and meta-analysis. Cancer Management and Research. 2018;**10**: 4881-4890. Available from: https://www.dovepress.com/effects-of-metformin-treatment-on-radiotherapy-efficacy-in-patients-wi-peer-reviewed-article-CMAR

[36] Skinner HD, Sandulache VC, Ow TJ, Meyn RE, Yordy JS, Beadle BM, et al. TP53 disruptive mutations lead to head and neck cancer treatment failure through inhibition of radiation-induced senescence. Clinical Cancer Research. 2012;**18**(1):290-300

[37] Fasih A, Elbaz HA, Hüttemann M, Konski AA, Zielske SP. Radiosensitization of pancreatic cancer cells by metformin through the AMPK pathway. Radiation Research. 2014; **182**(1):50-59. Available from: http://www.bioone.org/doi/10.1667/RR13568.1

[38] Chang PH, Yeh KY, Wang CH, Chen EYC, Yang SW, Chou WC, et al. Impact of metformin on patients with advanced head and neck cancer undergoing concurrent chemoradiotherapy. Head & Neck. 2017;**39**(8):1573-1577

[39] Bodmer M, Meier C, Krahenbuhl S, Jick SS, Meier CR. Long-term metformin use is associated with

decreased risk of breast cancer. Diabetes Care. 2010;**33**(6):1304-1308. Available from: http://care.diabetesjournals.org/cgi/doi/10.2337/dc09-1791

[40] Bosco JLF, Antonsen S, Sorensen HT, Pedersen L, Lash TL. Metformin and incident breast cancer among diabetic women: A population-based case-control study in Denmark. Cancer Epidemiology, Biomarkers & Prevention. 2011;**20**(1):101-111. Available from: http://cebp.aacrjournals.org/cgi/doi/10.1158/1055-9965.EPI-10-0817

[41] Campagnoli C, Pasanisi P, Abbà C, Ambroggio S, Biglia N, Brucato T, et al. Effect of different doses of metformin on serum testosterone and insulin in non-diabetic women with breast cancer: A randomized study. Clinical Breast Cancer. 2012;**12**(3):175-182. DOI: 10.1016/j.clbc.2012.03.004

[42] El-Haggar SM, El-Shitany NA, Mostafa MF, El-Bassiouny NA. Metformin may protect nondiabetic breast cancer women from metastasis. Clinical & Experimental Metastasis. 2016;**33**(4):339-357

[43] Goodwin PJ, Ligibel JA, Stambolic V. Metformin in breast cancer: Time for action. Journal of Clinical Oncology. 2009;**27**(20): 3271-3273. DOI: 10.1200/JCO.2009.22.1630

[44] Nanni O, Amadori D, De Censi A, Rocca A, Freschi A, Bologna A, et al. Metformin plus chemotherapy versus chemotherapy alone in the first-line treatment of HER2-negative metastatic breast cancer. The MYME randomized, phase 2 clinical trial. Breast Cancer Research and Treatment. 2019;**174**(2): 433-442. DOI: 10.1007/s10549-018-05070-2

[45] Jiralerspong S, Palla SL, Giordano SH, Meric-Bernstam F, Liedtke C, Barnett CM, et al. Metformin and pathologic complete responses to neoadjuvant chemotherapy in diabetic patients with breast cancer. Journal of Clinical Oncology. 2009;**27**(20): 3297-3302. Available from: http://ascopubs.org/doi/10.1200/JCO.2009.19.6410

[46] Niraula S, Dowling RJO, Ennis M, Chang MC, Done SJ, Hood N, et al. Metformin in early breast cancer: A prospective window of opportunity neoadjuvant study. Breast Cancer Research and Treatment. 2012;**135**(3): 821-830

[47] Hadad SM, Coates P, Jordan LB, Dowling RJO, Chang MC, Done SJ, et al. Evidence for biological effects of metformin in operable breast cancer: Biomarker analysis in a pre-operative window of opportunity randomized trial. Breast Cancer Research and Treatment. 2015;**150**(1):149-155

[48] Bonanni B, Puntoni M, Cazzaniga M, Pruneri G, Serrano D, Guerrieri-Gonzaga A, et al. Dual effect of metformin on breast cancer proliferation in a randomized presurgical trial. Journal of Clinical Oncology. 2012;**30**(21):2593-2600. Available from: http://ascopubs.org/doi/10.1200/JCO.2011.39.3769

[49] Bayraktar S, Hernadez-Aya LF, Lei X, Meric-Bernstam F, Litton JK, Hsu L, et al. Effect of metformin on survival outcomes in diabetic patients with triple receptor-negative breast cancer. Cancer. 2012;**118**(5):1202-1211. Available from: http://doi.wiley.com/10.1002/cncr.26439

[50] El-Benhawy SA, El-Sheredy HG. Metformin and survival in diabetic patients with breast cancer. The Journal of the Egyptian Public Health Association. 2014;**89**(3):148-153. Available from: http://content.wkhealth.com/linkback/openurl?sid=WKPTLP:landingpage&an=00004765-201412000-00007

[51] Hou G, Zhang S, Zhang X, Wang P, Hao X, Zhang J. Clinical pathological characteristics and prognostic analysis of 1,013 breast cancer patients with diabetes. Breast Cancer Research and Treatment. 2013;**137**(3): 807-816. Available from: http://link.springer.com/10.1007/s10549-012-2404-y

[52] Goodwin P, Pritchard K, Ennis M, Clemons M, Graham M, Fantus IG. Insulin-lowering effects of metformin in women with early breast cancer. Clinical Breast Cancer. 2008; **8**(6):501-505. DOI: 10.3816/CBC.2008.n.060

[53] He X, Esteva FJ, Ensor J, Hortobagyi GN, Lee MH, Yeung SCJ. Metformin and thiazolidinediones are associated with improved breast cancer-specific survival of diabetic women with HER2+ breast cancer. Annals of Oncology. 2012;**23**(7):1771-1780. Available from: https://academic.oup.com/annonc/article-lookup/doi/10.1093/annonc/mdr534

[54] Ferguson RD, Gallagher EJ, Cohen D, Tobin-Hess A, Alikhani N, Novosyadlyy R, et al. Hyperinsulinemia promotes metastasis to the lung in a mouse model of Her2-mediated breast cancer. Endocrine-Related Cancer. 2013; **20**(3):391-401. Available from: https://erc.bioscientifica.com/view/journals/erc/20/3/391.xml

[55] Rokkas T, Portincasa P. Colon neoplasia in patients with type 2 diabetes on metformin: A meta-analysis. European Journal of Internal Medicine. 2016;**33**:60-66. Available from: https://linkinghub.elsevier.com/retrieve/pii/S0953620516301431

[56] Hosono K, Endo H, Takahashi H, Sugiyama M, Sakai E, Uchiyama T, et al. Metformin suppresses colorectal aberrant crypt foci in a short-term clinical trial. Cancer Prevention Research. 2010;**3**(9):1077-1083

[57] Miranda VC, Braghiroli MI, Faria LD, Bariani G, Alex A, Bezerra Neto JE, et al. Phase 2 trial of metformin combined with 5-fluorouracil in patients with refractory metastatic colorectal cancer. Clinical Colorectal Cancer. 2016; **15**(4):321-328.e1. Available from: https://linkinghub.elsevier.com/retrieve/pii/S1533002816300597

[58] Garrett CR, Hassabo HM, Bhadkamkar NA, Wen S, Baladandayuthapani V, Kee BK, et al. Survival advantage observed with the use of metformin in patients with type II diabetes and colorectal cancer. British Journal of Cancer. 2012;**106**(8): 1374-1378. Available from: http://www.nature.com/articles/bjc201271

[59] Higurashi T, Hosono K, Takahashi H, Komiya Y, Umezawa S, Sakai E, et al. Metformin for chemoprevention of metachronous colorectal adenoma or polyps in post-polypectomy patients without diabetes: A multicentre double-blind, placebo-controlled, randomised phase 3 trial. The Lancet Oncology. 2016;**17**(4): 475-483. DOI: 10.1016/S1470-2045(15)00565-3

[60] Sivalingam VN, Kitson S, McVey R, Roberts C, Pemberton P, Gilmour K, et al. Measuring the biological effect of presurgical metformin treatment in endometrial cancer. British Journal of Cancer. 2016;**114**(3):281-289. DOI: 10.1038/bjc.2015.453

[61] Schuler KM, Rambally BS, Difurio MJ, Sampey BP, Gehrig PA, Makowski L, et al. Antiproliferative and metabolic effects of metformin in a preoperative window clinical trial for endometrial cancer. Cancer Medicine. 2015;**4**(2):161-173

[62] Laskov I, Drudi L, Beauchamp M-C, Yasmeen A, Ferenczy A, Pollak M, et al. Anti-diabetic doses of metformin decrease proliferation markers in tumors of patients with endometrial

cancer. Gynecologic Oncology. 2014; **134**(3):607-614. Available from: https://linkinghub.elsevier.com/retrieve/pii/S0090825814010543

[63] Mitsuhashi A, Sato Y, Kiyokawa T, Koshizaka M, Hanaoka H, Shozu M. Phase II study of medroxyprogesterone acetate plus metformin as a fertility-sparing treatment for atypical endometrial hyperplasia and endometrial cancer. Annals of Oncology. 2016;**27**(2):262-266. Available from: https://academic.oup.com/annonc/article-lookup/doi/10.1093/annonc/mdv539

[64] Ushijima K, Yahata H, Yoshikawa H, Konishi I, Yasugi T, Saito T, et al. Multicenter phase II study of fertility-sparing treatment with medroxyprogesterone acetate for endometrial carcinoma and atypical hyperplasia in young women. Journal of Clinical Oncology. 2007;**25**(19): 2798-2803. Available from: http://ascopubs.org/doi/10.1200/JCO.2006.08.8344

[65] Yates MS, Coletta AM, Zhang Q, Schmandt RE, Medepalli M, Nebgen D, et al. Prospective randomized biomarker study of metformin and lifestyle intervention for prevention in obese women at increased risk for endometrial cancer. Cancer Prevention Research. 2018;**11**(8):477-490. Available from: http://cancerpreventionresearch.aacrjournals.org/lookup/doi/10.1158/1940-6207.CAPR-17-0398

[66] Nevadunsky NS, Van Arsdale A, Strickler HD, Moadel A, Kaur G, Frimer M, et al. Metformin use and endometrial cancer survival. Gynecologic Oncology. 2014;**132**(1): 236-240. Available from: https://linkinghub.elsevier.com/retrieve/pii/S0090825813012754

[67] Ramos-Peñafiel C, Olarte-Carrillo I, Cerón-Maldonado R, Rozen-Fuller E, Kassack-Ipiña JJ, Meléndez-Mier G, et al. Effect of metformin on the survival of patients with ALL who express high levels of the ABCB1 drug resistance gene. Journal of Translational Medicine. 2018;**16**(1):245. DOI: 10.1186/s12967-018-1620-6

[68] Skinner HD, McCurdy MR, Echeverria AE, Lin SH, Welsh JW, O'Reilly MS, et al. Metformin use and improved response to therapy in esophageal adenocarcinoma. Acta Oncologica. 2013;**52**(5):1002-1009

[69] Leamm S, Lagarde SM, van Oijen MGH, Gisbertz SS, Wilmink JW, Hulshof MCCM, et al. Metformin use during treatment of potentially curable esophageal cancer patients is not associated with better outcomes. Annals of Surgical Oncology. 2015;**22**(S3): 766-771. Available from: http://link.springer.com/10.1245/s10434-015-4850-3

[70] Wright JL, Stanford JL. Metformin use and prostate cancer in Caucasian men: Results from a population-based case-control study. Cancer Causes & Control. 2009;**20**(9):1617-1622. Available from: http://link.springer.com/10.1007/s10552-009-9407-y

[71] Azoulay L, Dell'Aniello S, Gagnon B, Pollak M, Suissa S. Metformin and the incidence of prostate cancer in patients with type 2 diabetes. Cancer Epidemiology, Biomarkers & Prevention. 2011;**20**(2):337-344. Available from: http://cebp.aacrjournals.org/cgi/doi/10.1158/1055-9965.EPI-10-0940

[72] He XX, Tu SM, Lee MH, Yeung S-CJ. Thiazolidinediones and metformin associated with improved survival of diabetic prostate cancer patients. Annals of Oncology. 2011;**22**(12):2640-2645. Available from: https://academic.oup.com/annonc/article-lookup/doi/10.1093/annonc/mdr020

[73] Feng T, Sun X, Howard LE, Vidal AC, Gaines AR, Moreira DM, et al. Metformin use and risk of prostate cancer: Results from the REDUCE study. Cancer Prevention Research. 2015;**8**(11):1055-1060. Available from: http://cancerpreventionresearch.aacrjournals.org/cgi/doi/10.1158/1940-6207.CAPR-15-0141

[74] Rothermundt C, Hayoz S, Templeton AJ, Winterhalder R, Strebel RT, Bärtschi D, et al. Metformin in chemotherapy-naive castration-resistant prostate cancer: A multicenter phase 2 trial (SAKK 08/09). European Urology. 2014;**66**(3):468-474. Available from: https://linkinghub.elsevier.com/retrieve/pii/S0302283813014826

[75] Joshua AM, Zannella VE, Downes MR, Bowes B, Hersey K, Koritzinsky M, et al. A pilot 'window of opportunity' neoadjuvant study of metformin in localised prostate cancer. Prostate Cancer and Prostatic Diseases. 2014;**17**(3):252-258. DOI: 10.1038/pcan.2014.20

[76] Nguyen MM, Martinez JA, Hsu CH, Sokoloff M, Krouse RS, Gibson BA, et al. Bioactivity and prostate tissue distribution of metformin in a preprostatectomy prostate cancer cohort. European Journal of Cancer Prevention. 2018;**27**(6):557-562

[77] Rieken M, Kluth LA, Xylinas E, Fajkovic H, Becker A, Karakiewicz PI, et al. Association of diabetes mellitus and metformin use with biochemical recurrence in patients treated with radical prostatectomy for prostate cancer. World Journal of Urology. 2014;**32**(4):999-1005. Available from: http://link.springer.com/10.1007/s00345-013-1171-7

[78] Spratt DE, Zhang C, Zumsteg ZS, Pei X, Zhang Z, Zelefsky MJ. Metformin and prostate cancer: Reduced development of castration-resistant disease and prostate cancer mortality. European Urology. 2013;**63**(4):709-716. Available from: https://linkinghub.elsevier.com/retrieve/pii/S0302283812014728

[79] Janjetovic K, Vucicevic L, Misirkic M, Vilimanovich U, Tovilovic G, Zogovic N, et al. Metformin reduces cisplatin-mediated apoptotic death of cancer cells through AMPK-independent activation of Akt. European Journal of Pharmacology. 2011;**651**(1–3):41-50. Available from: https://linkinghub.elsevier.com/retrieve/pii/S001429991001126X

[80] Solano ME, Sander V, Wald MR, Motta AB. Dehydroepiandrosterone and metformin regulate proliferation of murine T lymphocytes. Clinical and Experimental Immunology. 2008;**153**(2):289-296. Available from: http://doi.wiley.com/10.1111/j.1365-2249.2008.03696.x

[81] Hirsch HA, Iliopoulos D, Tsichlis PN, Struhl K. Metformin selectively targets cancer stem cells, and acts together with chemotherapy to block tumor growth and prolong remission. Cancer Research. 2009;**69**(19):7507-7511. Available from: http://cancerres.aacrjournals.org/cgi/doi/10.1158/0008-5472.CAN-09-2994

[82] Zhu P, Davis M, Blackwelder AJ, Bachman N, Liu B, Edgerton S, et al. Metformin selectively targets tumor-initiating cells in ErbB2-overexpressing breast cancer models. Cancer Prevention Research. 2014;**7**(2):199-210. Available from: http://cancerpreventionresearch.aacrjournals.org/cgi/doi/10.1158/1940-6207.CAPR-13-0181

[83] Zhang Y, Guan M, Zheng Z, Zhang Q, Gao F, Xue Y. Effects of metformin on CD133+ colorectal cancer cells in diabetic patients. PLoS One. 2013;**8**(11):e81264. Available from:

https://dx.plos.org/10.1371/journal.pone.0081264

[84] Mohammed A, Janakiram NB, Brewer M, Ritchie RL, Marya A, Lightfoot S, et al. Antidiabetic drug metformin prevents progression of pancreatic cancer by targeting in part cancer stem cells and mTOR signaling. Translational Oncology. 2013;**6**(6):649-IN7. Available from: https://linkinghub.elsevier.com/retrieve/pii/S1936523313800046

[85] Montales MTE, Simmen RCM, Ferreira ES, Neves VA, Simmen FA. Metformin and soybean-derived bioactive molecules attenuate the expansion of stem cell-like epithelial subpopulation and confer apoptotic sensitivity in human colon cancer cells. Genes and Nutrition. 2015;**10**(6):49. Available from: http://link.springer.com/10.1007/s12263-015-0499-6

[86] Kuo SZ, Honda CO, Li WT, Honda TK, Kim E, Altuna X, et al. Metformin results in diametrically opposed effects by targeting non-stem cancer cells but protecting cancer stem cells in head and neck squamous cell carcinoma. International Journal of Molecular Sciences. 2019;**20**(1):193. Available from: https://www.mdpi.com/1422-0067/20/1/193

[87] Imamura K, Ogura T, Kishimoto A, Kaminishi M, Esumi H. Cell cycle regulation via p53 phosphorylation by a 5′-AMP activated protein kinase activator, 5-aminoimidazole-4-carboxamide-1-β–ribofuranoside, in a human hepatocellular carcinoma cell line. Biochemical and Biophysical Research Communications. 2001;**287**(2):562-567. Available from: https://linkinghub.elsevier.com/retrieve/pii/S0006291X0195627X

[88] Jones RG, Plas DR, Kubek S, Buzzai M, Mu J, Xu Y, et al. AMP-activated protein kinase induces a p53-dependent metabolic checkpoint. Molecular Cell. 2005;**18**(3):283-293. Available from: https://linkinghub.elsevier.com/retrieve/pii/S1097276505012207

[89] Zhou J, Huang W, Tao R, Ibaragi S, Lan F, Ido Y, et al. Inactivation of AMPK alters gene expression and promotes growth of prostate cancer cells. Oncogene. 2009;**28**(18):1993-2002. Available from: http://www.nature.com/articles/onc200963

Chapter 9

Metformin in Cervical Cancer: Metabolic Reprogramming

Malgorzata Tyszka-Czochara and Marcin Majka

Abstract

The reprogrammed metabolism plays a crucial role in intensively proliferating tumor cells to meet high energetic demands and adapt to metastasis and invasion. Metformin may counteract flexible metabolic phenotype of cervical cancer cells by restraining aerobic glycolysis (*Warburg effect*) and promoting mitochondrial-based metabolism. Metformin inhibits master oncogene c-Myc as well as hypoxia-inducible factor 1 (HIF-1α) and suppresses its downstream glycolytic regulatory enzymes and glucose transporters. Metformin targets bioenergetics of cervical cancer cells with aggressive phenotype and regulates the expression of enzymes controlling tricarboxylic acid cycle (TCA cycle) supplementation with substrates, glucose, and glutamine. The exposition of cervical tumor cells to Metformin alleviates their migratory capacity, restrains epithelial-to-mesenchymal transition (EMT) program implementation, and elucidates oxidative stress, which results in massive cell death due to apoptosis. The metabolic alterations caused by Metformin are specific to cancer cells. In summary, Metformin exerts antitumor effect in cervical cancer cells by regulating specific molecular targets in reprogrammed metabolism. Metformin selectively modulates metabolic pathways and thus may be potentially used in new precisely targeted therapeutic strategies for cervical cancer.

Keywords: Metformin, cancer, metabolism, metabolic reprogramming, *Warburg effect*, mitochondria, apoptosis, oncogenes, reactive oxygen species, epithelial-mesenchymal transition, targeted anticancer therapy

1. Introduction

The malignant transformation results in a specific rearrangement of metabolic processes called metabolic reprogramming of tumor cell. The altered metabolism causes a selective advantage to a transformed cell by facilitating its survival in a harsh environment and promoting the spread of tumor cells within the body.

Malignant cells very effectively adapt to high proliferation rate, metastasis, and invasion. Several molecular mechanisms were pointed out to drive such metabolic adaptation of cancer cells. The critical aspects of metabolic reprogramming in tumor cells substantially contribute to the *Warburg effect* [1], an increased catabolism of glucose to lactate in the presence of oxygen [2]. The altered metabolism of tumors results in elevated biosynthesis of macromolecules such as proteins, carbohydrates, and lipids and, in consequence, supports high proliferation rate of malignant cells [3].

In particular, the regulation of mitochondrial processes in cancer cells differs from normal counterparts, and it may be specific to the stage of tumor [4]. Therefore, cancer cells are sensitive to drugs that disrupt energy homeostasis, such as Metformin (1,1-dimethylbiguanide, Met) [5].

A generic drug, Metformin, has been widely used for treatment of *diabetes mellitus* in humans. However, it exerts pleiotropic effect in human organism. In particular, a great interest has been paid to Met, since retrospective analyses demonstrated that it significantly decreased the relative risk of cancer incidence in diabetic patients when compared with patients treated with other drugs. Clinical trials confirmed the epidemiological observations that Met exerted anticancer effects in humans [6]. It has been established that Met inhibits proliferation of various neoplastic cell lines in vitro, including breast, prostatic, colon, gastric, and cervical cancers [7, 8]. Currently, there is an intense ongoing research focused on molecular mechanisms behind these effects, since the implications of Met action in tumor cell are not completely understood [9].

To date, several molecular mechanisms were reported to play critical role in anticancer activity of Met. In particular, it was established that Met may affect energy metabolism of cancer cells by inhibition of complex I of mitochondrial electron transport chain (ETC) in mitochondria, which results in adenosine-5′-triphosphate (ATP) depletion and remodeling of the network of biosynthetic processes within the cell [9]. Met may act as an anticancer drug through the activation of the main energy regulator within the cell, adenosine 5′-monophosphate (AMP)-activated protein kinase (AMPK) [7], and inhibition of mechanistic target of rapamycin complex-1 (mTORC1) [10] in tumor cells. Some of the pharmacological effects of Met seem to be independent of its action on glycemia homeostasis. Several reports demonstrated that treatment of tumor cells with Met results in cell cycle perturbations and apoptosis [11, 12]. The intracellular targets affected by Met were comprehensively reviewed by Ikhlas and Ahmad [9] and Pierotti et al. [13].

Along with the advent of human papillomavirus (HPV) vaccines, the primary prevention of cervical cancer has become more successful, but cervical malignancy still remains the significant cause of cancer mortality in women worldwide. Currently, chemotherapy using cytostatic drugs (mainly cisplatin, cis-dichlorodiammineplatinum (II)) is still the primal regimen, despite low specificity and substantial toxicity in patients [14].

Aerobic glycolysis has been recognized as the most common metabolic feature of malignant cells. The alterations in metabolism of cancer cells combined with the overexpression of oncogenes (c-Myc) and transcription factors (hypoxia-inducible factor 1a, HIF 1a) confer a great advantage to malignant cells to avoid apoptosis induced by reactive oxygen species (ROS). In this study we focused on the effects of Met on metabolism of metastatic cervical tumor cells. Based on recent data, we reported that Met inhibited glycolytic phenotype of aggressive cervical cancer cells by regulation of expression of oncogenes and their downstream proteins, which led to cellular death. Furthermore, Met regulated mitochondrial metabolism, especially via supplementation of tricarboxylic acid cycle (TCA cycle, Krebs cycle) with pyruvate and glutamine. Met, by targeting epithelial and mesenchymal markers of tumor cells, alleviated invasive properties of cervical cancer cells.

This review summarizes recent findings on Met and cervical cancer underscoring new implications of this drug in regulation of peculiar metabolism of tumor cells. We discuss new perspectives about targeting specific alterations in cervical tumor metabolic pathways using Met.

2. Metformin regulates metabolism of metastatic cervical cancer cells in vitro study

A growing evidence suggests that the screening for molecular targets for anticancer therapeutic treatments should take into account the existing differences in tumor cell phenotypes. Therefore, the metabolic effects exerted by Met were studied using SiHa cells (American Type Culture Collection, ATCC designation HTB-35) originating from aggressive cervical tumor, which acquired malignant characteristics [15]. The regulation of apoptosis pathways in HTB-35 (SiHa) cells highly reflects the specificity of cervical tumor in vivo [16]. HTB-35 cells, even unstimulated with cytokines, have mesenchymal-like characteristics, especially high vimentin expression, along with enhancement of cell scattering and ability to move [17]. Another cell line, C-4I cells (ATCC, designation CRL1594) with epithelial phenotype, was derived from primary in situ tumor [18]. HTB-34 cells (ATCC designation MS751) were isolated from metastatic site in lymph node [19]. HTB-35, C-4I and HTB-34 are human squamous cell cervical carcinoma lines and it is worth noting that squamous cell cancer is the most common cervical cancer and accounts for almost 80% of cervical carcinomas in patients [14]. HeLa human cervical cancer cells (ATCC designation CCL2), which have been extensively used in mechanistic studies, expressed epithelial traits and were derived from *adenocarcinoma* [8].

2.1 Metformin hampers the expression of oncogenes controlling glycolytic phenotype of cervical cancer cells under hypoxic and normoxic conditions and promotes apoptosis

The reliance on glucose supply is linked to the aggressiveness of malignant cells. Such reprogrammed metabolism makes migrating cancer cells more robust and independent of environmental conditions. The dysregulation of glucose metabolism is caused by alterations in functioning of several oncogenes. Malignant cells may gain metabolic plasticity by upregulation of only few oncogenes, such as c-Myc, p53, phosphoinositide 3-kinase (PI3K) and the mammalian target of rapamycin (mTOR) [20]. Additionally, the activation of transcription factors, such as HIF-1α, makes malignant cells more resistant to hypoxia (decreased oxygen level in microenvironment), which is one of the main factors affecting tumor growth [20]. The activation of HIF-1α is one of the crucial processes that promote glycolysis to generate ATP along with the decrease of mitochondrial pathways' activity in aggressive tumors. What is more, the migrating tumor cells may avoid oxidative stress by relying on glucose catabolism. As a result, tumor cells have higher chance to survive detachment from extracellular matrix (ECM), whereas normal cells undergo programmed death due to anoikis in the absence of attachment to ECM [21]. Following detachment from primary tumor bed and transportation to plasma and lymph, malignant cells may spread within the body and form secondary tumors. Therefore, the reprogrammed metabolism plays a crucial role in facilitating tumor metastasis.

We found that Met may regulate glycolysis in aggressive cervical cancer cells. The glycolytic phenotype of tumor cells is triggered mainly by a master regulator HIF-1α and its downstream proteins. Our study showed that Met alleviated the hypoxia-induced activation of HIF-1α, which was followed by decreased expression of HIF-1α downstream protein effectors in HTB-35 cells, as demonstrated in [22]. In particular, Met downregulated GLUT transporters (solute carrier family 2 member receptors, SLC2A), specifically GLUT1 and GLUT3. Additionally, Met inhibited the regulatory enzymes of the glycolytic pathway, hexokinase 2 (HK2), bifunctional enzyme 6-phosphofructo-2-kinase/fructose-2,6-biphosphatase 4 (PFKFB4), pyruvate kinase (PKM), and lactate dehydrogenase (LDH) (**Figure 1**). Met exerted greater effect on regulatory proteins in HTB-35 cells exposed to decreased oxygen level in the air than normal conditions.

Recent studies have reported that overexpression of c-Myc oncogene plays a significant role in the formation of cervical cancer. The enhanced expression of c-Myc is also of particular relevance to promoting invasive phenotype of cancer cells. What is more, the upregulated c-Myc may collaborate with HIF to effectively induce glucose and glutamine consumption in tumor cells. As a result, mitochondrial oxidative phosphorylation decreases. In particular, the upregulated c-Myc enhances glutamine catabolism in tumor cells, since the oncogene controls glutaminase (GLS) expression [23]. As measured using qPCR analysis, Met decreased *c-MYC* transcript level in HTB-35 cells [22], which was in compliance with inhibition of GLS protein expression [11]. The treatment of cervical tumor cells with Met decreased mRNA level for another c-Myc downstream protein, *CCND1* (cyclin D1), which regulates cell cycle progression [22]. Zhang et al. [24] reported that Met caused a substantial decrease of cyclin D1 expression in bladder cancer cells. The overexpression of oncogene cyclin D1 is positively correlated with chemotherapeutic resistance and apoptosis avoidance in squamous cell cancers [23]. The inhibition of *CCND1* expression in aggressive cervical tumor cells resulted in enhanced apoptosis [22].

Met triggered another pro-apoptotic mechanism in cervical carcinoma cells via regulation of Bcl-2 (B-cell lymphoma 2) protein family members' expression [22]. Bcl-2 proteins are key players in the regulation of mitochondrial-dependent programmed cell death. The activation of BAX protein leads to disruption of mitochondrial membrane potential and apoptosis, whereas Bcl-2 acts as an apoptotic suppressor. The counterbalancing pro- and anti-apoptotic effectors of Bcl-2 protein family play a crucial role in the regulation of the mitochondrial apoptotic cascade within the cell and constitute another important apoptotic checkpoint [25]. However, the disturbance of BAX/Bcl-2 pathway may result in the resistance to apoptosis by inducing compensatory mechanisms, thereby influencing the efficacy of some therapeutic regimens [26]. The exposition of cervical tumor cells to Met

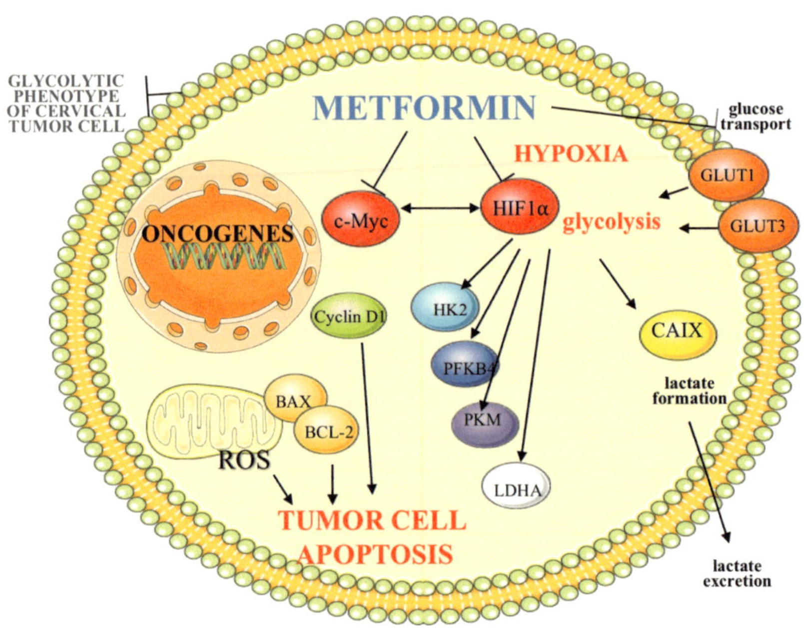

Figure 1.
Metformin inhibits glycolytic phenotype of cervical carcinoma cells (↑—activation, ⊢—inhibition) [11, 12, 21, 22].

significantly upregulated *BAX* transcript. It was found that the expression of *BAX* under hypoxic conditions was greater than in normoxia [22]. Additionally, Met downregulated transcript for *BCL-2* in HTB-35 cells in both, normoxic and hypoxic conditions.

The study using cervical cancer cells with metastatic phenotype cells showed that the downregulation of oncogenes/downstream regulatory proteins, together with the upregulation of pro-apoptotic BAX/Bcl-2, elucidated mitochondrial-dependent apoptosis in tumor cells. The obtained data suggest that Met was highly effective in facilitating cell death in cervical tumor cells [22], since it exerted its effect targeting independent events controlling mitochondrial apoptosis including the induction of ROS [11], the regulation of Bcl-2 protein family expression, and downregulation of cyclin D1. It should be emphasized that Met induced cell death solely in tumor cells, without causing detrimental effects to normal cells [11].

2.2 Metformin regulates TCA cycle supplementation in cervical cancer cells via pyruvate dehydrogenase (PDH) complex and generates oxidative stress in mitochondria

The reprogrammed metabolism of tumor cells not only meets high energetic demands but also provides intermediates for intensive proliferation. Therefore, glycolysis and mitochondrial oxidative phosphorylation may operate simultaneously in cancer cells. Many tumors may even switch between these pathways accordingly to the current requirements. Recent studies showed that most cancer cells have metabolically efficient mitochondria to provide intermediates for biosynthesis, generate reductive power (nicotinamide adenine dinucleotide phosphate, NADPH), and restore cofactor pool (e.g., nicotinamide adenine dinucleotide, NADH). In highly proliferating cancer cells, mitochondrial TCA cycle is active enough to sustain the biochemical reactions. Currently, the precise regulation of anabolic pathways and keeping their activities at adequate level is thought to play a key role in determination of "flexible" metabolic phenotype of cancer cells that enables their rapid division. Moreover, oxidative phosphorylation (OXPHOS) may represent a significant contribution to energy generation within malignant cell. On the other hand, inevitable products of OXPHOS are ROS and oxidative stress due to ROS overproduction may kill tumor cells [27].

It was demonstrated that the process of detachment of migrating squamous cancer cells from extracellular matrix (ECM) results in reprogramed metabolism toward glycolysis, particularly by PDH complex inhibition and following suppression of glucose respiration in mitochondria. Such metabolic phenotype of tumor cell enables efficient production of energy without excessive ROS generation. On the other hand, the stimulation of PDH activity may lead to increased anoikis sensitivity and attenuation of metastatic potential of cancer cells [28].

We found that Met may precisely regulate PDH metabolic checkpoint in cervical tumor cells (**Figure 2**). Met had great potency to activate oxidative decarboxylation of pyruvate to acetyl-CoA in HTB-35 cells expressing invasive phenotype, and it occurred via activation of PDH complex [11]. PDH complex plays a determinant role in the overall glucose disposal within the cell, since it funnels mitochondrial TCA cycle instead of lactate formation in cytosol. PDH activity is precisely regulated via covalent modification by the action of specific enzyme pyruvate dehydrogenase kinase (PDK). Several PDK activators were found to expand potent antitumor effect, also in cervical tumor HeLa cells [29]. We showed in aggressive cervical cancer HTB-35 cells that Met suppressed both PDK activity and the expression of gene encoding tumor-specific isoenzyme PDK1 [22]. This finding may have practical implications, since the screening strategy for PDK inhibitors should

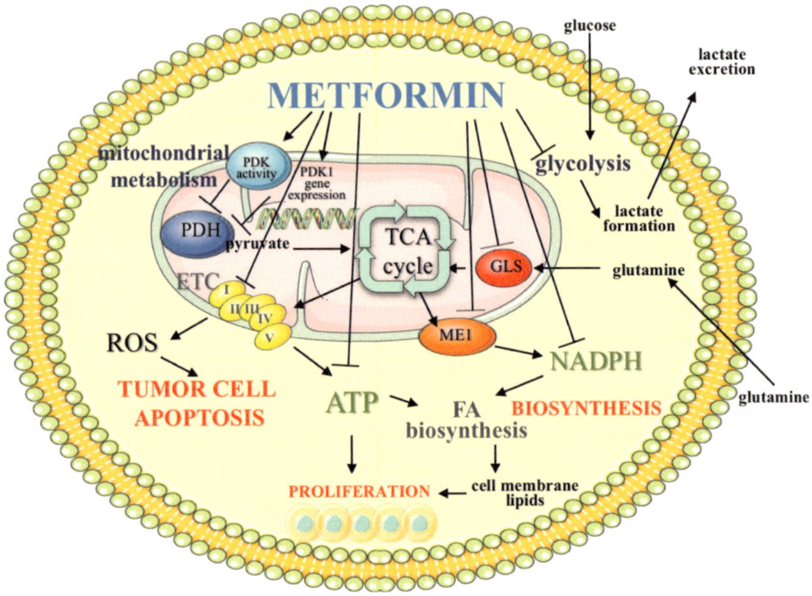

Figure 2.
Metformin regulates mitochondrial metabolism of cervical carcinoma cells (↑—activation, ⊢—inhibition) [11, 13, 22, 27, 30].

recognize the specificity among the PDK isoenzymes in order to avoid side effects in vivo [30]. Under hypoxic conditions inside tumors, the activation of HIF-1α decreases mitochondrial metabolism, which prevents the cell from oxidative stress and helps cancer cells avoid apoptosis [20, 23]. Our study showed that in aggressive cervical cancer cells Met counteracted these metabolic alterations by inhibiting PDK1, which is at the same time HIF-1α prime downstream effector. Furthermore, Met downregulated PDK1 gene expression also in normoxia [22].

In tumor cells that have functional mitochondria, the generation of oxidative stress may become an important therapeutic target [27, 30]. The imbalance of metabolic regulation and the resulting overproduction of ROS in mitochondrial ETC cause oxidative stress, which, at some point, becomes toxic to cancer cells, and that escalation of ROS elicits apoptosis-inducing factors and triggers death program through multiple mechanisms. In compliance, it has been newly reported that Met significantly increased ROS level, altered apoptosis-associated signaling, and induced cell death in human gastric adenocarcinoma cells [31] and human cervical cancer HeLa cells [32]. We found that in HTB-35 cervical cancer cells, Met caused excessive generation of mitochondrial ROS and elicited apoptosis [11, 22]. As shown in [22], the effect of Met was specific to tumor cells, and the formation of mitochondrial ROS was not affected in normal cells exposed to Met.

Met concomitantly targeted cytosolic glycolysis and mitochondrial pathways in HTB-35 cells, which increased apoptosis and suppressed survival of cervical tumor cells under normoxic and hypoxic conditions [22].

2.3 Met restrains glutamine entry into TCA cycle and inhibits cervical tumor cell proliferation

Glutamine may provide precursors to feed TCA cycle under limited flux of pyruvate from cytosolic glycolysis within tumor cells. The facilitated use of glutamine is a significant metabolic adaptation of cancer cell, besides enhanced glucose catabolism, and it provides intermediates sufficient for intensive biosynthesis and energy production [20]. Glutaminase (GLS) is a key regulator of glutamine entry to TCA [33], and the inhibition of the enzyme may suppress tumor cell growth [25].

As shown in [11], the exposition of cervical cancer cells with invasive phenotype to Met downregulated the expression of GLS, thereby protecting mitochondrial anabolism from additional carbon supply for synthesis of macromolecules. Additionally, the effect of Met on GLS expression was specific toward cervical cancer cells, and in normal cells drug did not change the expression of the enzyme [11].

Glutamine entry to tumor cell not only improves carbon supply for macromolecules buildup, but it also replenishes the pool of cellular NADPH, since the conversion of malate to pyruvate catalyzed by malic enzyme 1 (ME1) is accompanied by the reduction of $NADP^+$ (**Figure 2**). NADPH is used for biosynthesis, but it also plays a significant role in the antioxidant protection of tumor cell by reducing glutathione molecule. Met downregulated expression of ME1 and alleviated generation of NADPH in cells, which, in conditions of limited supplementation of HTB-35 cells with glucose (suppressed expression of GLUTs), resulted in hampering of biosynthesis and alleviation of ROS detoxification [11, 22].

Furthermore, Met treatment caused acute drop in ATP concentration in HTB-35 cells. This is in compliance with data obtained by Parker et al. [34] who demonstrated that non-small cell lung cancer (NSCLC) cells may be uniquely sensitized to metabolic stresses by the action of other biguanide, phenformin (1-(diaminomethylidene)-2-(2-phenylethyl)guanidine). The inhibition of ATP generation may block biosynthesis in cervical tumor cells which results in restraining of cell proliferation.

2.4 Alterations of fatty acid (FA) de novo synthesis in cervical tumor cells upon exposition to Metformin affect cell proliferation

The facilitated fatty acid (FA) de novo synthesis together with upregulated glycolysis was recognized as one of the prime metabolic alterations in such tumor cells [35]. The enhanced FA biosynthesis meets high demands of rapidly proliferating malignant cells (generating components for cell membranes and signaling molecules). We found that Met decreased unsaturated lipid content in aggressive cervical cancer cells (**Figure 2**). The mechanism of Met action included downregulation of regulatory enzyme elongase 6 (ELOVL6), which catalyzes elongation of fatty acid molecule. Met also suppressed stearoyl-CoA desaturase (SCD1), which controls desaturation of FA. It was shown by Fritz et al. [36] that pharmacologic inhibition of SCD1 activity impaired unsaturated FA synthesis, which resulted in decreased proliferation of both androgen-sensitive and androgen-resistant prostate cancer cells. The treatment of cervical cancer cell lines [22, 37] with Met decreased cervical tumor cell proliferation, but Met did not affect the growth of normal cells [11].

2.5 Metformin inhibits epithelial-to-mesenchymal transition (EMT) process and migration properties of cervical cancer cells

Emerging data indicate that the enhanced activity of enzymes regulating lipid de novo synthesis may contribute to activation of EMT process in tumor cells [36]. The activation of EMT program in epithelial cancer cells facilitates tumor progression, invasion, and metastasis. It has been shown in independent studies that Met inhibits EMT in various cancer cell lines [8, 37]. Recently, it has been reported that Met reversed EMT phenotype induced with *transforming growth factor beta 1* (TGF-β1) in breast, lung, and cervical cancer cells by targeting the mechanisms regulating the expression of E-cadherin. The exposition of tumor cells to Met resulted in suppression of their metastatic properties [8, 38].

In our study, EMT process was induced upon 48 h incubation of cervical cancer cells with 10 ng/mL of cytokine TGF-β1, as described in detail in [17]. HTB-35 cells, even unstimulated, expressed mesenchymal-like characteristics, and the incubation with TGF-β further enforced expression of mesenchymal marker, vimentin, along with enhancement of cell scattering and ability to move [17]. The study showed that Met was an effective suppressor of mesenchymal phenotype and, in particular, downregulated vimentin in HTB-35 cells (**Figure 3**). Recently, it was reported by Laskov et al. [39] that Met downregulated the expression of vimentin in endometrial cancers in vitro and in vivo in diabetic patients. The incubation of cervical cancer cell lines with Met reduced cells' ability to move, as shown using functional scratch test in C4-I and HTB-35 cells stimulated with TGF-β1 [17]. Mechanistic study revealed that Met inhibited the expression of transcription factors Snail-1, ZEB-1, and Twist-1. These mesenchymal markers facilitate EMT progress in cervical cancer cells.

Cheng and Hao [8] proposed another mechanism of Met action in cervical carcinoma cells via inhibition of mTOR/p70s6k signaling pathway and downregulation of glycolytic regulatory protein pyruvate kinase, isozyme M2 (PKM2), in HeLa cell line.

In order to clarify the molecular action of Met in cervical tumor cells with aggressive characteristics, the effect of the drug was tested in the hypoxic conditions. In cervical cancers, hypoxia and concomitant enhanced lactate formation result in acidification of microenvironment, which may promote the ability of metastatic cells to rapidly spread in tissue [41]. In such conditions, the activation of HIF1α induces its downstream protein carbonic anhydrase IX (CAIX). By regulation of tumor milieu pH, CAIX acts as a survival factor protecting malignant cells

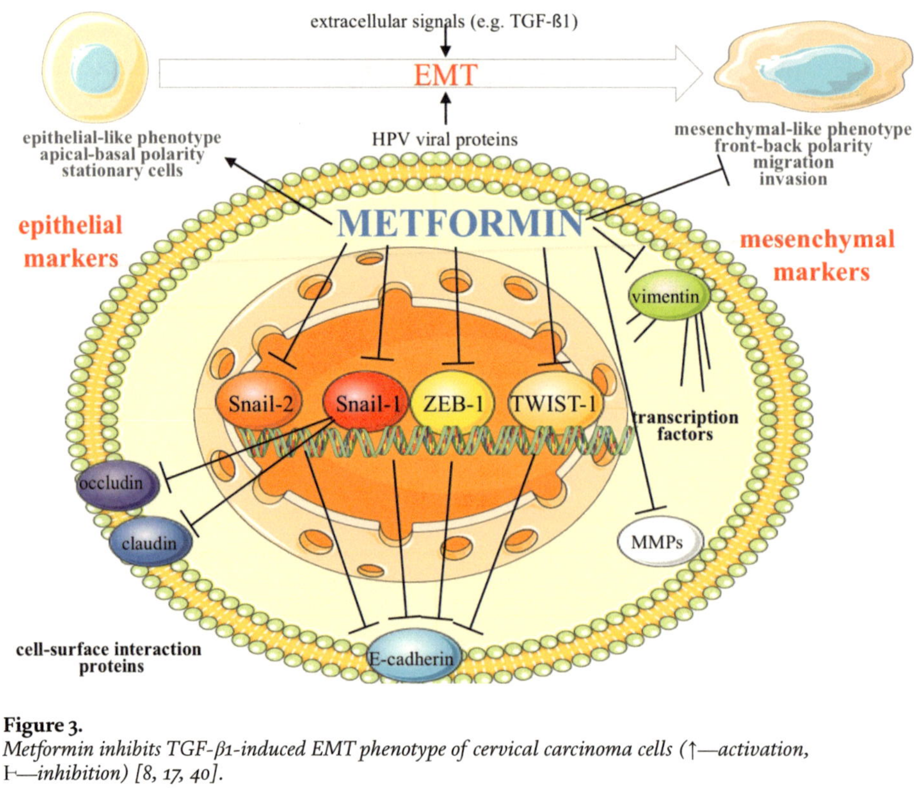

Figure 3.
Metformin inhibits TGF-β1-induced EMT phenotype of cervical carcinoma cells (↑—activation, ⊢—inhibition) [8, 17, 40].

against enhanced acidification of microenvironment. As a result, lactate damages adjacent normal cells and does not harm tumor cells [42]. Due to its relevant role in cell invasion, CAIX was proposed as a potential therapeutic target, also in cervical cancers [41, 42]. We showed that the exposition of HTB-35 cells to Met under hypoxia suppressed HIF-1α, which resulted in decreased transcription of *CAIX* gene, thereby alleviating invasive properties of cervical malignant cells [17].

3. In vivo findings related to the effect of Metformin

Recently, numerous beneficial activities of Met were reported. Met was shown to improve cardiovascular outcomes in humans [43], and the ability of Met to extend life-span in mammals has attracted great attention [44]. Emerging data indicate that Met may be applied as adjuvant in therapies aiming at combating diseases with high mortality rate, also in cervical cancer [45]. The clinical benefits of the use of Met in gynecologic oncology in humans were reviewed by Irie et al. [46] and Imai et al. [47]. Met also reduced the incidence of endometrial tumors and improved survival of patients with diagnosed local or advanced endometrial cancer [48]. Several clinical trials showed the potential of Met to elicit apoptosis in the uterus and prostate cancers in humans [49].

The potential pathological effects of Met have been well studied in long term in human population. One of the most undesirable effects in the context of peculiar metabolic alterations of cancer cell is the enhanced generation of lactic acid caused by biguanides. In fact, the application of phenformin (1-(diaminomethylidene)-2-(2-phenylethyl)guanidine) was associated with a much higher risk of lactic acidosis in patients, than Metformin. Therefore, the former drug was withdrawn from clinical use. Currently, the contraindication for the use of Met in patients is renal failure, since this group has greater risk of lactic acidosis. However, the concerns over lactic acidosis were shown to be largely unfounded, unless kidney disease was advanced. Yet, based on the recent data, Met can be safely used in patients with mild renal dysfunction, provided that patients are monitored appropriately [43, 50].

4. Conclusions

The exposition of aggressive cervical cancer cells to Met restrained the function of HIF-1α master regulator and downregulated HIF-1α downstream glycolytic genes. Met also downregulated glycolytic phenotype of HTB-35 cells through inhibition of oncogene *c-MYC* expression, which resulted in impairment of metabolic plasticity of cervical tumor cells, especially via downregulation of GLS.

Met precisely regulated PDH and GLS metabolic checkpoints in cervical tumor cells. In particular, in tumor cells Met targeted supplementation of mitochondrial pathways in pyruvate by downregulation of PDK1 gene expression and decreasing PDK activity. As a result, Met effectively enhanced TCA cycle flux in normoxic and hypoxic conditions. The downregulation of GLS and ME1 resulted in decreased regeneration of NADPH, the factor essential both for biosynthesis and cell protection against oxidative stress. The metabolic alterations of mitochondrial pathways caused by Met caused excessive generation of ROS which led to apoptosis. In cervical cancer cells, Met additionally induced apoptosis via upregulation of pro-apoptotic BAX protein expression and by downregulation of cyclin D1, oncogene *c-MYC* downstream protein. Met exerted its pro-apoptotic effect both in normal and decreased oxygen availability. This aspect of Met action may be important when designing anticancer therapies targeting cells in hypoxic milieu inside solid tumors.

It is also important to highlight another cellular mechanism of Met action, namely, the suppression of EMT process in cervical tumor cells. EMT seems implicated into invasiveness and metastasis of cancer, and Met was able to inhibit EMT pathways. In cervical tumor cells stimulated with TGF-β1 as well as in unstimulated ones, Met decreased the expression of the main mesenchymal marker vimentin and reduced motility of cells. In addition, Met downregulated adaptive enzyme *CAIX* in tumor cells under hypoxia. CAIX promoted migration of malignant cells and acted as an important survival factor, and thus it has recently been proposed as therapeutic target in cervical cancers. Met might be considered as a potential factor targeting CAIX to hamper cervical tumor invasiveness.

These findings provide a new insight into regulation of glycolysis and mitochondrial pathways in cervical tumor cells using nontoxic and well-studied drug, Metformin, indicating the future prospect about utilization of this molecule in clinical oncological routine. The identification and targeting of specific alterations in tumor metabolic pathways may constitute a sole basis to design new precise therapeutic strategies in cervical malignancy. To date, very few innovative therapies against cervical malignancy are being tested in clinical trials; thus more specific and effective intervention is highly required.

The artworks were prepared using elements from Servier Medical Art.

Author details

Malgorzata Tyszka-Czochara[1*] and Marcin Majka[2*]

1 Department of Food Chemistry and Nutrition, Faculty of Pharmacy, Jagiellonian University Medical College, Krakow, Poland

2 Department of Transplantation, Faculty of Medicine, Jagiellonian University Medical College, Krakow, Poland

*Address all correspondence to: malgorzata.tyszka-czochara@uj.edu.pl and mmajka@cm-uj.krakow.pl

References

[1] Liberti MV, Locasale JW. The Warburg effect: How does it benefit cancer cells? Trends in Biochemical Sciences. 2016;**41**:211-218. DOI: 10.1016/j.tibs.2015.12.001

[2] Wilde L, Roche M, Domingo-Vidal M, Tanson K, Philp N, Curry J, et al. Metabolic coupling and the reverse Warburg effect in cancer: Implications for novel biomarker and anticancer agent development. Seminars in Oncology. 2017;**44**:198-203. DOI: 10.1053/j.seminoncol.2017.10.004

[3] Cairns RA, Harris IS, Mak TW. Regulation of cancer cell metabolism. Nature Reviews. Cancer. 2011;**11**:85-95

[4] Rodríguez-Enríquez S, Carreño-Fuentes L, Gallardo-Pérez JC, Saavedra E, Quezada H, Vega A, et al. Oxidative phosphorylation is impaired by prolonged hypoxia in breast and possibly in cervix carcinoma. The International Journal of Biochemistry & Cell Biology. 2010;**42**:1744-1751

[5] Bost F, Decoux-Poullot A, Tanti J, Clavel S. Energy disruptors: Rising stars in anticancer therapy? Oncogene. 2016;**5**:1-8

[6] Kim HJ, Lee S, Chun KH, Jeon JY, Han SJ, Kim DJ, et al. Metformin reduces the risk of cancer in patients with type 2 diabetes: An analysis based on the Korean National Diabetes Program Cohort. Medicine (Baltimore). 2018;**97**:e0036

[7] Lin SC, Hardie DGAMPK. Sensing glucose as well as cellular energy status. Cell Metabolism. 2018;**27**:299-313. DOI: 10.1016/j.cmet.2017.10.009

[8] Cheng K, Hao M. Metformin inhibits TGF-β1-induced epithelial-to-mesenchymal transition via PKM2 relative-mTOR/p70s6k signaling pathway in cervical carcinoma cells. International Journal of Molecular Sciences. 2016;**17**:e2000. DOI: 10.3390/ijms17122000

[9] Ikhlas S, Metformin AM. Insights into its anticancer potential with special reference to AMPK dependent and independent pathways. Life Sciences. 2017;**185**:53-62

[10] Barrière G, Tartary M, Rigaud M. Metformin: A rising star to fight the epithelial mesenchymal transition in oncology. Anti-Cancer Agents in Medicinal Chemistry. 2013;**13**:333-340

[11] Tyszka-Czochara M, Bukowska-Strakova K, Majka M. Metformin and caffeic acid regulate metabolic reprogramming in human cervical carcinoma SiHa/HTB-35 cells and augment anticancer activity of cisplatin via cell cycle regulation. Food and Chemical Toxicology. 2017;**106**:260-272

[12] Sacco F, Calderone A, Castagnoli L, Cesareni G. The cell-autonomous mechanisms underlying the activity of metformin as an anticancer drug. British Journal of Cancer. 2016;**115**:1451-1456

[13] Pierotti MA, Berrino F, Gariboldi M, Melani C, Mogavero A, Negri T, et al. Targeting metabolism for cancer treatment and prevention: Metformin, an old drug with multi-faceted effects. Oncogene. 2013;**32**:1475-1487. DOI: 10.1038/onc.2012.181

[14] Small W Jr, Baco MA, Bajaj A, et al. Cervical cancer: A global health crisis. Cancer. 2017;**123**:2404-2412

[15] Miekus K, Pawlowska M, Sekuła M, Drabik G, Madeja Z, Adamek D, et al. MET receptor is a potential therapeutic target in high grade cervical cancer. Oncotarget. 2015;**12**:10086-10101

[16] Carlson MW, Iyer VR, Marcotte EM. Quantitative gene expression assessment identifies appropriate cell line models for individual cervical cancer pathways. BMC Genomics. 2007;**10**:2-13

[17] Tyszka-Czochara M, Lasota M, Majka M. Caffeic acid and Metformin inhibit invasive phenotype induced by TGF-β1 in C-4I and HTB-35/SiHa human cervical squamous carcinoma cells by acting on different molecular targets. International Journal of Molecular Sciences. 2018;**19**:e266

[18] Auersperg N. Histogenetic behavior of tumors. I. Morphologic variation in vitro and in vivo of two related human carcinoma cell lines. Journal of the National Cancer Institute. 1969;**43**:151-173

[19] Available from: https://www.lgcstandards-atcc.org

[20] Pavlova NN, Thompson CB. The emerging hallmarks of cancer metabolism. Cell Metabolism. 2016;**23**:27-47

[21] Paoli P, Giannoni E, Chiarugi P. Anoikis molecular pathways and its role in cancer progression. Biochimica et Biophysica Acta. 1833;**2013**:3481-3498

[22] Tyszka-Czochara M, Bukowska-Strakova K, Kocemba-Pilarczyk KA, Majka M. Caffeic acid targets AMPK signaling and regulates tricarboxylic acid cycle anaplerosis while Metformin downregulates HIF-1α-induced glycolytic enzymes in human cervical squamous cell carcinoma lines. Nutrients. 2018;**10**:pii: E841

[23] Dang CVA. Time for MYC: Metabolism and therapy. Cold Spring Harbor Symposia on Quantitative Biology. 2016;**81**:79-83. DOI: 10.1101/sqb.2016.81.031153

[24] Zhang JW, Zhao F, Sun Q. Metformin synergizes with rapamycin to inhibit the growth of pancreatic cancer in vitro and in vivo. Oncology Letters. 2018;**15**:1811-1816

[25] Green DR, Galluzzi L, Kroemer G. Cell biology. Metabolic control of cell death. Science. 2014;**345**:1250256

[26] Indran IR, Tufo G, Pervaiz S, Brenner C. Recent advances in apoptosis, mitochondria and drug resistance in cancer cells. Biochimica et Biophysica Acta. 1807;**2011**:735-745A

[27] Zhao Y, Butler EB, Tan M. Targeting cellular metabolism to improve cancer therapeutics. Cell Death & Disease. 2013;**4**:e532

[28] Kamarajugadda L, Stemboroski Q, Cai NE, Simpson S, Nayak M, Tan JL. Glucose oxidation modulates anoikis and tumor metastasis. Molecular and Cellular Biology. 2012;**32**:1893-1907

[29] Choi YW, Lim IK. Sensitization of metformin-cytotoxicity by dichloroacetate via reprogramming glucose metabolism in cancer cells. Cancer Letters. 2014;**346**:300-308

[30] Luengo A, Gui DY, Vander Heiden MG. Targeting metabolism for cancer therapy. Cell Chemical Biology. 2017;**24**:1161-1180. DOI: 10.1016/j.chembiol.2017.08.028

[31] Lu CC, Chiang JH, Tsai FJ, Hsu YM, Juan YN, Yang JS, et al. Metformin triggers the intrinsic apoptotic response in human AGS gastric adenocarcinoma cells by activating AMPK and suppressing mTOR/AKT signaling. International Journal of Oncology. 2019;**54**;1271-1281. DOI: 10.3892/ijo.2019.4704

[32] Tang ZY, Sheng MJ, Qi YX, Wang LY, He DY. Metformin enhances inhibitive effects of carboplatin on HeLa cell proliferation and increases sensitivity to carboplatin by activating mitochondrial associated apoptosis

signaling pathway. European Review for Medical and Pharmacological Sciences. 2018;**22**:8104-8112

[33] Li Y, Erickson JW, Stalnecker CA, Katt WP, Huang Q, Cerione RA, et al. Mechanistic basis of glutaminase activation: A key enzyme that promotes glutamine metabolism in cancer cells. The Journal of Biological Chemistry. 2016;**291**:20900-20910

[34] Parker SJ, Svensson RU, Divakaruni AS, Lefebvre AE, Murphy AN, Shaw RJ, et al. LKB1 promotes metabolic flexibility in response to energy stress. Metabolic Engineering. 2017;**43**(Pt B):208-217

[35] Currie A, Schulze A, Zechner R, Walther TC, Farese R Jr. Cellular fatty acid metabolism and cancer. Cell Metabolism. 2013;**18**:153-161

[36] Fritz V, Benfodda Z, Rodier G, Henriquet C, Iborra F, Avancès C, et al. Abrogation of de novo lipogenesis by stearoyl-CoA desaturase 1 inhibition interferes with oncogenic signaling and blocks prostate cancer progression in mice. Molecular Cancer Therapeutics. 2010;**9**:1740-1754

[37] Tyszka-Czochara M, Konieczny P, Majka M. Caffeic acid expands anti-tumor effect of metformin in human metastatic cervical carcinoma HTB-34 cells: Implications of AMPK activation and impairment of fatty acids de novo biosynthesis. International Journal of Molecular Sciences. 2017;**18**:E462

[38] Koeck S, Amann A, Huber JM, Gamerith G, Hilbe W, Zwierzina H. The impact of Metformin and salinomycin on transforming growth factor β-induced epithelial-to-mesenchymal transition in non-small cell lung cancer cell lines. Oncology Letters. 2016;**11**:2946-2952

[39] Laskov I, Abou-Nader P, Amin O, Philip CA, Beauchamp MC, Yasmeen A, et al. Metformin increases E-cadherin in tumors of diabetic patients with endometrial cancer and suppresses epithelial-mesenchymal transition in endometrial cancer cell lines. International Journal of Gynecological Cancer. 2016;**26**:1213-1221

[40] Lee MY, Shen MR. Epithelial-mesenchymal transition in cervical carcinoma. American Journal of Translational Research. 2012;**4**:1-13

[41] Svastova E, Pastorekova S. Carbonic anhydrase IX: A hypoxia-controlled "catalyst" of cell migration. Cell Adhesion & Migration. 2013;**7**:226-231

[42] Pastorek J, Pastorekova S. Hypoxia-induced carbonic anhydrase IX as a target for cancer therapy: From biology to clinical use. Seminars in Cancer Biology. 2015;**31**:52-64

[43] Lipska KJ, Flory JH, Hennessy S, Inzucchi SE. Citizen petition to the US Food and Drug Administration to change prescribing guidelines: The Metformin experience. Circulation. 2016;**134**:1405-1408

[44] Martin-Montalvo A, Mercken EM, Mitchell SJ, Palacios HH, Mote PL, Scheibye-Knudsen M, et al. Metformin improves healthspan and lifespan in mice. Nature Communications. 2013;**4**:2192

[45] Uehara T, Mitsuhashi A, Tsuruoka N, Shozu M. Metformin potentiates the anticancer effects of cisplatin under normoxic conditions in vitro. Oncology Reports. 2015;**33**:744-750. DOI: 10.3892/or.2014.3611

[46] Irie H, Banno K, Yanokura M, Iida M, Adachi M, Nakamura K, et al. Metformin: A candidate for the treatment of gynecological tumors based on drug repositioning. Oncology Letters. 2016;**11**:1287-1293

[47] Imai A, Ichigo S, Matsunami K, Takagi H, Yasuda K. Clinical benefits

of Metformin in gynecologic oncology. Oncology Letters. 2015;**10**:577-582

[48] Tang YL, Zhu LY, Li Y, Yu J, Wang J, Zeng XX, et al. Metformin use is associated with reduced incidence and improved survival of endometrial cancer: A meta-analysis. BioMed Research International. 2017;**2017**:5905384. DOI: 10.1155/2017/5905384

[49] Vancura A, Bu P, Bhagwat M, Zeng J, Vancurova I. Metformin as an anticancer agent. Trends in Pharmacological Sciences. 2018;**39**:867-878. DOI: 10.1016/j.tips.2018.07.006

[50] Imam TH. Changes in metformin use in chronic kidney disease. Clinical Kidney Journal. 2017;**10**:301-304

Chapter 10

Antitumoral Effects of Metformin in Ovarian Cancer

Maritza P. Garrido, Margarita Vega and Carmen Romero

Abstract

In the last years, the antidiabetic drug metformin has received considerable attention in pursuing new drugs for anticancer treatments. Several reports have shown that metformin would have antitumor effects, not only attributable to its systemic effects but also due to direct effects on tumor cells. It has been proposed that metformin could be a suitable alternative for the treatment of gynecological cancers, such as ovarian cancer. This disease is characterized by high cell proliferation and angiogenesis potential, because ovarian cancer cells overexpress most oncogenic molecules including growth factors. The aim of the present chapter is to discuss the molecular mechanism by which metformin would affect tumor cells, with focus on epithelial ovarian cancer.

Keywords: metformin, ovarian cancer, cell proliferation, angiogenesis, growth factors, AMPK

1. Introduction

Metformin or 1,1-dimethylbiguanide is a derivate of isoamylene guanidine, a substance found in the plant *Galega officinalis* [1]. This drug is widely used in metabolic disorders as type 2 diabetes mellitus, metabolic syndrome, and gestational diabetes [2, 3]. Besides, metformin is used as a treatment for polycystic ovarian syndrome [4], which is characterized by the dysfunction of reproductive tissues such as the ovary and endometrium. In this context, metformin improves ovarian follicle dynamics and frequency of ovulation [5, 6], and it increases the expression of endometrial GLUT4 (insulin-regulated glucose transporter), which may improve endometrial physiology in these patients [7].

In the last decades, metformin has been studied in the context of cancer, especially after an initial report by Evans et al., performed with a Scottish database, who found that metformin intake reduces the risk of cancer in type 2 diabetic patients [8].

Type 2 diabetes and obesity affect a significant percentage of the world population [9, 10] whose food habits and lifestyle have been changing in the last decades. Both obesity and type 2 diabetes are pathologies associated with increased incidence and poor prognosis of ovarian cancer by several authors [11–13]. These observations could be explained because obesity and type 2 diabetes are characterized by molecular changes that could encourage tumoral transformation and progression, such as hyperinsulinemia, hyperglycemia, dyslipidemia, increased insulin-like growth factors (IGF), adipose tissue factors, and inflammatory components [14–19].

IntechOpen

By its chemical nature, metformin gets into the cell through organic cation transporters (OCTs) and multidrug and toxin extrusion transporters [20]. Because metformin cannot be metabolized, almost its entirety is excreted by the kidneys; the plasmatic levels of this drug do not reflect its intracellular concentration, mainly by its high apparent volume of distribution and prolonged half-life [21, 22]. Therefore, metformin is accumulated in tissues, and its plasmatic concentration is probably lower than of organs that express OCT transporters. This observation supports most *in vitro* studies that use high concentrations of metformin to study its antitumoral properties. Importantly, these transporters are present in the ovary [23, 24], so ovarian cancer cells could be a target for metformin action.

2. Indirect antitumoral effects of metformin in cancer

It is discussed that metformin could display direct and indirect antitumoral effects. The systemic effects of this drug include the decrease of blood glucose and insulin levels by action in its classical target organs: liver, muscle, and fat tissues. In humans, metformin decreases the hepatic gluconeogenesis and the release of glucose from hepatic reserves, which produces an increase in the peripheral uptake of glucose and its metabolism, decreasing patients' hyperglycemia and hyperinsulinemia [1, 2, 25]. These conditions (hyperglycemia and hyperinsulinemia) favor tumoral growth and are associated with cancer incidence, by two possible mechanisms: (1) high availability of glucose for cancer cells and (2) high levels of insulin, which could act in insulin-like growth factor (IGF) receptors [14–16]. IGF/IGF receptors display an important role in the ovary, because 100% of the ovarian carcinomas express IGF receptors [26].

In fat tissue, metformin decreases the activity of lipogenic enzymes such as HMG-CoA reductase, acetyl-CoA carboxylase (ACC), and fatty acid synthase, decreasing the endogen production of cholesterol and the fatty acid synthesis [1, 27, 28]. This produces a decrease in the plasma levels of lipids in patients using metformin [29–32], which in addition to metformin-hypoglycemic properties, decreases the readiness of energy substrates of tumoral cells.

All these metformin-mediated changes impair survival and mitogenic signaling and decrease nutrient availability for ovarian cancer cells.

3. Effects of metformin in ovarian cancer

3.1 Direct effects of metformin in ovarian cancer cells: role of AMPK

Several studies have shown that metformin displays direct antitumoral effects. Most of these studies have been performed in ovarian cancer cell lines, where metformin impairs cell proliferation, migration, and angiogenesis potential and enhances the chemotherapy sensibility [33–36].

The direct antitumoral effects of metformin are commanded by metabolic changes in cancer cells. Because metformin is a drug with pleiotropic effects, several molecular targets at different levels of the tumoral cell have been described. One of the most studied targets for metformin is the adenosine monophosphate-activated protein kinase (AMPK), a key sensor of the energetic status of the cell [37], and it was described that metformin treatment can activate AMPK in *in vitro* and *in vivo* experiments of ovarian cancer models [33, 38]. The activation of AMPK occurs by increasing the AMP/ATP ratio [39] which exposes the activation loop of AMPK to be phosphorylated in the residue threonine 172 by serine/threonine kinases such as liver kinase B1 (LKB1) [40]. Activated AMPK phosphorylates several proteins; the phosphorylation can either activate or repress protein function at the cellular level [41, 42]. Despite that an important part of the studies indicates that the antitumoral effect of metformin could be AMPK-dependent; in the absence of AMPK, metformin preserves most of its antitumoral effects [43], indicating that the mechanism of this drug is more complex.

3.2 Antiproliferative mechanism of metformin in ovarian cancer cells

One of the characteristic hallmarks of cancer cells is an increased cell proliferation. To do so, ovarian cancer cells overexpress several growth factors and its receptors, which produce an enhanced cell signaling related with survival and proliferation in these cells [44–46].

In ovarian cancer, growth factors can activate protein kinase B (AKT) and the extracellular signal-regulated kinase (ERK) signaling pathways, among others [47–49]. These signaling pathways are associated with an increase of cell proliferation in most kinds of cancer cells [50, 51]. Some studies have shown that metformin treatment decreases IGF-1 and insulin levels, in a mice model with ovarian cancer [51], and also metformin treatment blocks the pro-tumoral effects of the nerve growth factor (NGF) in epithelial ovarian cancer cells [35] or the insulin/IGF-I signaling in uterine serous carcinoma [52].

The activation by growth factors of AKT and ERK signaling in ovarian cancer cells induces the activation of mechanistic target of rapamycin complex 1 (mTORC1), which controls protein translation and cell growth [53–55]. It is described that metformin-activated AMPK inhibits mTORC1 signaling in ovarian cancer cells [56, 57], which could impair its cell potential to proliferate and fend it in unfavorable conditions. Additionally, one key point in the antitumoral effect of metformin is that AMPK decreases the signaling pathways mediated by AKT and ERK in several types of cells, including cancer cells [38, 57, 58]. These signaling pathways are associated with the increase of most oncoproteins, for example, the transcription factor c-MYC and the inhibitory apoptotic protein survivin (BIRC5) [59–62]. c-MYC is a proto-oncogene that controls several genes related with cell growth and cell proliferation, and some reports show that metformin decreases c-MYC protein levels in ovarian cancer cell lines [63, 64]. In addition, metformin decreases the mRNA levels of survivin in metastatic ovarian cancer cells [65].

According to current evidences, c-MYC controls the transcription and cell cycle inhibitors [66]. In agreement with the metformin-depending decrease of c-MYC in ovarian cancer cells, metformin induces the degradation of cyclin D1 [33, 38], a protein required for progression from G1 to S phase of the cell cycle, and increases p21 expression (a negative regulator of cell cycle) [67]. These results are consistent with experiments performed in primary ovarian cancer cell cultures and ovarian cancer cell lines, which show that metformin induces cell cycle arrest in the G0/G1 phase and decreases the percentage of cells in S phase of the cellular cycle [35, 68, 69]. These findings highly suggest that metformin decreases the progression of the cell cycle in ovarian cancer cells.

Even more, several authors have shown that metformin can elicit cytostatic or cytotoxic effects in ovarian cancer cells. A key point for a better understanding of these differences is that metformin inhibits tumor cell proliferation in the presence of glucose (with a cytostatic effect) but induces apoptosis in low-glucose conditions [70]. For example, ovarian cancer cells are more sensitive to metformin at concentrations of 2.5 millimolar than in 25 millimolar of glucose (found in culture conditions). This is a consequence of reactive oxygen species accumulation, which increase cell apoptosis and endoplasmic reticulum stress and decrease of c-MYC protein levels [63, 70].

3.3 Effect of metformin in lipid metabolism of ovarian cancer cells

For cell proliferation, the cancer cell has high requirements of substrates for synthesis of structural components and signaling. One target of AMPK is the sterol regulatory element-binding protein 1 (SREBP1), a lipogenic transcription factor [71], which increases cellular biosynthesis of fatty acids and cholesterol by transcription of the enzymes ACC, HMG-CoA reductase, and fatty acid synthase [72], not only in fat tissue but also in ovarian cancer cells [73]. Because ACC is involved in the taxol-mediated cytotoxic effect of ovarian cancer cells [74], besides the fact that the inhibition of ACC suppresses ovarian cancer cell growth *in vivo* and *in vitro* [75], it is possible to conclude that ACC inhibition could contribute to an important part of the antitumoral effects of metformin.

3.4 Anti-angiogenic activity of metformin in ovarian cancer

Angiogenesis, defined as the generation of new blood vessels from preexisting ones [76], is an essential process to supply oxygen and nutrients to normal and tumoral ovarian cells. Unfortunately, this process is exacerbated in ovarian cancer cells, which overexpress some growth factors, such as vascular endothelial growth factor (VEGF) or NGF [77, 78] which promotes angiogenesis.

The relevance of metformin in the vascular context is recognized; however, its action depends on the cell type, metabolic status, and nutrient availability. For example, some pro-angiogenic properties have been attributed to metformin under hypoxia and hyperglycemia, similar characteristics to myocardial infarction in diabetic patients. In this context, metformin enhances endothelial cell survival, migration, and apoptosis inhibition [79, 80]; this strongly suggests that the use of metformin could be beneficial in the context of cardiovascular diseases in diabetic patients. On the other hand, metformin could have an opposite effect in endothelial cells under hypoglycemic conditions (as tumor endothelial cells), where metformin produces an inhibition of its cell proliferation and angiogenesis potential, as will be discussed later.

In the ovary, the correct formation and regression of blood vessels during each ovarian cycle is indispensable for proper follicular development, ovulation, and corpus luteum formation, so that angiogenesis displays a key role in ovarian homeostasis and pathogenesis [81]. In patients with polycystic ovary syndrome, an increased expression of VEGF is described, and it is hypothesized that part of the beneficial metformin-associated effects will be mediated by a decrease or normalization of its VEGF levels. For example, it is described that in a rat model with dehydroepiandrosterone-induced polycystic ovaries, metformin administration restores the ovarian-increased levels of VEGF and angiopoietin 1, both angiogenic factors [82]. In addition, women with polycystic ovarian syndrome who take metformin have decreased their levels of plasmatic endothelin 1 and plasminogen activator inhibitor-1 [83, 84], molecules that also promote angiogenesis.

The angioprotection is an antitumoral mechanism that has been explored in ovarian cancer. Considering that the most studied angiogenic factor is VEGF, a monoclonal antibody against VEGF called bevacizumab has been developed and was approved for the use in advanced stages of ovarian cancer [85, 86]. In ovarian cancer models, the main knowledge of anti-angiogenic characteristics of metformin comes from VEGF modulation. Several *in vitro* models have shown that metformin decreases both VEGF mRNA and protein levels in ovarian cancer cell lines and then, its angiogenic potential [33, 64]. In a mice model with ovarian cancer, metformin decreases VEGF levels in plasma and ascitic fluid, with a consistent decrease of the ovarian tumor growth [51]. Interestingly, metformin reduces the vascular density (showed by CD31 staining) of ovarian cancer xenografts in mice, and metformin-/cisplatin-treated mice have significantly less vascular density than either metformin or cisplatin alone [33]. Because cisplatin/carboplatin and paclitaxel are drugs used in the first-line chemotherapy in ovarian cancer [87, 88], these results suggest that metformin could potentiate the anti-angiogenic effects of chemotherapy during ovarian cancer treatment.

On the other hand, metformin treatment (in millimolar concentrations) displays direct effects in the endothelial cells, by reducing cell proliferation in human umbilical vein endothelial cells (HUVEC) and endothelial progenitor cells [89, 90]. Similar results were replicated by our group where metformin decreases cell proliferation of the endothelial cell line EA.hy926, in a dose-dependent manner [35], as well as, the endothelial cell differentiation (**Figure 1**). These results suggest that metformin affects in a direct manner the angiogenesis potential of endothelial cells.

3.5 Posttranscriptional regulation by metformin in ovarian cancer cells

In the ovarian cell, posttranscriptional regulations control gene expression at RNA level [91]. The micro-RNAs (miRs) are short non-codificant RNAs that regulate the expression of approximately 60% of protein-coding genes of the human genome [92]. miRs bind to a messenger RNA target, producing its degradation or translational repression depending of complementary degree [93]. The machinery for expression, processing, and exportation of miRs depends on several proteins as RNAse III DICER and exportins [93]. It is described that DICER downregulation is an oncogenic event that enhances epithelial-mesenchymal transition (EMT) and metastatic dissemination in cancer cells [94]. An important antecedent is that metformin elicits anticancer effects through the sequential modulation of DICER and c-MYC in breast cancer cells, increasing oncosuppressor miRs [95]. These mechanisms have not been investigated in ovarian cancer cells; nevertheless, preliminary results from our group show that metformin increases the oncosuppressor miRs 23-b and miR-145 in the epithelial ovarian cells [96].

As already mentioned in point 3.3, the activation of AMPK by metformin produces an inhibitory phosphorylation of acetyl-CoA carboxylase, an enzyme that regulates lipid metabolism. Importantly, intermediaries of lipid metabolism participate in cell signaling and chromatin structure, modulating processes as cell histone acetylation that depends on cytosolic acetyl-CoA [97]. The decrease of the

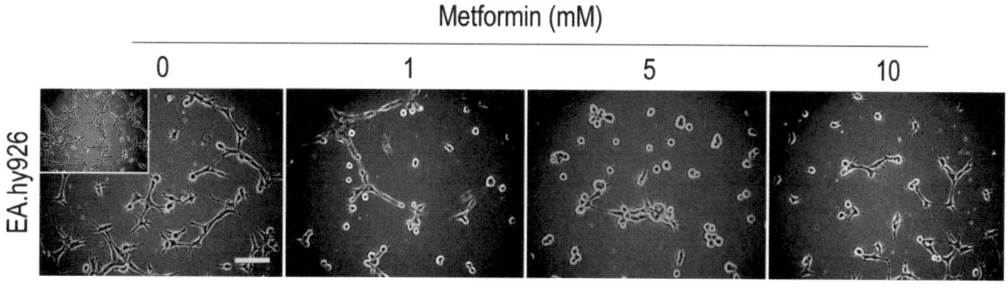

Figure 1.
Effect of metformin on the differentiation of endothelial cells. Metformin reduces the multicellular junctions and polygonal structures of endothelial cells EA.hy926 in a matrigel assay (4 h). Upper insert: positive control (NGF 100 ng/ml). Magnification bar: 50 μm.

conversion of acetyl-CoA to malonyl-CoA leads to an increase in the acetylation of histones in the chromatin and altered gene expression in ovarian cancer cells [67]. Because acetylation of nucleosomal histones is linked to nuclear processes as transcription, replication, and repair among other functions [98], it is possible that several antitumoral effects of metformin could be regulated by protein acetylation and transcriptional regulation of several oncosuppressor proteins.

The summary of the main studied antitumoral effects of metformin is shown in **Figure 2**.

3.6 Studies of metformin in diabetic patients with ovarian cancer

A recent meta-analysis shows that among available studies of relationship between metformin intake with ovarian cancer incidence and prognosis in diabetic patients, the majority of the studies indicate a negative correlation between the use of metformin and the incidence of ovarian cancer, as well as, a positive correlation with better prognosis [99]. The same study shows that metformin treatment in diabetic patients has a reduction of 24% risk of ovarian cancer occurrence and also a 42% of reduction in mortality [99]. The main studies that showed metformin benefits in the context of ovarian cancer diabetic patients are summarized in **Table 1**.

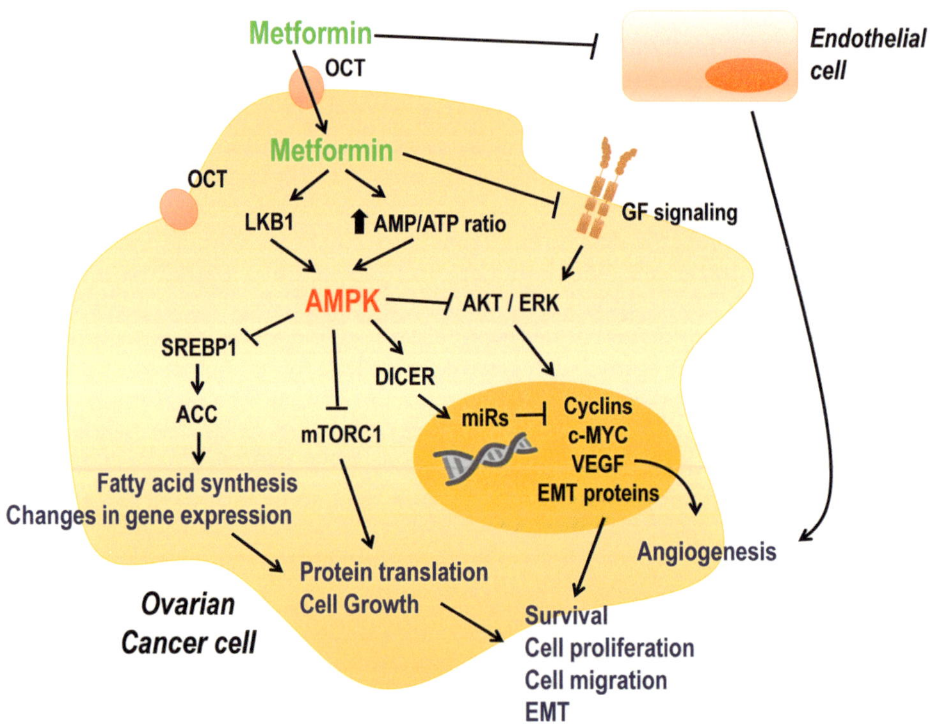

Figure 2.

Main antitumoral mechanism of metformin in ovarian cancer cells. Metformin enters the cell through organic cationic transporters (OCT) and produces the activation of liver kinase B1 (LKB1) and an increase of AMP/ATP ratio, which results in the activation of AMPK. This kinase has several targets as sterol regulatory element-binding protein 1 (SREBP) and acetyl-CoA carboxylase (ACC); the mechanistic target of rapamycin complex 1 (mTORC1) and AKT/ERK signaling; key proteins in the fatty acid synthesis and cell growth, survival, proliferation, and migration; and the processes of epithelial-mesenchymal transition (EMT). On the other hand, metformin can block the growth factor (GF) signaling dependent or independent of AMPK activation. Also metformin decreases the angiogenic potential of ovarian cancer cells, impairs the expression of vascular endothelial growth factor (VEGF), or acts directly on the endothelial cells.

Research	Study and population	Main finding
Wang et al. [12]	Retrospective cohort study N = 568, China	• Metformin group of OvCa patients had longer median PFS* than non-metformin, nondiabetic, and metformin-discontinued groups • Similar PFS* in dose (500 or 1000 mg of metformin) • Metformin treatment must be continuous to obtain beneficial effects
Bar et al. [114]	Retrospective cohort study N = 143, Israel	• Metformin was associated with a reduced risk of recurrence of OvCa (lower PFS*), and this association was stronger in diabetic patients
Tseng et al. [115]	Retrospective cohort study N = 479,475, China	• 601 metformin ever-users and 2600 never-users developed OvCa (incidence of 49.4 and 146.4 per 100,000 person-years) • Metformin use was associated with a decreased risk of OvCa
Kumar et al. [116]	Case-control study 72 cases (OvCa, metformin users), 142 controls (OvCa, non-metformin) USA	• Metformin was associated with a better survival in OvCa patients • 5-year DSS** was higher in metformin group • Metformin was an independent predictor of survival
Romero et al. [102]	Retrospective cohort study N = 341, USA	• Metformin group had a longer PFS* and overall survival of OvCa compared to nonusers or nondiabetic patients • Metformin group decreased hazard for disease recurrence
Bodmer et al. [117]	Case-control study 1611 cases (OvCa) and 9170 controls (non-OvCa), UK	Metformin use was associated with a decreased of risk of OvCa

**PFS: progression-free survival (length of time during and after the treatment of OvCa that a patient lives with the disease but it does not get worse).*
***DSS: disease-specific survival (percentage of people in a study or treatment group who have not died from OvCa in a defined period of time).*

Table 1.
Summary of studies that evaluated incidence and prognosis of ovarian cancer (OvCa) patients using and not using metformin.

Although several observational studies show positive effects of metformin in diabetic patients, it has not yet been elucidated if metformin could be beneficial in nondiabetic patients. In addition, ovarian cancer has a low incidence, and the number of participants in some of the available studies is low; therefore, the evidence should be interpreted with caution.

Because of the increased interest in the possible use of metformin in nondiabetic patients, there are currently six clinical trials inscribed in NIH ClinicalTrials.gov database to study metformin intake in association with carboplatin and paclitaxel (first-line chemotherapy) in nondiabetic woman with ovarian cancer (NCT02312661, NCT02437812, NCT03378297, NCT02122185, NCT01579812, and NCT02201381) from phase 0 to phase III of the study. The results of one of these trials show that metformin was well tolerated and the outcome results were favorable, because tumors from metformin-treated women have a threefold decrease in specific subpopulations of ovarian cancer stem cells with an increased sensitivity to cisplatin *in vitro* [100], supporting the use of metformin in the following phases of the study.

3.7 Role of metformin in metastasis and chemoresistance

Besides the abovementioned benefits, metformin treatment has a relevant role in the metastasis and chemoresistance prevention of several ovarian cancer models. For example, *in vitro* experiments have shown that metformin decreases the adhesion capacity, invasion, and migration of ovarian cancer cell lines [101]. In rodents, metformin treatment inhibits the growth of metastatic nodules in the lung product of ovarian cancer [33], and importantly, the use of metformin in diabetic women decreases the probability of disease recurrence [102].

The cancer stem cells, recently called "tumor-initiating cells," are a tumoral cell subpopulation with critical role in therapy resistance and metastasis [103–105]. There are several markers to identify them, as lactate dehydrogenase (LDH), aldehyde dehydrogenase (ALDH), or cell-surface antigens as CD44, CD133, or CD117 [106–108]. Metformin treatment decreases the abundance of ovarian cancer LDH+ and decreases its ability to form tumor spheres, an attachment-independent growth characteristic of these kinds of cells [109]. At the same time, a low dose of metformin (micromolar concentration) decreases the abundance of CD44+/CD117+ ovarian cancer cells selectively, whereas CD133+ or ALDH+ cell subpopulation were more sensitive to millimolar concentration of this drug [109, 110].

Another key point is that metformin decreases the expression of classical markers related with EMT. This process is necessary to confer an increased migratory capacity to tumor cells, participating in the intra-/extravasation and hence, in the tumor cell dissemination. In CD44+/CD117+ ovarian cancer cells, metformin treatment decreases snail2, twist, and vimentin protein levels (these are mesenchymal markers), increasing E-cadherin protein levels (a known epithelial marker) [110]. These observations are related with a study performed in diabetic patients with endometrial cancer, where in the biopsies of these patients using metformin were found increased levels of E-cadherin [111]. These findings suggest that metformin decreases the process of EMT in ovarian cancer cells, affecting preferentially tumor-initiating cells, which constitutes a relevant advantage, because this type of cells is not affected by traditional chemotherapy.

One important aspect in ovarian cancer treatment is the high percentage of chemoresistance developed by patients. In this context, metformin stands as a promising drug, since several studies showed that it could increase the susceptibility of ovarian cancer cells to chemotherapy and revert its acquired chemoresistance [34, 112, 113]. One recent study performed in ovarian cancer cell lines treated for 6 months with cisplatin and paclitaxel (for the acquirement of chemoresistance phenotype) shows that metformin treatment increases drug sensitivity and reduces migratory abilities of these ovarian cancer cells. In addition, the same study shows that metformin decrease the ovarian cancer stem cell population and the expression of specific biomarkers of pluripotent genes [112].

3.8 Main conclusions

Metformin is an antidiabetic drug that displays antitumoral effects in several *in vivo* and *in vitro* models of cancer, including ovarian cancer. The mechanism of its antitumoral effects could be either dependent or independent of AMPK, a key sensor of the cell energetic status. Metformin has several cell targets which include transcription factors and cell cycle regulators; wherewith it impairs cell proliferation by the arrest of the cell cycle. In addition, metformin modulates enzymes of metabolic pathways and lipid metabolism, as well as epigenetic and posttranscriptional regulation of the ovarian cancer cells, which can explain its pleiotropic actions. Another important point is that metformin regulates angiogenesis in the ovarian cancer cells, mainly decreasing VEGF expression, which impairs the angiogenic potential of these cells. On the other hand, metformin acts directly in endothelial cells, decreasing its proliferation, migration and differentiation, which complement its anti-angiogenic effect.

An important niche for metformin treatment could be its selective effect in ovarian cancer cells with stem cell phenotype, which are responsible for ovarian cancer dissemination and chemotherapy resistance. Several studies show that metformin reduces ovarian cancer stem cells abundance and that it could have a chemosensitivity role when used in combination with first-line chemotherapy agents. This opens the possibility to the potential use of metformin as a coadjuvant agent in ovarian cancer treatment.

Finally, there are several observational studies in diabetic women with ovarian cancer which show that metformin is associated with less ovarian cancer incidence and better prognosis. However, it is important to consider that the number of participants using metformin in some of these studies is low and that several *in vitro* experiments have shown that metformin action depends on the metabolic context and nutrient and oxygen availability of ovarian cancer cells. For these reasons, the use of metformin in nondiabetic women with ovarian cancer should be considered with caution.

Currently, there are several clinical trials performed in women with ovarian cancer. These trials are studying the effect of metformin treatment together with standard chemotherapy in the ovarian cancer prognosis and clinic-pathological markers, which could be helpful to elucidate whether this drug could be considered as a coadjuvant alternative in the treatment of ovarian cancer.

Acknowledgements

The authors would like to thank the National Fund for Scientific and Technological Development (FONDECYT) #1160139.

Conflict of interest

The authors declare no conflict of interest.

Appendices and nomenclature

ACC	acetyl-CoA carboxylase
AKT	activate protein kinase B
AMPK	adenosine monophosphate-activated protein kinase
ALDH	aldehyde dehydrogenase
EMT	epithelial-mesenchymal transition
ERK	extracellular signal-regulated kinase
HUVEC	human umbilical vein endothelial cells
IGF	insulin-like growth factor
LDH	lactate dehydrogenase
LKB1	liver kinase B1
mTORC1	mechanistic target of rapamycin complex 1
miRs	micro-RNAs
NGF	nerve growth factor
OCTs	organic cationic transporters
SREBP1	sterol regulatory element-binding protein 1
VEGF	vascular endothelial growth factor

Author details

Maritza P. Garrido, Margarita Vega and Carmen Romero*
Laboratory of Endocrinology and Reproduction Biology, Clinical Hospital University of Chile, Obstetrics and Gynecology Department, Faculty of Medicine, University of Chile, Santiago, Chile

*Address all correspondence to: cromero@hcuch.cl

References

[1] Rena G, Hardie DG, Pearson ER. The mechanisms of action of metformin. Diabetologia. 2017;**60**(9):1577-1585

[2] Scarpello JH, Howlett HC. Metformin therapy and clinical uses. Diabetes & Vascular Disease Research. 2008;**5**(3):157-167

[3] Kelley KW, Carroll DG, Meyer A. A review of current treatment strategies for gestational diabetes mellitus. Drugs Context. 2015;**4**:212282

[4] Mathur R, Alexander CJ, Yano J, Trivax B, Azziz R. Use of metformin in polycystic ovary syndrome. American Journal of Obstetrics and Gynecology. 2008;**199**(6):596-609

[5] Pirwany IR, Yates RW, Cameron IT, Fleming R. Effects of the insulin sensitizing drug metformin on ovarian function, follicular growth and ovulation rate in obese women with oligomenorrhoea. Human Reproduction. 1999;**14**(12):2963-2968

[6] Mahamed RR, Maganhin CC, Sasso GRS, de Jesus Simoes M, Baracat MCP, Baracat EC, et al. Metformin improves ovarian follicle dynamics by reducing theca cell proliferation and CYP-17 expression in an androgenized rat model. Journal of Ovarian Research. 2018;**11**(1):18

[7] Carvajal R, Rosas C, Kohan K, Gabler F, Vantman D, Romero C, et al. Metformin augments the levels of molecules that regulate the expression of the insulin-dependent glucose transporter GLUT4 in the endometria of hyperinsulinemic PCOS patients. Human Reproduction. 2013;**28**(8):2235-2244

[8] Evans JM, Donnelly LA, Emslie-Smith AM, Alessi DR, Morris AD. Metformin and reduced risk of cancer in diabetic patients. BMJ. 2005;**330**(7503):1304-1305

[9] NCD_Risk_Factor_Collaboration_ (NCD-RisC). Worldwide trends in body-mass index, underweight, overweight, and obesity from 1975 to 2016: A pooled analysis of 2416 population-based measurement studies in 128.9 million children, adolescents, and adults. Lancet. 2017;**390**(10113):2627-2642

[10] Unnikrishnan R, Pradeepa R, Joshi SR, Mohan V. Type 2 diabetes: Demystifying the global epidemic. Diabetes. 2017;**66**(6):1432-1442

[11] Beral V, Hermon C, Peto R, Reeves G, Brinton L, Marchbanks P, et al. Ovarian cancer and body size: Individual participant meta-analysis including 25,157 women with ovarian cancer from 47 epidemiological studies. PLoS Medicine. 2012;**9**(4):e1001200

[12] Wang SB, Lei KJ, Liu JP, Jia YM. Continuous use of metformin can improve survival in type 2 diabetic patients with ovarian cancer: A retrospective study. Medicine (Baltimore). 2017;**96**(29):e7605

[13] AkhavanS,Ghahghaei-NezamabadiA, Modaresgilani M, Mousavi AS, Sepidarkish M, Tehranian A, et al. Impact of diabetes mellitus on epithelial ovarian cancer survival. BMC Cancer. 2018;**18**(1):1246

[14] Perseghin G, Calori G, Lattuada G, Ragogna F, Dugnani E, Garancini MP, et al. Insulin resistance/hyperinsulinemia and cancer mortality: The Cremona study at the 15th year of follow-up. Acta Diabetologica. 2012;**49**(6):421-428

[15] Tsujimoto T, Kajio H, Sugiyama T. Association between hyperinsulinemia and increased risk of cancer death

in nonobese and obese people: A population-based observational study. International Journal of Cancer. 2017;**141**(1):102-111

[16] Ryu TY, Park J, Scherer PE. Hyperglycemia as a risk factor for cancer progression. Diabetes and Metabolism Journal. 2014;**38**(5):330-336

[17] Furstenberger G, Senn HJ. Insulin-like growth factors and cancer. The Lancet Oncology. 2002;**3**(5):298-302

[18] Duong MN, Geneste A, Fallone F, Li X, Dumontet C, Muller C. The fat and the bad: Mature adipocytes, key actors in tumour progression and resistance. Oncotarget. 2017;**8**(34):57622-57641

[19] Murata M. Inflammation and cancer. Environmental Health and Preventive Medicine. 2018;**23**(1):50

[20] Gong L, Goswami S, Giacomini KM, Altman RB, Klein TE. Metformin pathways: Pharmacokinetics and pharmacodynamics. Pharmacogenetics and Genomics. 2012;**22**(11):820-827

[21] Funk RS, Krise JP. Cationic amphiphilic drugs cause a marked expansion of apparent lysosomal volume: Implications for an intracellular distribution-based drug interaction. Molecular Pharmaceutics. 2012;**9**(5):1384-1395

[22] Wilcock C, Bailey CJ. Accumulation of metformin by tissues of the normal and diabetic mouse. Xenobiotica. 1994;**24**(1):49-57

[23] Andreev E, Brosseau N, Carmona E, Mes-Masson AM, Ramotar D. The human organic cation transporter OCT1 mediates high affinity uptake of the anticancer drug daunorubicin. Scientific Reports. 2016;**6**:20508

[24] Ota K, Ito K, Akahira J, Sato N, Onogawa T, Moriya T, et al. Expression of organic cation transporter SLC22A16 in human epithelial ovarian cancer: A possible role of the adriamycin importer. International Journal of Gynecological Pathology. 2007;**26**(3):334-340

[25] Bromage DI, Yellon DM. The pleiotropic effects of metformin: Time for prospective studies. Cardiovascular Diabetology. 2015;**14**:109

[26] Ouban A, Muraca P, Yeatman T, Coppola D. Expression and distribution of insulin-like growth factor-1 receptor in human carcinomas. Human Pathology. 2003;**34**(8):803-808

[27] Tokubuchi I, Tajiri Y, Iwata S, Hara K, Wada N, Hashinaga T, et al. Beneficial effects of metformin on energy metabolism and visceral fat volume through a possible mechanism of fatty acid oxidation in human subjects and rats. PLoS One. 2017;**12**(2):e0171293

[28] Sharma A, Bandyopadhayaya S, Chowdhury K, Sharma T, Maheshwari R, Das A, et al. Metformin exhibited anticancer activity by lowering cellular cholesterol content in breast cancer cells. PLoS One. 2019;**14**(1):e0209435

[29] Gregorio F, Ambrosi F, Manfrini S, Santucci A, Filipponi P. Meformin, plasma glucose and free fatty acids in type II diabetic out-patients: Results of a clinical study. Diabetes Research and Clinical Practice. 1997;**37**(1):21-33

[30] Castro Cabezas M, van Wijk JP, Elte JW, Klop B. Effects of metformin on the regulation of free fatty acids in insulin resistance: A double-blind, placebo-controlled study. Journal of Nutrition and Metabolism. 2012;**2012**:394623

[31] Pentikainen PJ, Voutilainen E, Aro A, Uusitupa M, Penttila I, Vapaatalo H. Cholesterol lowering effect of metformin in combined

hyperlipidemia: Placebo controlled double blind trial. Annals of Medicine. 1990;**22**(5):307-312

[32] Lin SH, Cheng PC, Tu ST, Hsu SR, Cheng YC, Liu YH. Effect of metformin monotherapy on serum lipid profile in statin-naive individuals with newly diagnosed type 2 diabetes mellitus: A cohort study. PeerJ. 2018;**6**:e4578

[33] Rattan R, Graham RP, Maguire JL, Giri S, Shridhar V. Metformin suppresses ovarian cancer growth and metastasis with enhancement of cisplatin cytotoxicity *in vivo*. Neoplasia. 2011;**13**(5):483-491

[34] Dos Santos Guimaraes I, Ladislau-Magescky T, Tessarollo NG, Dos Santos DZ, Gimba ERP, Sternberg C, et al. Chemosensitizing effects of metformin on cisplatin- and paclitaxel-resistant ovarian cancer cell lines. Pharmacological Reports. 2018;**70**(3):409-417

[35] Garrido MP, Vera C, Vega M, Quest AFG, Romero C. Metformin prevents nerve growth factor-dependent proliferative and proangiogenic effects in epithelial ovarian cancer cells and endothelial cells. Therapeutic Advances in Medical Oncology. 2018;**10**:1758835918770984

[36] Zheng Y, Zhu J, Zhang H, Liu Y, Sun H. Metformin inhibits ovarian cancer growth and migration *in vitro* and *in vivo* by enhancing cisplatin cytotoxicity. American Journal of Translational Research. 2018;**10**(10):3086-3098

[37] Hardie DG, Ross FA, Hawley SA. AMPK: A nutrient and energy sensor that maintains energy homeostasis. Nature Reviews. Molecular Cell Biology. 2012;**13**(4):251-262

[38] Gwak H, Kim Y, An H, Dhanasekaran DN, Song YS. Metformin induces degradation of cyclin D1 via AMPK/GSK3beta axis in ovarian cancer. Molecular Carcinogenesis. 2017;**56**(2):349-358

[39] Wheaton WW, Weinberg SE, Hamanaka RB, Soberanes S, Sullivan LB, Anso E, et al. Metformin inhibits mitochondrial complex I of cancer cells to reduce tumourigenesis. eLife. 2014;**3**:e02242

[40] Shaw RJ, Kosmatka M, Bardeesy N, Hurley RL, Witters LA, DePinho RA, et al. The tumour suppressor LKB1 kinase directly activates AMP-activated kinase and regulates apoptosis in response to energy stress. Proceedings of the National Academy of Sciences of the United States of America. 2004;**101**(10):3329-3335

[41] Luo Z, Zang M, Guo W. AMPK as a metabolic tumour suppressor: Control of metabolism and cell growth. Future Oncology. 2010;**6**(3):457-470

[42] Li W, Saud SM, Young MR, Chen G, Hua B. Targeting AMPK for cancer prevention and treatment. Oncotarget. 2015;**6**(10):7365-7378

[43] Rattan R, Giri S, Hartmann LC, Shridhar V. Metformin attenuates ovarian cancer cell growth in an AMP-kinase dispensable manner. Journal of Cellular and Molecular Medicine. 2011;**15**(1):166-178

[44] Owens OJ, Stewart C, Leake RE. Growth factors in ovarian cancer. British Journal of Cancer. 1991;**64**(6):1177-1181

[45] Zhou L, Leung BS. Growth regulation of ovarian cancer cells by epidermal growth factor and transforming growth factors alpha and beta 1. Biochimica et Biophysica Acta. 1992;**1180**(2):130-136

[46] Vera C, Tapia V, Vega M, Romero C. Role of nerve growth factor and its TRKA receptor in normal ovarian and epithelial ovarian cancer

angiogenesis. Journal of Ovarian Research. 2014;7:82

[47] Urzua U, Tapia V, Geraldo MP, Selman A, Vega M, Romero C. Nerve growth factor stimulates cellular proliferation of human epithelial ovarian cancer. Hormone and Metabolic Research. 2012;**44**(9):656-661

[48] Liefers-Visser JAL, Meijering RAM, Reyners AKL, van der Zee AGJ, de Jong S. IGF system targeted therapy: Therapeutic opportunities for ovarian cancer. Cancer Treatment Reviews. 2017;**60**:90-99

[49] Khabele D, Kabir SM, Dong Y, Lee E, Rice VM, Son DS. Preferential effect of akt2-dependent signaling on the cellular viability of ovarian cancer cells in response to EGF. Journal of Cancer. 2014;**5**(8):670-678

[50] Sever R, Brugge JS. Signal transduction in cancer. Cold Spring Harbor Perspectives in Medicine. 2015;**5**(4):a006098

[51] Al-Wahab Z, Mert I, Tebbe C, Chhina J, Hijaz M, Morris RT, et al. Metformin prevents aggressive ovarian cancer growth driven by high-energy diet: Similarity with calorie restriction. Oncotarget. 2015;**6**(13):10908-10923

[52] Sarfstein R, Friedman Y, Attias-Geva Z, Fishman A, Bruchim I, Werner H. Metformin downregulates the insulin/IGF-I signaling pathway and inhibits different uterine serous carcinoma (USC) cells proliferation and migration in p53-dependent or -independent manners. PLoS One. 2013;**8**(4):e61537

[53] Jewell JL, Guan KL. Nutrient signaling to mTOR and cell growth. Trends in Biochemical Sciences. 2013;**38**(5):233-242

[54] Tian T, Li X, Zhang J. mTOR signaling in cancer and mTOR inhibitors in solid tumour targeting therapy. International Journal of Molecular Sciences. 2019;**20**(3):755

[55] Populo H, Lopes JM, Soares P. The mTOR signalling pathway in human cancer. International Journal of Molecular Sciences. 2012;**13**(2):1886-1918

[56] Rattan R, Giri S, Shridhar V. Metformin inhibits ovarian cancer cell growth in an AMP-kinase dependent manner and inhibiting mTOR pathway. Cancer Research. 2008;**68** (9 Suppl):1469

[57] Li C, Liu VW, Chan DW, Yao KM, Ngan HY. LY294002 and metformin cooperatively enhance the inhibition of growth and the induction of apoptosis of ovarian cancer cells. International Journal of Gynecological Cancer. 2012;**22**(1):15-22

[58] Dang JH, Jin ZJ, Liu XJ, Hu D, Wang J, Luo Y, et al. Metformin in combination with cisplatin inhibits cell viability and induces apoptosis of human ovarian cancer cells by inactivating ERK 1/2. Oncology Letters. 2017;**14**(6):7557-7564

[59] Tsai WB, Aiba I, Long Y, Lin HK, Feun L, Savaraj N, et al. Activation of Ras/PI3K/ERK pathway induces c-Myc stabilization to upregulate argininosuccinate synthetase, leading to arginine deiminase resistance in melanoma cells. Cancer Research. 2012;**72**(10):2622-2633

[60] Zhao Q, Assimopoulou AN, Klauck SM, Damianakos H, Chinou I, Kretschmer N, et al. Inhibition of c-MYC with involvement of ERK/JNK/MAPK and AKT pathways as a novel mechanism for shikonin and its derivatives in killing leukemia cells. Oncotarget. 2015;**6**(36):38934-38951

[61] Zhao P, Meng Q, Liu LZ, You YP, Liu N, Jiang BH. Regulation of survivin

by PI3K/Akt/p70S6K1 pathway. Biochemical and Biophysical Research Communications. 2010;**395**(2):219-224

[62] Ye Q, Cai W, Zheng Y, Evers BM, She QB. ERK and AKT signaling cooperate to translationally regulate survivin expression for metastatic progression of colorectal cancer. Oncogene. 2014;**33**(14):1828-1839

[63] Litchfield LM, Mukherjee A, Eckert MA, Johnson A, Mills KA, Pan S, et al. Hyperglycemia-induced metabolic compensation inhibits metformin sensitivity in ovarian cancer. Oncotarget. 2015;**6**(27):23548-23560

[64] Garrido MP, Hernandez A, Saldaña C, Vega M, Carmen R. PO-026 metformin inhibits the NGF-induced increase c-MYC and VEGF levels in ovarian cancer cells. ESMO Open. 2018;**3**(Suppl. 2):A237-A2A8

[65] Rogalska A, Forma E, Ciesielski P, Brys M, Krzeslak A, Marczak A. Effect of metformin on apoptosis induction in ovarian cancer cells. Przeglad Menopauzalny. 2014;**13**(3):155-161

[66] Hanson KD, Shichiri M, Follansbee MR, Sedivy JM. Effects of c-myc expression on cell cycle progression. Molecular and Cellular Biology. 1994;**14**(9):5748-5755

[67] Galdieri L, Gatla H, Vancurova I, Vancura A. Activation of AMP-activated protein kinase by metformin induces protein acetylation in prostate and ovarian cancer cells. The Journal of Biological Chemistry. 2016;**291**(48):25154-25166

[68] Patel S, Singh N, Kumar L. Evaluation of effects of metformin in primary ovarian cancer cells. Asian Pacific Journal of Cancer Prevention. 2015;**16**(16):6973-6979

[69] Fu YL, Zhang QH, Wang XW, He H. Antidiabetic drug metformin mitigates ovarian cancer SKOV3 cell growth by triggering G2/M cell cycle arrest and inhibition of m-TOR/PI3K/Akt signaling pathway. European Review for Medical and Pharmacological Sciences. 2017;**21**(5):1169-1175

[70] Ma L, Wei J, Wan J, Wang W, Wang L, Yuan Y, et al. Low glucose and metformin-induced apoptosis of human ovarian cancer cells is connected to ASK1 via mitochondrial and endoplasmic reticulum stress-associated pathways. Journal of Experimental & Clinical Cancer Research. 2019;**38**(1):77

[71] Li Y, Xu S, Mihaylova MM, Zheng B, Hou X, Jiang B, et al. AMPK phosphorylates and inhibits SREBP activity to attenuate hepatic steatosis and atherosclerosis in diet-induced insulin-resistant mice. Cell Metabolism. 2011;**13**(4):376-388

[72] Xu X, So JS, Park JG, Lee AH. Transcriptional control of hepatic lipid metabolism by SREBP and ChREBP. Seminars in Liver Disease. 2013;**33**(4):301-311

[73] Nie LY, Lu QT, Li WH, Yang N, Dongol S, Zhang X, et al. Sterol regulatory element-binding protein 1 is required for ovarian tumour growth. Oncology Reports. 2013;**30**(3):1346-1354

[74] Wu J, Ji F, Di W, Chen H, Wan Y. Activation of acetyl-coenzyme A carboxylase is involved in Taxol-induced ovarian cancer cell death. Oncology Letters. 2011;**2**(3):543-547

[75] Li S, Qiu L, Wu B, Shen H, Zhu J, Zhou L, et al. TOFA suppresses ovarian cancer cell growth *in vitro* and *in vivo*. Molecular Medicine Reports. 2013;**8**(2):373-378

[76] Klagsbrun M, Moses MA. Molecular angiogenesis. Chemistry & Biology. 1999;**6**(8):R217-R224

[77] Folkman J. Role of angiogenesis in tumour growth and metastasis. Seminars in Oncology. 2002;**29**(6 Suppl. 16):15-18

[78] Tapia V, Gabler F, Munoz M, Yazigi R, Paredes A, Selman A, et al. Tyrosine kinase A receptor (trkA): A potential marker in epithelial ovarian cancer. Gynecologic Oncology. 2011;**121**(1):13-23

[79] Bakhashab S, Ahmed F, Schulten HJ, Ahmed FW, Glanville M, Al-Qahtani MH, et al. Proangiogenic effect of metformin in endothelial cells is via upregulation of VEGFR1/2 and their signaling under hyperglycemia-hypoxia. International Journal of Molecular Sciences. 2018;**19**(1):293

[80] Detaille D, Guigas B, Chauvin C, Batandier C, Fontaine E, Wiernsperger N, et al. Metformin prevents high-glucose-induced endothelial cell death through a mitochondrial permeability transition-dependent process. Diabetes. 2005;**54**(7):2179-2187

[81] Di Pietro M, Pascuali N, Parborell F, Abramovich D. Ovarian angiogenesis in polycystic ovary syndrome. Reproduction. 2018;**155**(5):R199-R209

[82] Di Pietro M, Parborell F, Irusta G, Pascuali N, Bas D, Bianchi MS, et al. Metformin regulates ovarian angiogenesis and follicular development in a female polycystic ovary syndrome rat model. Endocrinology. 2015;**156**(4):1453-1463

[83] Velazquez EM, Mendoza SG, Wang P, Glueck CJ. Metformin therapy is associated with a decrease in plasma plasminogen activator inhibitor-1, lipoprotein(a), and immunoreactive insulin levels in patients with the polycystic ovary syndrome. Metabolism. 1997;**46**(4):454-457

[84] Diamanti-Kandarakis E, Spina G, Kouli C, Migdalis I. Increased endothelin-1 levels in women with polycystic ovary syndrome and the beneficial effect of metformin therapy. The Journal of Clinical Endocrinology and Metabolism. 2001;**86**(10):4666-4673

[85] FDA. FDA Approves Bevacizumab in Combination with Chemotherapy for Ovarian Cancer [online]. 2018. Available from: https://www.fda.gov/drugs/resources-information-approved-drugs/fda-approves-bevacizumab-combination-chemotherapy-ovarian-cancer [Accessed: 05 July 2019]

[86] Burger RA,Brady MF, Bookman MA, Fleming GF, Monk BJ, Huang H, et al. Incorporation of bevacizumab in the primary treatment of ovarian cancer. The New England Journal of Medicine. 2011;**365**(26):2473-2483

[87] Raja FA, Chopra N, Ledermann JA. Optimal first-line treatment in ovarian cancer. Annals of Oncology. 2012;**23**(Suppl. 10):x118-x127

[88] Ledermann JA. First-line treatment of ovarian cancer: Questions and controversies to address. Therapeutic Advances in Medical Oncology. 2018;**10**:1758835918768232

[89] Esfahanian N, Shakiba Y, Nikbin B, Soraya H, Maleki-Dizaji N, Ghazi-Khansari M, et al. Effect of metformin on the proliferation, migration, and MMP-2 and -9 expression of human umbilical vein endothelial cells. Molecular Medicine Reports. 2012;5(4):1068-1074

[90] Li WD, Li NP, Song DD, Rong JJ, Qian AM, Li XQ. Metformin inhibits endothelial progenitor cell migration by decreasing matrix metalloproteinases, MMP-2 and MMP-9, via the AMPK/mTOR/autophagy pathway. International Journal of Molecular Medicine. 2017;**39**(5):1262-1268

[91] Alberts B, Johnson A, Lewis J, Raff M, Roberts K, Walter P. Posttranscriptional controls. In: Molecular Biology of the Cell. 4th ed. New York: Garland Science; 2002

[92] Babiarz JE, Blelloch R. Small RNAs - their biogenesis, regulation and function in embryonic stem cells. In: StemBook. 2009 May 31. Cambridge (MA): Harvard Stem Cell Institute; 2008

[93] O'Brien J, Hayder H, Zayed Y, Peng C. Overview of microRNA biogenesis, mechanisms of actions, and circulation. Frontiers in Endocrinology (Lausanne). 2018;**9**:402

[94] Martello G, Rosato A, Ferrari F, Manfrin A, Cordenonsi M, Dupont S, et al. A microRNA targeting dicer for metastasis control. Cell. 2010;**141**(7):1195-1207

[95] Blandino G, Valerio M, Cioce M, Mori F, Casadei L, Pulito C, et al. Metformin elicits anticancer effects through the sequential modulation of DICER and c-MYC. Nature Communications. 2012;**3**:865

[96] Garrido MP, Valenzuela M, Vallejos C, Salvatierra R, Hernández A, Vega M, et al, editors. Metformin decreases NGF-induced cell proliferation of ovarian cancer cells by modulation of c-MYC and β-catenin/TCF-Lef transcriptional activity and oncosuppressors micro-RNAs. In: 23rd International Symposium on Molecular Medicine; 28-30 March 2019; Bangkok, Thailand; 2019

[97] Takahashi H, McCaffery JM, Irizarry RA, Boeke JD. Nucleocytosolic acetyl-coenzyme A synthetase is required for histone acetylation and global transcription. Molecular Cell. 2006;**23**(2):207-217

[98] Ehrenhofer-Murray A. Chromatin acetylation. In: Encyclopedic Reference of Genomics and Proteomics in Molecular Medicine. Berlin, Heidelberg: Springer Berlin Heidelberg; 2006. pp. 266-268

[99] Shi J, Liu B, Wang H, Zhang T, Yang L. Association of metformin use with ovarian cancer incidence and prognosis: A systematic review and meta-analysis. International Journal of Gynecological Cancer. 2019;**29**(1):140-146

[100] Buckanovich RJ, Brown J, Shank J, Griffith K, Reynolds K, Johnston C, et al. A phase II clinical trial of metformin as a cancer stem cell targeting agent in stage IIc/III/IV ovarian, fallopian tube, and primary peritoneal cancer. Journal of Clinical Oncology. 2017;**35**(15_suppl):5556

[101] Wu B, Li S, Sheng L, Zhu J, Gu L, Shen H, et al. Metformin inhibits the development and metastasis of ovarian cancer. Oncology Reports. 2012;**28**(3):903-908

[102] Romero IL, McCormick A, McEwen KA, Park S, Karrison T, Yamada SD, et al. Relationship of type II diabetes and metformin use to ovarian cancer progression, survival, and chemosensitivity. Obstetrics and Gynecology. 2012;**119**(1):61-67

[103] Prieto-Vila M, Takahashi RU, Usuba W, Kohama I, Ochiya T. Drug resistance driven by cancer stem cells and their niche. International Journal of Molecular Sciences. 2017;**18**(12):2574

[104] Lu W, Kang Y. Epithelial-mesenchymal plasticity in cancer progression and metastasis. Developmental Cell. 2019;**49**(3):361-374

[105] Motohara T, Katabuchi H. Ovarian cancer stemness: Biological and clinical implications for metastasis and chemotherapy resistance. Cancers (Basel). 2019;**11**(7):907

[106] Suraneni MV, Badeaux MD. Tumour-initiating cells, cancer metastasis and therapeutic implications. In: Madame Curie Bioscience Database. Austin: Landes Bioscience; 2000-2013

[107] Kryczek I, Liu S, Roh M, Vatan L, Szeliga W, Wei S, et al. Expression of aldehyde dehydrogenase and CD133 defines ovarian cancer stem cells. International Journal of Cancer. 2012;**130**(1):29-39

[108] Parte SC, Batra SK, Kakar SS. Characterization of stem cell and cancer stem cell populations in ovary and ovarian tumours. Journal of Ovarian Research. 2018;**11**(1):69

[109] Shank JJ, Yang K, Ghannam J, Cabrera L, Johnston CJ, Reynolds RK, et al. Metformin targets ovarian cancer stem cells *in vitro* and *in vivo*. Gynecologic Oncology. 2012;**127**(2):390-397

[110] Zhang R, Zhang P, Wang H, Hou D, Li W, Xiao G, et al. Inhibitory effects of metformin at low concentration on epithelial-mesenchymal transition of CD44(+)CD117(+) ovarian cancer stem cells. Stem Cell Research & Therapy. 2015;**6**:262

[111] Laskov I, Abou-Nader P, Amin O, Philip CA, Beauchamp MC, Yasmeen A, et al. Metformin increases E-cadherin in tumours of diabetic patients with endometrial cancer and suppresses epithelial-mesenchymal transition in endometrial cancer cell lines. International Journal of Gynecological Cancer. 2016;**26**(7):1213-1221

[112] Bishnu A, Sakpal A, Ghosh N, Choudhury P, Chaudhury K, Ray P. Long term treatment of metformin impedes development of chemoresistance by regulating cancer stem cell differentiation through taurine generation in ovarian cancer cells. The International Journal of Biochemistry & Cell Biology. 2019;**107**:116-127

[113] Kim NY, Lee HY, Lee C. Metformin targets Axl and Tyro3 receptor tyrosine kinases to inhibit cell proliferation and overcome chemoresistance in ovarian cancer cells. International Journal of Oncology. 2015;**47**(1):353-360

[114] Bar D, Lavie O, Stein N, Feferkorn I, Shai A. The effect of metabolic comorbidities and commonly used drugs on the prognosis of patients with ovarian cancer. European Journal of Obstetrics, Gynecology, and Reproductive Biology. 2016;**207**:227-231

[115] Tseng CH. Metformin reduces ovarian cancer risk in Taiwanese women with type 2 diabetes mellitus. Diabetes/Metabolism Research and Reviews. 2015;**31**(6):619-626

[116] Kumar S, Meuter A, Thapa P, Langstraat C, Giri S, Chien J, et al. Metformin intake is associated with better survival in ovarian cancer: A case-control study. Cancer. 2013;**119**(3):555-562

[117] Bodmer M, Becker C, Meier C, Jick SS, Meier CR. Use of metformin and the risk of ovarian cancer: A case-control analysis. Gynecologic Oncology. 2011;**123**(2):200-204

Chapter 11

Metformin Activity against Breast Cancer: Mechanistic Differences by Molecular Subtype and Metabolic Conditions

Reema S. Wahdan-Alaswad and Ann D. Thor

Abstract

Obesity and type 2 diabetes increase the risk of and reduce survival in breast cancer (BC) patients. Metformin is the only anti-diabetic drug that alters this risk, with a reduction in BC incidence and improved outcomes. Metformin has AMP-kinase (AMPK) dependent and independent mechanisms of action, most notably affecting the liver and skeletal muscle. We and others have shown that metformin also downregulates protein and lipid synthesis; deactivates various receptor tyrosine kinases; alters cell cycle transcription/translation; modulates mitochondrial respiration and miRNA activation; targets key metabolic molecules; induces stem cell death and may induce apoptosis or autophagy in BC cells. Many of these anti-cancer effects are molecular subtype-specific. Metformin is most potent against triple negative (basal), followed by luminal BCs. The efficacy of metformin, as well as dose needed for the activity, is also modulated by the extracellular glucose concentration, cellular expression of the glucose transporter protein 1 (GLUT1), and the organic cation transporter protein 1 (OCT1, which transports metformin into cells). This chapter summarizes the diverse clinical and preclinical data related to the anti-cancer effects of metformin, focused against breast cancer.

Keywords: metformin, breast cancer, TGF-β, STAT3, and PI3K/AKT/mTOR, FASN, MiR-193b, cancer stem cells, EGFR, cholesterol, glucose

1. Introduction

Metabolic dysregulation of carbohydrate and lipid metabolism is frequent in cancer cells, facilitating growth and survival through adaptive mechanisms. Otto Warburg was the first to recognize that cancer cells favor glycolysis as compared to oxidative phosphorylation for the generation of energy (ATP) [1]. While the former is less efficient in terms of energy production per molecule of glucose, it also generates precursor molecules (amino acids, fatty acids, etc.) for replication and facilitates survival under oxidative stress [2]. This is in contrast to normal cells, which typically use oxidative metabolism to derive more energy (ATP) per molecule of glucose [3, 4]. Nearly a century later, we now recognize that cancer cells may utilize either aerobic or anaerobic respiration. The majority of cancer cells also have alterations of mitochondrial respiration, further providing a selective advantage to

IntechOpen

facilitate cancer growth and survival [5]. More specifically, it may increase intracellular reactive oxygen species by disruption of the mitochondrial electron transport chain to reduce the mitochondrial membrane potential in BC or act directly to inhibit the mitochondrial respiratory-chain complex 1 (MRCC1) [6–8].

Chronic energy excess and physical inactivity lead to systemic alterations of carbohydrate and fatty acid metabolism characterized by systemic hyperglycemia, hyperinsulinemia with insulin resistance followed by hypoinsulinemia, an increase in inflammatory cytokines and adipokines, alterations of steroid and growth hormones, and downregulation of immune surveillance and tissue oxygenation [3, 9, 10]. These changes are frequent but variable in patients with obesity and type 2 diabetes and can be modified by drugs, exercise, body weight, socioeconomic factors, access to healthcare, genetic risk, and other factors. Patients with these disorders are at an increased risk of cardiovascular disease, cancer, and other diseases associated with significant morbidity and mortality. In the U.S., there are ~13.8 million type 2 diabetics, 5 million undiagnosed diabetics, and 41 million persons with prediabetes/metabolic syndrome [11–13]. Obesity is a frequent comorbidity, often proceeding diabetes by years or decades.

Energy-sensing systems are integral to maintaining homeostasis in normal and transformed cells. Energy deprivation is frequent in cancer cells due to an inadequate vascular supply to meet the needs of increased cell replication.
In energy-stressed cells, AMPK is allosterically modified by binding to AMP and ADP, rendering them targetable by AMPK kinases. AMPK activation induces signaling, upregulates energy production, and inhibits energy programming for cell growth and motility. In cancerous cells, this shift often fails to occur even with stress. As a result, cancer cells typically prioritize replication and motility to favor cancer growth and metastasis. Drugs that activate AMPK, most notably metformin, reengage the AMPK failsafe to inhibit proliferation and motility. Thus, metformin provides a unique and generally less-toxic approach to combat the emergence or growth of cancers through inhibition of cell replication. This is particularly important for patients with obesity and type 2 diabetes, who lack homeostasis and experience wide swings in systemic glucose, insulin, and other energy precursors and growth factors that contribute to systemic energy stress.

2. Metabolic dysregulation, breast cancer, and metformin

Abundant epidemiologic and clinical data have shown that obesity and type 2 diabetes increase the risk and severity of cardiovascular disease and human cancer. Each of these chronic metabolic disorders as a single variable significantly increases the risk of breast cancer (BC) [10, 14]. In combination, the risk is increased by 20–50%, depending on the severity of disease and other variables. It is highest in women with abdominal (central) obesity in the postmenopausal setting, in women of all ethnic backgrounds [15–17]. Obesity also promotes BC in premenopausal women of color, especially African Americans and Latinos [18–23]. In patients with obesity and diabetes, BC also presents at a higher disease stage and is more resistant to treatment, resulting in a shorter disease-free interval and a significantly higher mortality rate [24, 25].

Steroid receptor-positive BC (luminal A) and basal (triple negative) BC cells are the most responsive to extracellular glucose at or above 7 mM of glucose to promote cell replication, tumor growth, and motility. In contrast, steroid receptor-positive BC cells that also express high HER2 (luminal B) and steroid receptor-negative, HER2 positive (the HER2 subtype) are less responsive to hyperglycemia, even at levels associated with untreated type 2 diabetes (10 mM glucose or higher) [26].

Glucose directly promotes signaling in epithelial cells or can act indirectly by interacting with molecular signaling proteins, such as the insulin-like growth factor (IGF-1), sex hormones, and adipokines [3, 27, 28]. Insulin and insulin-like growth factors are frequently increased in newly diagnosed BC patients [28–31]. These potent growth factors promote BC growth and are associated with a worse prognosis, both in overweight and 'normal' weight women [24, 29, 32–34]. Epidemiological and clinical data show that obesity and type 2 diabetes are particularly associated with luminal A (estrogen and progesterone responsive) as well as triple negative BCs [19, 21, 27, 35, 36].

Metformin (N′, N′-dimethylbiguanide) is the most frequently used drug to treat patients with metabolic syndrome (prediabetes) and type 2 diabetes worldwide. It has been used successfully for over six decades and has a very favorable benefit-risk profile [37]. Metformin is stable at room temperature with a long shelf life, is inexpensive and orally administered, and has low rates of significant toxicity or drug-drug interaction. Metformin is best known for its effects on liver and skeletal muscle cells, where it downregulates insulin resistance, lowers serum insulin, stimulates insulin receptor tyrosine kinase activity, inhibits hepatic glucose output (thus lowering A1C), increases glucose uptake by skeletal muscle cells, and can alter fatty acid metabolism.

Epidemiologic data show a significant lowering of cancer risk in patients with metabolic dysregulation (obesity, diabetes, or metabolic syndrome) who take metformin [29, 34, 38, 39]. Metformin use by BC patients has also been associated with improved treatment response and survival. In one meta-analytic study of BC patients with diabetes, metformin use was associated with a 65% improvement in BC-specific survival as compared to nonusers [40]. The anticancer properties of metformin are in contrast to other antidiabetic agents, including sulfonylureas and insulin, which promote cancer growth [9].

It is also taken for its 'antiaging' properties in individuals without obesity or metabolic dysregulation, particularly outside of the US [10, 41, 42].

Numerous clinical trials are currently underway in BC patients to evaluate the benefit of metformin combined with or following the administration of other therapeutic agents [29, 32, 33, 43–46]. Studies designed to test the benefit of metformin in patients in only specific molecular subtypes of BC have not been performed, although some have looked at molecular cohort interactions as a secondary goal [30, 47–51]. There are limited data on the use of metformin in metabolically 'normal' BC patients. However, our preclinical data suggest that metformin is most active in all molecular subtypes with physiological levels of extracellular glucose [26]. This evidence provides a rationale for testing metformin in otherwise healthy BC patients.

3. AMPK-dependent mechanisms of metformin action in BC

Cellular uptake of metformin requires expression and functionality of the organic cation transporter 1 (OCT1) protein, which in some individuals or BCs may be altered (more or less effective in transporting metformin into the cell) by polymorphism or genetic error [52]. Polymorphisms have also been associated with a decrease in metformin efficacy in diabetic patients [53–55]. In BC cells, we have demonstrated that OCT1 expression is associated with the anticancer activity *in vivo* [44]. Once inside the cell, metformin may directly interact with the metabolic sensor AMPK to induce activation, restoring homeostasis and blocking cellular replication and motility under low energy (stress) conditions. The AMPK 'switch' is also influenced by the intracellular AMP:ATP ratio, which in turn is influenced by fatty acid oxidation and glucose metabolism. Thus, metformin can indirectly affect AMPK, through reduction of gluconeogenesis and thus changing of the AMP:ATP ratio. These mechanisms are represented in **Figure 1**. These processes are modulated by P53 status. It is mutated in many BCs, particularly tumors that are high grade, late-stage or nonluminal in subtype. In BCs that are P53 competent, AMPK activation (from metformin or other triggers) upregulates P53 tumor suppressor activity as a downstream target. This induces activation of cell cycle checkpoint proteins, to inhibit cell proliferation [56]. In P53 incompetent cells, AMPK activation from metformin may be less effective through P53 mechanisms. Given the numerous other actions of metformin, as well as the molecular subtype specificity of the drug, we postulated that P53 status alone would not have a major impact on anticancer effects of metformin. We have demonstrated that this is the case in preclinical studies of numerous BC cell lines [57]. In other cells, metformin may induce cell cycle arrest and death through activation of apoptotic pathways and downregulation of p53 [58, 59] or PARP cleavage, especially in triple negative BC [60, 61].

Activation of mTOR-dependent protein synthesis and cell growth (downstream of the PI3K/Akt signaling axis), along with AMPK, provides a robust signaling platform for BC cell growth, proliferation, and chemotherapy resistance. In addition to activating AMPK, metformin inhibits mTOR and downstream signaling components of this critical pathway. Mutation of the PI3K catalytic subunit (PIK3CA) occurs in 20-35% of BCs [62, 63]. Mutation or loss of the tumor suppressor gene PTEN has also been demonstrated in 40% of BC [64, 65]. Metformin can also inhibit gluconeogenesis and mTOR signaling independent of AMPK and the tuberous sclerosis 2 (TSC2) gene in some experimental systems (in hepatic cells that lack AMPK or its kinase, LKB1). In this model system, metformin induces

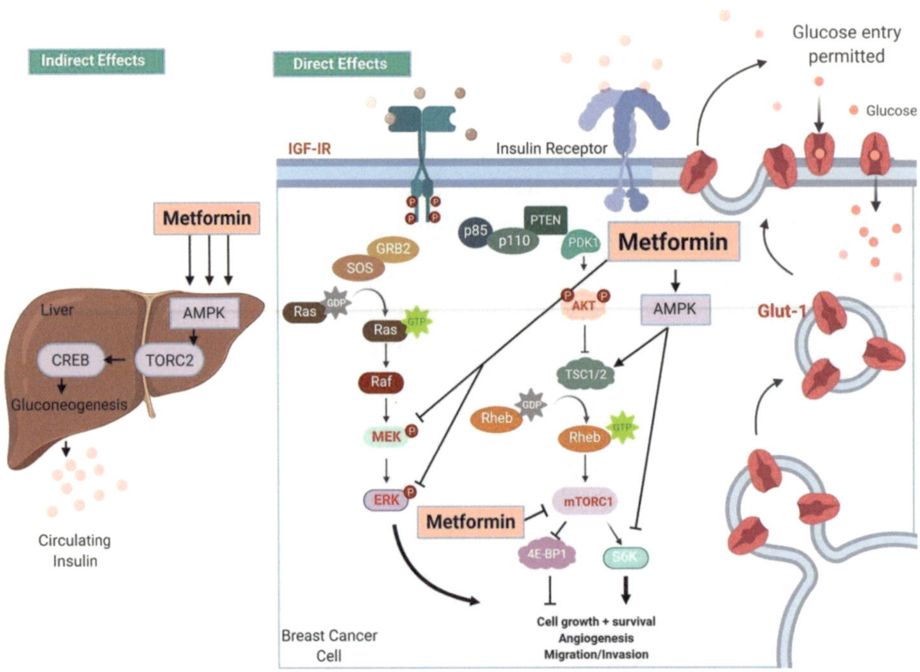

Figure 1.
Metformin AMPK-dependent mechanism of action on breast cancer. Metformin activates AMPK directly through insulin-like growth factor (IGF-I) or insulin receptor, which in turn can activate PI3K/Akt/mTOR or RAS/Raf/MEK/ERK to increase cell growth, survival, angiogenesis, migration, and invasion. Metformin indirectly activates AMPK, which activates mTORC2, CREB, and gluconeogenesis. Lastly, glucose can enter BC cell through GLUT-1, and metformin can directly downregulate GLUT-1 receptor.

downregulation of hepatic gluconeogenesis through non-AMPK–associated mechanisms [66, 67].

Signaling systems and thus metformin sensitivity by dose or mechanism vary by the molecular subtype of BC as well as unique genomic changes in each patient's BC. For example, we have shown that metformin-induced partial S phase arrest increased P-AMPK and reduced P-EGFR, P-MAPK, P-Src, cyclin D1, and cyclin E, with the induction of PARP cleavage and apoptosis only in triple negative BCs [44]. In this tumor subtype, metformin specifically targets Stat3 and is not dependent on mTOR signaling [44]. In non-triple negative BCs (luminal and HER2), metformin induces partial cell cycle arrest at the G1 checkpoint, reduces cyclin D1 and E2F1 expression, and inhibits AMPK, MAPK, Akt, and mTOR activity [44, 57, 68]. Metformin-associated AMPK activation may also inactivate the insulin receptor substrate 1 (IRS1), which in turn regulates IGF-IR and PI3K/Akt signaling pathways to block the progrowth effects of hyperinsulinemia and insulin-like growth factors typically associated with type 2 diabetes [66, 67, 69].

Metformin is unique in the breadth and complexity of AMPK-dependent direct and indirect targets that inhibit cancer. Several new mechanisms fall into the rapidly expanding field of immuno-oncology. Metformin-induced activation of AMPK activates the programmed death ligand-1 (PDL-1) at S195, reducing stability and membrane localization and thus increasing PDL-1 degradation [70]. Metformin also promotes cytotoxic T cell lymphocyte activity in tumor tissue and enhances tumor-associated immune surveillance [6, 70, 71]. Additionally, metformin upregulates pro-inflammatory cytokines (tumor necrosis factor alpha (TNFα), interleukin-6 (IL-6), IL-1β, the nuclear factor kappa-light-chain-enhancer of activated B-cells (NF-κB), the hypoxia-inducible factor 1-alpha (HIF-1α), and the vascular endothelial growth factor (VEGF), reviewed in [72, 73]).

AMPK-dependent mechanisms of action have been validated using clinical trial–derived BC samples as well as preclinical model systems, reviewed in detail elsewhere [43]. Some of these were especially important to spur the expansion of metformin use in BC patients. The timing, dose, and duration of metformin treatment in BC patients with or without other chemotherapy are actively under investigation. Neoadjuvant metformin, in particular, has shown benefit with a higher rate of complete pathological response, as compared to similar BC patients [74].

3.1 Metformin targets cell cycle proteins in AMPK-dependent manner in breast cancer

AMPK plays an integral role in the regulation of cell cycle and cell division. The ability of metformin to activate AMPK thus has a significant inhibitory effect on cell-cycle associated proteins. This mechanism is represented in **Figure 2**. Expression profiling of BC derived from metformin-treated patients as compared to controls has shown consistent downregulation of many gene encoding proteins involved in mitosis, including kinesins, tubulins, histones, Aurora, as well as Polo-like kinases and ribosomal proteins (critical for protein and macromolecular biosynthesis, respectively) [75]. Given the targeted effects of metformin, it is not surprising that its actions are synergistic with drugs like paclitaxel that induce defects in mitotic spindle assembly, chromosome segregation, and cell division. In combination, metformin and paclitaxel dramatically increase the number of cells arrested in G2-M and apoptosis, as compared to either agent alone [76]. Metformin may also induce GO/G1 arrest due to activation of AMPK, downregulation of cyclin D1, and enhanced binding of CDK2 by $p27^{Kip1}$ and $p21^{cip1}$ [60, 61], especially in non-triple negative cells. Some have shown that metformin sensitivity to GO/G1

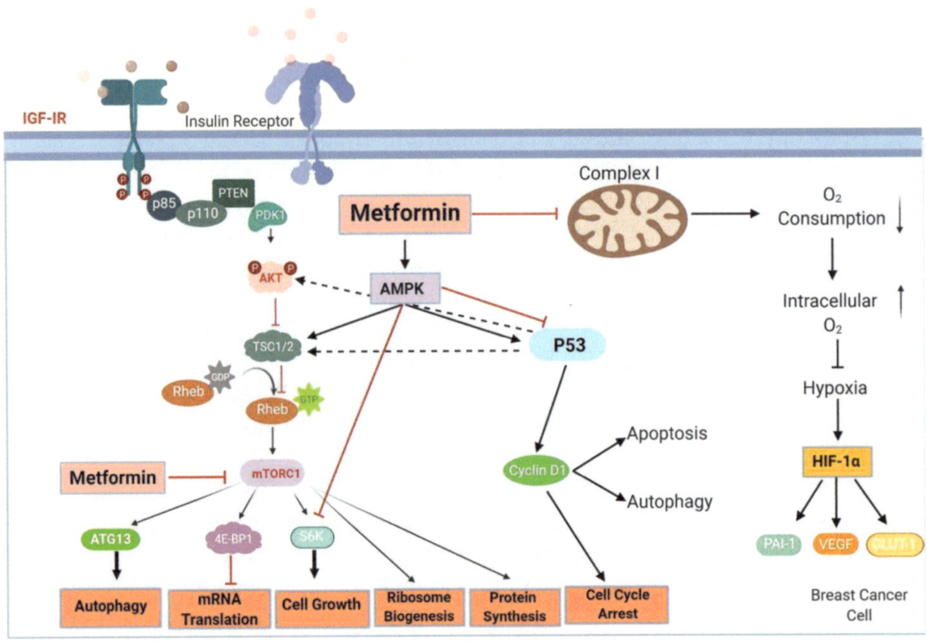

Figure 2.
AMPK-dependent action on cell cycle and alternate mechanisms. Metformin activates AMPK directly through insulin-like growth factor (IGF-I) or insulin receptor, which in turn can activate PI3K/Akt/mTOR or RAS/Raf/MEK/ERK signaling pathway. Metformin can also inhibit downstream signaling intermediates to attenuate autophagy, mRNA translation, cell growth, ribosome biogenesis, protein synthesis, and cell cycle growth. Metformin can also activate AMPK, which blocks P53 and induces cell cycle arrest. Lastly, metformin can block complex I of mitochondrial biogenesis to increase intracellular O2, which can block HIF-1 and VEGF production.

arrest is linked to overexpression of $p27^{Kip1}$ $p21^{cip1}$ [60, 61]. We have demonstrated that metformin induces cycle arrest at the G1 checkpoint in luminal A, B and HER2 BC [75] associated with a reduction of cyclin D1 and E2F1 expression, with no changes in $p27^{Kip1}$ or $p21^{waf1}$. While these authors describe how metformin can increase CDK chemical inhibitors to control BC growth [57, 61], others have utilized cell cycle-dependent kinases (CDK) inhibitors with metformin and report that this combination should be used with caution [77].

In addition to downregulating cell replication under stress, metformin upregulates the cellular DNA-damage response, resulting in a decline in the mutational burden for those cancer cells that survive. Mechanisms underlying this effect include selective activation of the ataxia telangiectasia mutated (ATM) gene as well as ATM targets, such as protein kinase CHK2 gene and attenuation of reactive oxygen species ROS that result in DNA damage [78]. Algire et al. have postulated that downregulation of ROS production and thus somatic mutation are likely contributing mechanisms for the reduction in cancer risk associated with metformin use [8].

In summary, AMPK plays a central regulatory role in human cells, including BC where it regulates energy metabolism, cell growth and motility, response to insulin and growth factors, and estrogen production. Metformin induces AMPK activation in a robust manner, to affect numerous target pathways and intermediate molecules. The activity of AMPK and thus metformin can be modified by interacting factors including hormones, growth factors, and energy sensors. Selective targeting of AMPK-dependent pathways has shown less efficacy than metformin alone against BC [79], consistent with the findings that not all mechanisms of metformin action are AMPK dependent.

4. AMP-independent mechanisms of action on metformin

4.1 Metformin action on glucose and metabolism

Upregulation of bioavailable glucose, insulin, and other growth factors increase the risk and promote BC aggression [16, 23, 27, 80, 81]. In addition to shifts in host metabolism, glycolytic reprogramming occurs in breast epithelial cells during malignant transformation. This process is accentuated by systemic dysregulation of carbohydrate and lipid metabolism, as bioavailable sugars and fat typically increase in these patients. Glycolytic reprogramming includes dependence on aerobic respiration, providing less-efficient energy (ATP) production per molecule of glucose from and incomplete oxidative phosphorylation. Cancer cell reprogramming includes activation of numerous signaling intermediaries, including phosphatidylinositide 3-kinase (PI3K), protein kinase B (Akt), mammalian target of rapamycin (mTOR), phosphatase and tensin homolog (PTEN), and AMPK [82–84]. Changes in other factors including c-MYC, hypoxia-inducible factor 1-alpha (HIF1α), epidermal growth factor receptor (EGFR), tumor protein 53 (P53), and the Met receptor may also facilitate cancer cell dependence on aerobic glycolysis [16, 85–87].

We have focused on the effects of extracellular glucose and other carbohydrates, combined with or without metformin using BC cell lines and animal models of obesity, metabolic syndrome, and mammary tumorigenesis, summarized in **Figure 3** and detailed elsewhere [26, 47, 49, 52, 57, 68, 88–93]. Importantly, most *in vitro* studies of metformin use commercially purchased media containing ~17 mM glucose (incompatible with human life, above concentrations achieved in diabetes). This is significantly higher than serum derived from normal persons (~5 mM), metabolic syndrome patients (~7 mM), or uncontrolled diabetes (~10 mM) [26]. We have shown that all molecular subtypes of BC cells grown with high glucose media require significantly more metformin to achieve the same anticancer efficacy (i.e., much higher EC50 of metformin) [26]. Normalization of glucose concentration in the culture media significantly reduced the EC50 of metformin for all BC cell types to induce BC growth inhibition or death. This hyperglycemic override of metformin action by dose makes biologic sense, given the ability of glucose to enter cells and promote many of the same pathways we have shown that are critical to metformin action. Similar issues may arise in animal models, particularly if the animals are overfed or obese. In both mouse and rat model systems, we have achieved plasma metformin concentrations equivalent to the normal range in humans, by providing it in the drinking water. We have also shown that metformin accumulates in the cytoplasm, markedly higher than serum levels in mammary tumor cells with functional and sufficient OCT1 protein [26].

Luminal A and some subsets of triple negative BC cell lines show the greatest increase in proliferation when cultured in media with supraphysiologic glucose or insulin. In contrast, luminal B and HER2 BC cells were significantly less responsive to glucose or insulin, even at the highest concentrations examined. This responsivity pattern was similar to the cellular response to metformin by molecular BC subtype, with triple negative being the most responsive. From a molecular standpoint, triple negative BC cell responsivity to high glucose and metformin by dose was unique (efficacy at lower EC50s). Triple negative BC cells are especially dependent on glucose/glucosamine (metabolized through glycolysis) and lipids for energy and building block production, cell division, phenotypic aggression, and motility [94]. When grown with media containing supraphysiologic glucose, they upregulate specific genes, including EGFR, P-EGFR, IGF1R, P-IGF1R, IRS2, cyclin D1, and cyclin E expression, and inhibit AMPK/P-AMPK and p38 in a dose-dependent manner [26]. With the addition of metformin, there is a downregulation of these

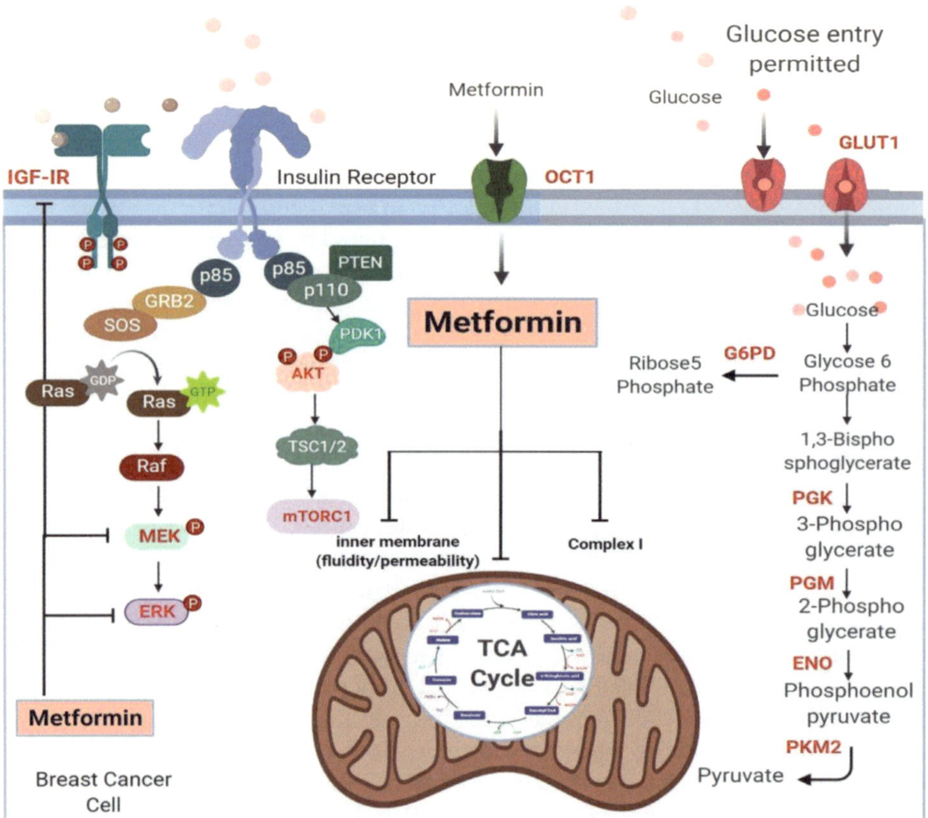

Figure 3.
Metformin action on glucose and metabolism breast cancer. Metformin enters the BC cell through OCT 1 transporter to attenuate inner membrane fluidity/permeability, the Krebs cycle (TCA), and complex I of the mitochondria. Metformin can also block downstream signaling intermediates involved in the PI3K/Akt/mTOR or RAS/Raf/MEK/ERK signaling pathways, which can control BC cell growth. Lastly, metformin blocks GLUT1 transporter and key enzymes that are involved in carbohydrate synthesis.

genes and the upregulation of genes associated with cell killing and growth control [49, 94]. Our report showed that glucose promotes phenotypic aggression and reduces metformin efficacy by targeting key enzymes that are required for glucose metabolism in TNBC. Such enzymes include G6PD, Fructose-2-6-BP, PGK, PGM, ENO, PKM2, and LDH-A (shown in **Figure 3** and reviewed in [49]). Further, we reported that metformin attenuated the expression of over 20 critical genes involved in glucose metabolism, glucose transporters, gluconeogenesis, and tricarboxylic acid cycle [49]. Metformin-associated gene expression changes also reduced phenotypic aggressiveness and stem-like progenitor cell pool [26, 49, 90, 92]. Metformin treatment also restricted cell proliferation with S phase arrest, motility (through downregulation of intermediate filament proteins), and increased apoptosis (through activation of both the intrinsic and extrinsic pathways) [26, 47, 57, 88, 89, 92]. Metformin significantly inhibits carbohydrate induced pro-oncogenic metabolic and biologic characteristics of triple negative BC cells [26]. Altogether, metformin's ability to target key glucose transporters, such a GLUT1, along with key genes involved in glucose and carbohydrate metabolism, highlights the role that this agent may play to control highly aggressive malignant BC cells via downregulation of the cellular metabolic machinery.

We have also shown that inhibition of lipid biosynthesis was requisite to the anticancer effects of metformin in triple negative BC cells. It downregulates both fatty acid synthase (FASN) and the cholesterol biosynthesis pathway, as detailed below. Other studies have focused on interactions between obesity, weight gain, hormonal status, and BC, and more specifically if metformin could be used to disrupt this process. Using a rat model of mammary tumor development after exposure to a carcinogen, animals were overfed and then segregated into lean and obese. Both subsets were subjected to ovary removal, half were given metformin, and they were followed for the development and progression of mammary tumors [52, 93, 95]. Obese rats experienced marked changes in metabolism, akin to metabolic syndrome. Mammary tumors from these obese rats showed enhanced tumor growth and tumor-associated glucose uptake, 50% higher than nonobese rats in association with upregulation of the progesterone receptor. In contrast, the lean rats preferentially deposited excess nutrients in mammary (nontumor) and peripheral tissues. Metformin abrogated systemic metabolic dysregulation, reduced tumorigenesis, tumor progression, and tumor-associated PR expression in obese rats. Similar changes in body weight and obesity are frequent after female menopause has been observed in BC of postmenopausal females with obesity, providing additional clues for the use and timing of metformin associated with BC risk and treatment for future study.

4.2 Metformin action on cholesterol, EGFR signaling, and lipid rafts

The mevalonate pathway, also known as the β-hydroxy β-methylglutaryl-CoA (HMG-CoA) reductase pathway, is critical for cancer cell survival. Inhibition of the pathway by statins or other agents has been shown to have anticancer effects [96, 97]. In contrast, elevated cholesterol has been strongly associated with BC risk, a worse BC-associated outcome and chemotherapeutic resistance. This reflects the pivotal role of lipids including cholesterol in cancer survival and growth, including upregulation of signaling through membrane-bound receptors, facilitation of intracellular signaling pathways, and serving as an anchor for intracytoplasmic filaments to promote motility and invasion and as a precursor for cellular metabolism to generate energy and facilitate replication [98, 99]. We have shown that triple negative BC cells are especially dependent on the upregulation of lipid and cholesterol biosynthesis [100].

Statins are widely prescribed for patients with high cholesterol or lipid abnormalities, most often to reduce the risk of cardiovascular disease. Statins also benefit women to reduce the risk and disease progression of BC. Two population-based studies from Northern Europe are particularly compelling. A Finnish study involving over 30,000 women showed that statin use, pre- or post-BC diagnosis, reduced BC-specific mortality by about 50% [101]. A large Danish study showed a benefit for BC patients as well, with significantly lower recurrence rates in statin users as compared to nonusers. They also reported that lipophilic statins (rather than hydrophilic satins) had the most anti-BC activity [102]. A recent study from MD Anderson Cancer Center suggests that statin use is particularly beneficial for BC patients with triple negative tumors, especially in patients with higher stage disease [95]. Their data are consistent with our preclinical data, showing significant upregulation of lipid metabolism-associated gene triple negative BC as compared to other molecular subtypes. See for further discussion elsewhere [103]. A major issue with statin use is toxicity, which reportedly occurs in up to half of patients. Some statin drugs are also expensive and thus may be unaffordable by many patients.

Metformin, in contrast, is relatively nontoxic and inexpensive. We have demonstrated that metformin has potent effects in lipid and cholesterol biosynthesis in BC cells. More specifically, it inhibits transcriptional activation of HMGCo-A (the enzyme targeted by statins), as well as over 20 other genes in the cholesterol biosynthesis pathway. We have also shown that it induces translational activation of downstream signaling, including the genes ACAA2, HMGCS1, HMGCR, MVK, MVD, LSS, and DHCR24 (**Figure 4**). Through broad inhibition of cholesterol biosynthesis in triple negative BC, metformin induces a significant reduction of membrane-associated and intracellular cholesterol and reduces GM1 lipid rafts through decreased synthesis and destabilization (disassociation). GM1 lipid raft stability has a profound effect on some receptors that rely on GM1 lipid rafts (like EGFR) for stability, ligand binding, and thus activation, resulting in downstream signaling. We have shown that metformin inhibits cholesterol biosynthesis and raft production, reducing membranous EGFR and its activation associated with downstream signaling in TNBC [91]. We have also shown that in combination, metformin and the statin-mimetic MβCD were synergistic in attenuating cholesterol biosynthesis and cell proliferation [91]. Others have validated our observation that metformin downregulates genes involved in cholesterol biosynthesis, reporting downregulation of HMGCR, LDLR, and SREBP1 [104]. A particularly exciting corollary of these findings is the potential of metformin to synergize with receptor tyrosine kinase inhibitors (RTKIs) against BC. This is an underexplored area of breast oncology research with tremendous translational potential, given the growing use of RTKIs against BC.

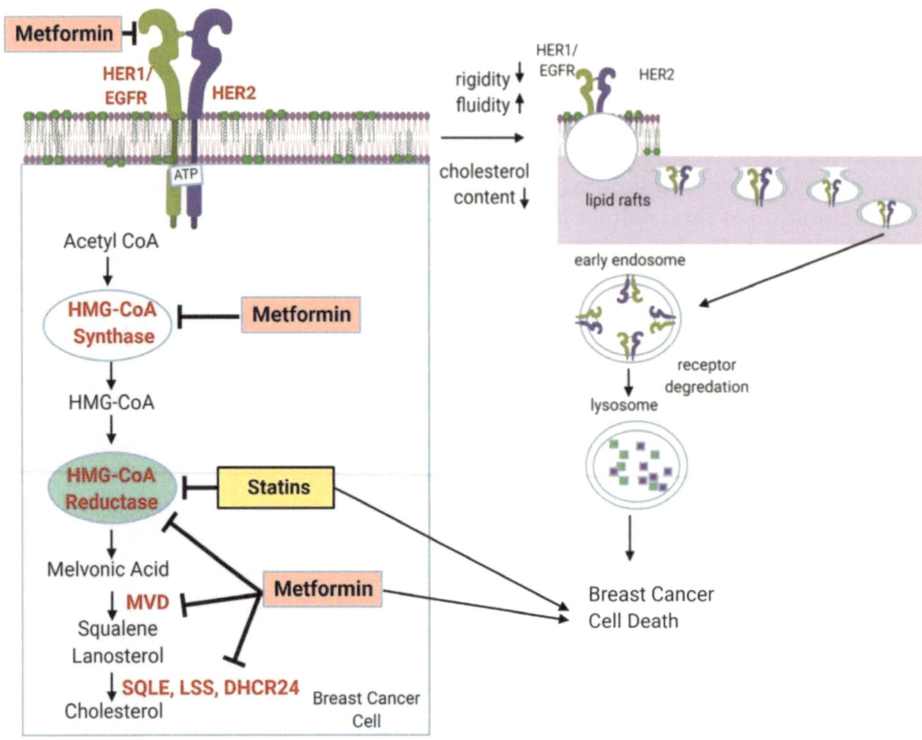

Figure 4.
Metformin action on cholesterol synthesis and lipid rafts. Metformin blocks epidermal growth factor receptor (EGFR), human epidermal growth factor receptors 2/3 (HER2/HER3), which in turn can block key enzymes involved in cholesterol synthesis pathway. Metformin and statins both can inhibit rate limiting step HMG-CoA Reductase, HMGCR. Metformin can also decrease cellular membrane rigidity, increase fluidity, and decrease cholesterol content to allow for the internalization of EGFR, HER2, or HER3 receptors. Internalization of these receptors is through GM1 lipid rafts, which are degraded and allow for BC cell death.

4.3 Metformin action on miRNA and FASN signaling

MiRNAs are endogenous, short (21-25) nucleotide sequences that control gene expression during post-transcriptional translation. It has previously been reported that more than half of human genes are regulated by miRNAs [105]. A growing body of evidence has highlighted the role of miRNAs as master regulators of metabolic processes, such as lipid and cholesterol synthesis [92, 105, 106]. Perturbations of these processes are important for tumor development. Modulation of these regulators using synthetic antagomirs to block the activity of specific miRNAs is an important new area of breast research. Metformin exerts some of its anticancer activity through modulation of miRNAs that target genes in metabolic and other pathways (**Figure 5**) [92, 107, 108]. miRNAs have been reported to be potential biomarkers for BC (i.e., *miR-9, miR-10b,* and *miR-17-5p*), whereas others reportedly have prognostic (i.e., *miR-148a* and *miR-335*) or predictive relevance (i.e., *miR-26a, miR-30c, miR-187,* and *miR-339-5p*) [109].

We have shown that metformin increases several members of the miR-193 family. It upregulates miR-193b, which in turn targets and downregulates the FASN 3'UTR. FASN is an important component of *de novo* fatty acid synthesis. Using an miR-193b mimetic, we induced a drastic reduction in fatty acid synthase (FASN) protein expression as well as increased growth inhibition and apoptosis of TNBC [92]. A separate expression profiling study of metformin-treated TNBC cells has shown similar results [106]. These data show that inhibition of FASN and fatty acid biosynthesis contributes to the potency of metformin against BC cells.

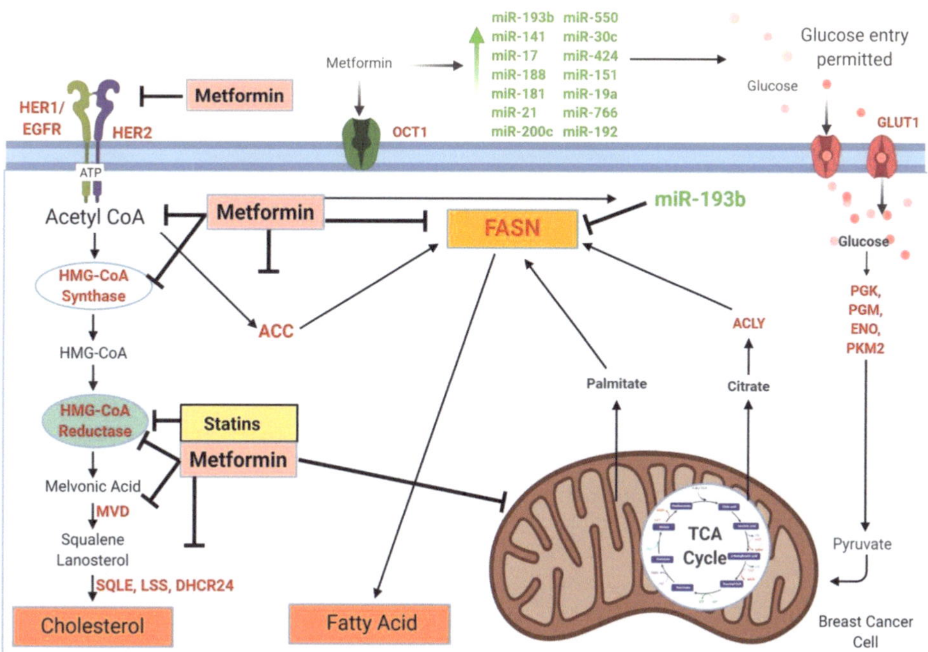

Figure 5.
Metformin action on lipid synthesis and miRNAs metformin blocks EGFR, HER2, and HER3, which in turn can block key enzymes involved in cholesterol synthesis pathway as described in ***Figure 4****. Metformin can also block acetyl-CoA carboxylase (ACC), which in turn can decrease fatty acid synthase (FASN). Metformin can also increase a myriad of miRNAS (shown in green). One of these miRNAs (miR-193b) can target FASN, which can decrease fatty acid synthesis in BC cells. Additionally metformin can block FASN and increase BC cell death.*

4.4 Metformin action on PI3K/Akt/mTOR signaling in breast cancer

The PI3K/Akt/mTOR pathway plays a central role in regulating protein synthesis, cell proliferation, tumorigenesis, angiogenesis, tumor growth, and metastasis [63]. While AMPK-dependent phosphorylation is frequently described in metformin-mediated inhibition of the PI3K/Akt/mTOR signaling pathway, AMPK activation is not mandatory for these effects; see schematic in **Figure 6** [57]. We have shown that metformin inhibits Akt and mTOR and inhibits cellular proliferation and colony formation and causes a partial G1 cell cycle arrest in all ER-positive, HER2 normal or abnormal BC cell lines examined [57]. Metformin-mediated inhibition of the PI3K/Akt/mTOR signaling pathway has also been shown to induce inhibition of cell replication, S phase arrest, and apoptosis, with a reduction in E2F1 and cyclin D1 expression in triple negative BC cell lines [57].

4.5 Metformin action in STAT3 signaling

TNBC shows high activation of the signal transducer and activator of transcription 3 (STAT3) signaling pathway, which in turn promotes cell growth, invasion, migration, metastasis, angiogenesis, immune evasion, and drug resistance and inhibits apoptosis [88]. We have shown that metformin specifically targets STAT3 signaling to reduce P-STAT3 at both Ser727 and Tyr705 phosphorylation sites but not STAT3 expression in TNBC, schematically represented in **Figure 6**. In combination with a Stat3 inhibitor, metformin significantly downregulated STAT3

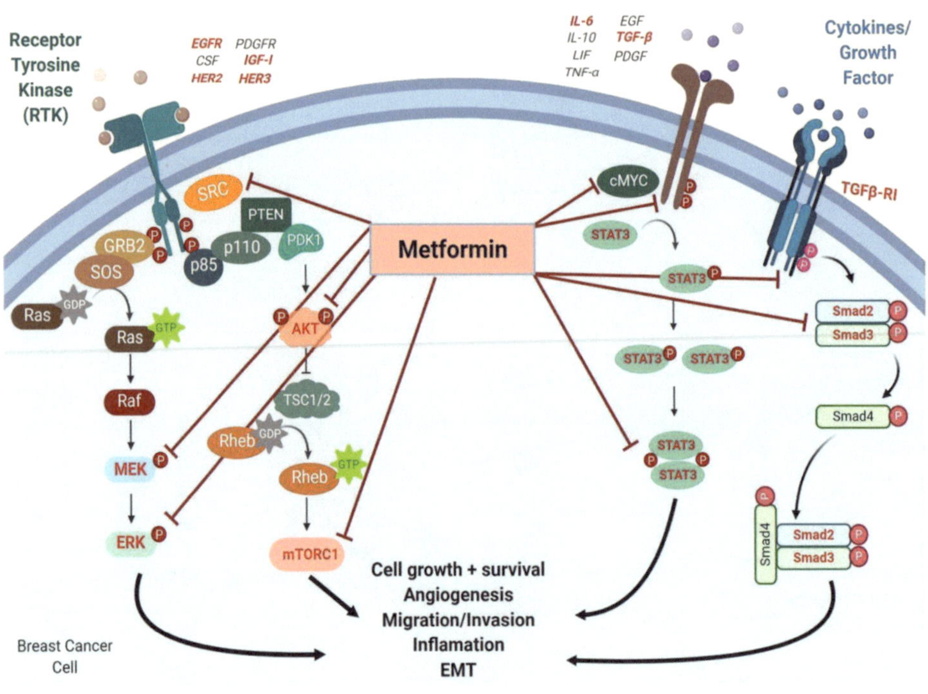

Figure 6.
Metformin action in breast cancer. Metformin can block receptor tyrosine kinase (RTK), such as EGFR, HER2, and HER3. Metformin further blocks downstream signaling intermediates involved in PI3K/Akt/mTOR or RAS/Raf/MEK/ERK signaling pathway, such as AKT, mTOR, MEK, or ERK, which can decrease cell growth, angiogenesis, and migration/invasion. Further, metformin can further block cytokine and growth factor receptors such as the TGF-RII. Metformin can block IL-6/STAT3 pathway and TGF-signaling pathway, which in turn can decrease cell growth, angiogenesis, migration/invasion, inflammation, and EMT.

expression and was synergistic in reducing cell growth and the induction of apoptosis in TNBC [88]. Given that TNBC also shows an upregulation/activation of the PI3K/Akt/mTOR signaling pathways, we then combined metformin with an mTOR inhibitor rapamycin, to determine if it would reduce metformin efficacy. Significant interactions with metformin were not observed; thus, mechanisms underlying its effects are not dependent on mTOR.

The JAK/STAT pathway is upregulated by obesity-associated mechanisms that promote BC growth. Others have demonstrated that metformin attenuates Janus kinase (JAK)/STAT3 signaling at Ser515 and Ser518 within the Src homology 2 domain of JAK1 [110]. Metformin has also been shown to preferentially inhibit nuclear translocation of NK-κB and phosphorylation of STAT3 in cancer stem cells (CSCs) as compared to non-CSCs [111]. Given the procarcinogenic and prometastatic role that JAK/STAT pathways play in TNBC, the development of therapeutic strategies to attenuate these pathways using metformin may provide benefit with limited toxicity.

4.6 Metformin and TGF-β signaling in TNBC

A subset of TNBC subclassified as mesenchymal-stem like/claudin-low (MSL/CL) characteristically shows high expression and activation of TGF-β signaling, phenotypic aggression, and a worse outcome. In addition to TGF-β receptor 2 expression, BC in this group shows upregulation of Smad2, Smad3, ID1, and ID3 [90]. They are especially responsive to TGF-β ligand 1 (TGF-β1), resulting in cell proliferation, migration, and invasion. MSL/CL cell lines also demonstrate downregulation of several growth factor receptors in response to metformin, including fibroblast growth factor receptors (FGFR2 and FGFR3), hormone receptors (AR, ESR1, and PGR), and claudin integral membrane proteins of tight junctions (CLDN3, CLDN4, and CLDN7) in the MSL/CL BC subtypes [90]. Metformin directly attenuated TGF-β signaling pathway by downregulating activation of Smad2/Smad3, ID1, and ID3 (**Figure 6**). In combination with TGF-β inhibitors (TβRI-KIs; LY2197s299 or SB431542), metformin synergistically enhanced cell death in MSL/CL BC cells [90]. Overall, these data suggest that targeting TGF-β signaling using metformin with or without a TGF-β inhibitor may provide benefit for patients with MSL/CL BCs.

The process of epithelial-mesenchymal transition (EMT) is also common in TNBC and has been associated with biologic aggression and stem-like properties. Metformin reportedly inhibits EMT in a metastatic canine model of mammary cancer [112]. Others have shown that metformin reduces EMT through blockade of transcription factors like ZEB1, TWIST1, and SNAIL (Slug) [113–115]. Given that TGF-β pathway activation and EMT promote breast cancer stem cells (BCSC), therapeutic resistance, dormancy, and a poor outcome [113], and that metformin has been shown to block these in TNBC, inhibitors against TGF-β-induced EMT combined with metformin may provide benefit in some TNBC patients.

4.7 Metformin action on breast cancer and angiogenesis, and the microenvironment

Clinical studies have demonstrated that diabetic patients treated with metformin are less likely to develop cardiovascular disease, independent of glycemic control. It is unclear whether this outcome reflects downregulation of hyperglycemia and systemic inflammatory triggers or vascular damage, or whether metformin has a direct effect on endothelial cells, vascular resistance, elasticity, and damage

[12, 80, 116]. In the context of breast cancer, it has long been demonstrated that high-stage and grade cancers with a worse prognosis have the capacity to upregulate peri- and intratumoral neo-angiogenesis [117]. The induction of new vessels provides metabolic and oxygen delivery advantages to the cancer cells, facilitating survival and growth. Neo-angiogenesis is also associated with an increased capacity of the BC to metastasize, particularly to distant sites including the visceral organs and brain. We have demonstrated a reduction in vascular density and growth, in association with metformin treatment in preclinical models. Others have shown that metformin is associated with reduced tumor angiogenesis in many different cancer cell types. Metformin and alternate biguanides, such as phenformin, downregulate VEGF-dependent activation of ERK1, inhibiting neo-angiogenesis and reducing microvessel density (MVD) [118]. Wang et al. have shown that metformin also downregulates the expression of two other genes, platelet-derived growth factor B (PDGF-B) and fibroblast growth factor (FGF-2), to reduce angiogenesis [119]. Downregulation of PDGF-B also restricts BC cell proliferation, survival, and migration, [117]. Metformin's effect on the microenvironment and angiogenesis has also been shown to enhance chemo-sensitivity, via a reduction in MVD leakage and cancer cell hypoxia *in vivo* [117]. Thus, metformin's effects go beyond the cancer cell itself and include the peri- and intratumoral microenvironment and neovasculature.

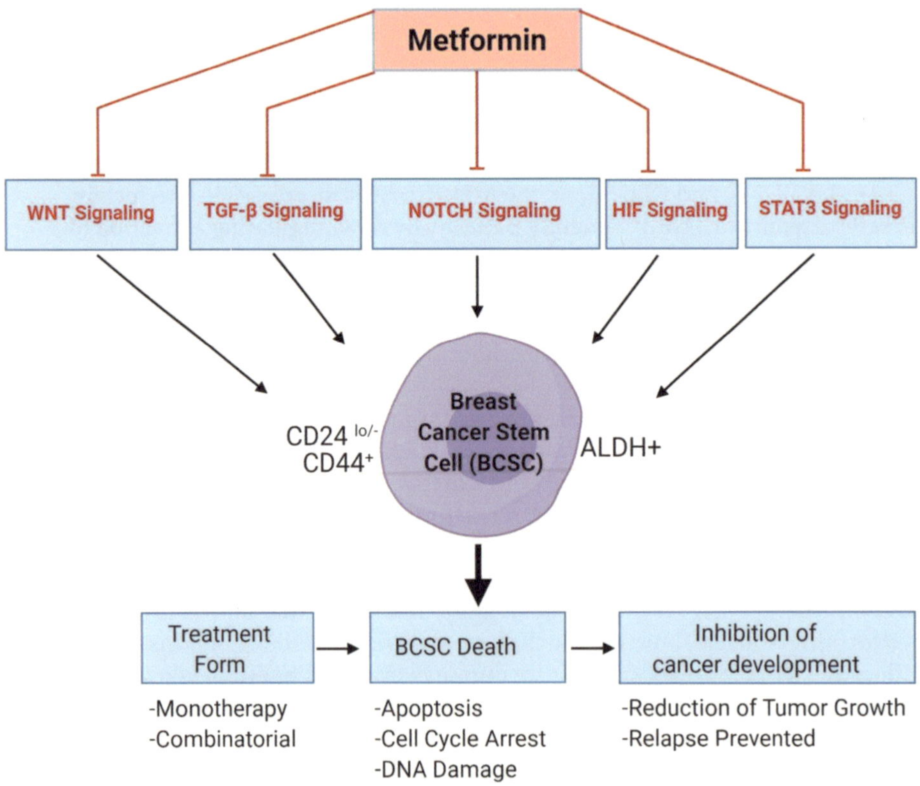

Figure 7.
Metformin action on breast cancer stem cells. Metformin can block a myriad of signaling pathways involved in BCSCs, including WNT, transforming growth factor (TGF), NOTCH, hypoxia inducible factor (HIF), and STAT3 signaling pathways. These pathways are thought to enrich for BCSC through the enrichment of CD44 positive receptor and aldehyde dehydrogenase (ALDH+) and decrease in CD24 expression. Metformin can be given as a monotherapy or combinatorial therapy with alternate chemotherapeutic agents, which in turn can induce BCSC death with an increase in apoptosis, cell cycle arrest, and DNA damage. Overall, reduction in BCSCs can result in reduction of tumor growth and prevention in therapy-mediated relapse.

4.8 Metformin action on breast cancer stem cells

Cancer stem cells (CSCs), also known as tumor-initiating cells (TICs), are the progenitor cells that give rise to BC as well as heterogeneity within transformed populations. CSCs are maintained as a subpopulation within the neoplasm that perpetuates clonal expansion and may facilitate dormancy, metastasis, chemoresistance, and relapse. Among the molecular BC subtypes, TNBC shows the highest enrichment of CSCs, identified by expression patterns with flow cytometry as CD44+, CD24−/low CSC [120]. BC CSCs are particularly sensitive to metformin, which induces rapid cell death facilitated through a number of pathways involved in cell differentiation, renewal, metastasis, and metabolism (**Figure** 7). It directly targets key CSC gene signatures such as Notch 1, NFκB, Sox2, KLF-4, Oct4, Lin28, MMP-9, and MMP-2 [121]. Metformin attenuates CSCs in resistant BC, through repression of let-7 miRNA [121]. Its ability to attenuate key metabolic genes, such as FASN via upregulation of miR-193b, also contributes to its anti-CSC activity as stem cells are heavily dependent on aerobic glycolysis [92].

The capacity of metformin to induce CSC cell death has significant clinical relevance, given their role in therapeutic resistance, dormancy, and disease progression. Metformin reduces cancer recurrence through the preferential killing of differentiated rather than undifferentiated CSCs [122]. In combination with chemotherapy, metformin is especially active against BC CSCs [111]. In studies of trastuzumab-resistant BC cells as well as xenograft models, the combination of trastuzumab and metformin significantly reduced CD44+, CD24−/low CSC subpopulations and reduced tumor volume [111, 123, 124]. In combination with doxorubicin, paclitaxel, or carboplatin, metformin can also eradicate CSCs and reduce the effective dosage required of the highly toxic chemotherapeutic agents, minimizing patient risk [111, 123].

5. Clinical evidence with metformin in breast cancer prevention and treatment

The pleiotropic oncostatic effects of metformin have been explored as an adjuvant therapeutic option for the management of BC [43, 125, 126]. Epidemiological studies have demonstrated associations between metformin use in patients with type 2 diabetes and decreased cancer incidence and cancer-related mortality [10]. Several observational and randomized trials have evaluated a number of biomarker changes after metformin administration, increasing the footage of metformin as an off-label agent for BC. Over 11 ongoing and 13 completed clinical trials have tested the efficacy of metformin as a monotherapy or in combination with chemotherapy and/or radiotherapy for the management of BC (reviewed in [43, 127]). Goodwin *et al.* have shown that after six months of metformin treatment, a reduction in insulin by 22% had improved metabolic indices, such as insulin sensitivity, body weight, and cholesterol levels in nondiabetic patients with early-stage BC [29]. This information suggests that metformin is effective in the nondiabetic population. These data and other clinical trials further provide support in using metformin as an adjuvant agent as it is the only agent that does not promote BC but actually retards tumor growth. In addition, these clinical trials further support the need to screen for metabolic dysfunction and evaluate whether or not metformin should be integrated into the treatment for BC therapy. Further, BC patients receiving 1500 mg/day of metformin showed a significant reduction in insulin levels and insulin resistance [44, 128]. The effect of metformin in response to neoadjuvant chemotherapy has been examined in diabetic BC patients. This study included 2529 women with BC and confirmed that metformin could achieve higher pathological complete response with neoadjuvant therapy relative to non-metformin users [129]. Dowling et al. have further examined neoadjuvant metformin in a prospective window of opportunity study [32]. Clinical and biological effects of metformin on nondiabetic BC patients were evaluated. These patients were treated with 500 mg of metformin three times daily for 2 weeks. Significant attenuated expression of the insulin receptor was observed in treated breast tumors and had high expression of OCT1 (organic cation transporter 1) [32]. The effect of metformin in nondiabetic BC patients was previously reviewed [43]. Systemic reviews and meta-analyses, highlighting a summary of studies involving metformin therapy in nondiabetic patients and diabetic patients, were reviewed in [43].

5.1 Metformin dose recommended for breast cancer patients

Pharmacokinetic profiling of mouse tumors provided preclinical analysis of appropriate human doses to provide efficient inhibition of tumor growth [130]. Based on this evidence, metformin-mediated activation of AMPK and antitumor function was dependent on cellular uptake of the drug, which is primarily controlled by membrane transporters OCT1, OCT2, and OCT3 [131]. Based on the high expression of OCT transporters, 850 mg/day of metformin is required to inhibit tumor growth efficiently. If a tumor expresses low levels of OCT transporter, then 2250 mg/day is recommended [132]. Additionally, a dose of metformin of 500–850 mg/day is typically recommended with standard chemotherapy (including anthracyclines, platinum, taxanes, and capecitabine) for first- or second-line therapy (please see https://www.drugbank.ca/drugs/DB00331). The combination of metformin with a chemotherapeutic agent is recommended for a number of cycles until progression is unacceptable or toxicity develops.

5.2 Indications and contraindications for metformin use for breast cancer

Metformin is not approved for clinical use by the FDA and is still considered investigational for the treatment for BC. While metformin is well established as an inexpensive, well-tolerated, and effective for the treatment of diabetes, adjuvant use of metformin for BC remains to be defined. Current clinical trials have not outlined indications and contraindications for metformin use as adjuvant therapy for BC. Generally, metformin hydrochloride tablets are contraindicated in patients with (1) severe renal impairment (eGFR below 30 mL/min/1.73 m2), (2) hypersensitivity to metformin, and (3) acute or chronic metabolic acidosis including diabetic ketoacidosis. Additionally, current clinical trials with metformin have been listed (https://clinicaltrials.gov/ct2/show/NCT01310231 and https://clinicaltrials.gov/ct2/show/NCT01101438). The NCIC CTG MA.32 Phase III randomized clinical trial has completed enrollment of 3649 nondiabetic women receiving standard surgical, chemotherapeutic, hormonal, biologic, and radiation treatment for T1-3, N0-3, M0 breast cancer. This trial has provided preliminary findings [33] and has not defined clear indications and/or contraindications for metformin use as adjuvant therapy for breast cancer.

6. Conclusions

A preponderance of clinical, epidemiological, and scientific evidence indicates that metabolic dysregulation of carbohydrate and lipid metabolism promote BC pathogenesis and a worse outcome, for women who have the disease [9, 10, 30, 40, 45, 129, 133].

One of the therapeutic agents commonly used in patients with metabolic syndrome or type 2 diabetes, metformin, has demonstrated significant anti-BC activity. Metformin inhibits gluconeogenesis, reduces circulating levels of glucose, increases insulin sensitivity, and reduces hyperinsulinemia associated with insulin [134]. These factors have been associated with BC prognosis. Several mechanisms of metformin action involve AMPK-dependent and AMPK-independent signaling pathways, and these effects are remarkably broad and potent. Its ability to target metabolic dysregulation of carbohydrate and lipid metabolism as well as cancer stem cells appear to be equally important in its anticancer activity against BC [129, 133–137]. Furthermore, the effects of metformin are unique among molecular subsets of BC. A better understanding of these mechanisms will facilitate targeted applications in patients with specific subtypes, fostering the goal of more personalized cancer care.

A number of clinical trials are underway to evaluate metformin in BC patients [30, 44–46, 50, 136]. Most have been designed to evaluate its efficacy, in combination with various chemo- or radiotherapy agents; see (https://clinicaltrials.gov/ct2/results?term=+cancer+AND+metformin). Most ongoing or completed clinical trials have evaluated metformin's effect on cellular proliferation or death, pathological response rate, progression-free or overall survival. Some have also sought to compare its efficacy in patients with or without metabolic dysregulation, as a secondary aim. None have specifically been designed to evaluate interactions with CSCs, or in selected molecular subtypes, although correlative studies have provided some data in this regard. The ALTTO trial has shown that metformin improves outcomes for patients with diabetes and either HER2+ or hormone receptor positive BC [30]. The NCIC Clinical Trials Group (NCIC CTG) MA.32 has shown benefit from metformin, as compared to placebo on outcomes in early stage BC [33]. It demonstrated efficacy with improvements in body weight, insulin, glucose, and leptin levels in BC patients examined, regardless of baseline BMI or fasting insulin levels [33].

In conclusion, metformin is a unique drug with a long track record of human use, which has demonstrated robust efficacy against type 2 diabetes and metabolic dysregulation. Epidemiologic data show independent and significant benefit in preventing cardiovascular disease and cancer in these patients. Metformin is an inexpensive oral agent that is currently available worldwide. It is generally well tolerated and has a low risk:benefit ratio. Epidemiological and clinical data have shown that metformin reduces BC incidence and mortality in women with metabolic dysregulation, obesity, and type 2 diabetes. This subpopulation of woman is at significantly higher risk for BC, particularly in the postmenopausal setting. Preclinical and clinical evidence shows that metformin inhibits BC cell replication and tumor growth, decreases tumor aggression, reduces the stem cell pool, and slows motility/metastasis and can promote cell death through apoptosis, autophagy, or upregulation of immunity. Metformin has unique effects on molecular subsets of BC, with the aggressive triple negative BC showing the most sensitivity and lowest EC50 data. TNBC is particularly sensitive to metformin's downregulation of fatty acid and cholesterol biosynthesis, glucose transport, and carbohydrate metabolism. This cancer subtype is typically the most aggressive and is less responsive to traditional chemotherapy; thus, metformin's potency may provide significant benefit especially in these patients.

Acknowledgements

Grant support provided in part by Susan G Komen for the Cure K100575 to RSW, SME, and ADT; ACS-IRG 16-184-56 RSW from the American Cancer Society; CCL-C92110 RSW and ADT from the Colorado Cancer League.

Conflict of interest

The authors have declared that no conflict of interest exists.

Abbreviations

ACAA2	Acetyl-coenzyme A acetyltransferase 2
ADP	Adenosine di-phosphate
AKT	Protein kinase B
ALTTO	Adjuvant lapatinib and/or trastuzumab treatment optimization
AMP	Adenosine monophosphate
AMPK	AMP-activated protein kinase
AMPKK	AMP-activated protein kinase kinase
ATP	Adenosine triphosphate
AR	Androgen receptor
BC	Breast cancer
BCSCs	Breast cancer stem cells
CDK	Cyclin-dependent kinase
CL	Claudin-low
CLDN	Claudin integral membrane proteins of tight junctions
CSC	Cancer stem cells
DHCR24	24-dehydrocholesterol reductase
ESR1	Estrogen receptor
HIF-1α	Hypoxia-inducible factor 1-alpha
EC	Effective concentration/Inhibitory concentration
EGFR	Epidermal growth factor receptor
EMT	Epithelial mesenchymal transition
FASN	Fatty acid synthase
FDA	Food and Drug Administration
FGFR2	Fibroblast growth factor receptor 2
FGFR3	Fibroblast growth factor receptor 3
GLUT1	Glucose transporter 1
GM1	GM1 gangliosidosis marker
HER2	Human epidermal growth factor receptor 2
HER3:	Human epidermal growth factor receptor 3
HMGCo-A	β-Hydroxy β-methylglutaryl-CoA
HMGCS1	Hydroxymethylglutaryl-CoA synthase
HMGCR	3-Hydroxy-3-Methylglutaryl-CoA Reductase
ID1	Inhibitor of differentiation-1
IGFIR	Insulin-like growth factor receptor
IGF1	Insulin-like growth factor-1
IRS1	Insulin receptor substrate 1
IL-1β	Interleukin 1 beta
IL-6	Interleukin-like 6
JAK	Janus kinase
LDLR	Low-density lipoprotein receptor
LKB1	Liver kinase B1
LSS	Lanosterol synthase
MAPK	Mitogen-activated protein kinases
MβCD	Methyl-β-cyclodextrin
MTOR	Mammalian target of rapamycin
MRCC1	Mitochondrial respiratory-chain complex 1

MSL	Mesenchymal stem-like
MVD	Mevalonate diphosphate decarboxylase
MVK	Mevalonate kinase
NCIC CTG	NCIC Clinical Trials Group
NF-κB	Nuclear factor kappa-light-chain-enhancer of activated B-cells
OCT1	Organic cation transporter 1
OCT2	Organic cation transporter 2
OCT3	Organic cation transporter 2
P-	Phosphorylated
P53	Tumor protein 53
PARP	Poly (ADP-ribose) polymerase
PGR	Progesterone receptor
PI3K	Phosphatidyl-inositide 3-kinase
PTEN	Phosphatase and tensin homolog
RNA	Ribonucleic acid
ROS	Reactive oxygen species
SRC	Proto-oncogene c-Src
SREBP1	Sterol regulatory element-binding transcription factor 1
STAT3	Signal transducer and activator of transcription 3
TGF-β	Transforming growth factor beta
TNBC	Triple negative breast cancer
TNF-α	Tumor necrosis factor alpha
TSC2	Tuberous sclerosis complex 2
US	United States
VEGF	Vascular endothelial growth factor

Author details

Reema S. Wahdan-Alaswad and Ann D. Thor*
Department of Pathology, University of Colorado Anschutz Medical Campus, Aurora, Colorado, United States of America

*Address all correspondence to: ann.thor@cuanschutz.edu

References

[1] Warburg O. On the origin of cancer cells. Science. 1956;**123**(3191):309-314

[2] Warburg O, Wind F, Negelein E. The metabolism of tumors in the body. The Journal of General Physiology. 1927;**8**(6):519-530

[3] Young CD, Anderson SM. Sugar and fat - that's where it's at: Metabolic changes in tumors. Breast Cancer Research. 2008;**10**(1):202

[4] Warburg O, Geissler AW, Lorenz S. On growth of cancer cells in media in which glucose is replaced by galactose. Hoppe-Seyler's Zeitschrift für Physiologische Chemie. 1967;**348**(12):1686-1687

[5] Gatenby RA, Gillies RJ. Why do cancers have high aerobic glycolysis? Nature Reviews. Cancer. 2004;**4**(11):891-899

[6] Viollet B et al. Cellular and molecular mechanisms of metformin: An overview. Clinical Science. 2012;**122**(6):253-270

[7] Zhou G et al. Role of AMP-activated protein kinase in mechanism of metformin action. The Journal of Clinical Investigation. 2001;**108**(8):1167-1174

[8] Algire C et al. Metformin reduces endogenous reactive oxygen species and associated DNA damage. Cancer Prevention Research. 2012;**5**(4):536-543

[9] Bowker SL et al. Increased cancer-related mortality for patients with type 2 diabetes who use sulfonylureas or insulin. Diabetes Care. 2006;**29**(2):254-258

[10] Evans JM et al. Metformin and reduced risk of cancer in diabetic patients. BMJ. 2005;**330**(7503):1304-1305

[11] Centers for Disease Control and Prevention. National Diabetes Statistics Report, 2017. Atlanta, GA: Centers for Disease Control and Prevention, U.S. Dept of Health and Human Services; 2017. p. 2017

[12] Center for Disease Control and Prevention. National Diabetes Fact Sheet: General Information and National Estimates on Diabetes in the United States, 2005. Atlanta: U. S. Department of Health and Human Services, Center for Disese Control and Prevention; 2005

[13] Bloomgarden ZT. Developments in diabetes and insulin resistance. Diabetes Care. 2006;**29**(1):161-167

[14] Pasanisi P et al. Metabolic syndrome as a prognostic factor for breast cancer recurrences. International Journal of Cancer. 2006;**119**(1):236-238

[15] Vona-Davis L, Howard-McNatt M, Rose DP. Adiposity, type 2 diabetes and the metabolic syndrome in breast cancer. Obesity Reviews. 2007;**8**(5):395-408

[16] Wani B et al. Metabolic syndrome and breast cancer risk. Indian Journal of Medical and Paediatric Oncology. 2017;**38**(4):434-439

[17] Xue F, Michels KB. Diabetes, metabolic syndrome, and breast cancer: A review of the current evidence. The American Journal of Clinical Nutrition. 2007;**86**(3):s823-s835

[18] Schapira DV et al. Abdominal obesity and breast cancer risk. Annals of Internal Medicine. 1990;**112**(3):182-186

[19] Stoll BA. Upper abdominal obesity, insulin resistance and breast cancer risk. International Journal of Obesity and Related Metabolic Disorders. 2002;**26**(6):747-753

[20] Barnett GC et al. Risk factors for the incidence of breast cancer: Do they affect survival from the disease? Journal of Clinical Oncology. 2008;**26**(20):3310-3316

[21] Barnett JB. The relationship between obesity and breast cancer risk and mortality. Nutrition Reviews. 2003;**61**(2):73-76

[22] Fernandez JR, Allison DB. Understanding racial differences in obesity and metabolic syndrome traits. Nutrition Reviews. 2003;**61**(9):316-319

[23] Harvie M, Hooper L, Howell AH. Central obesity and breast cancer risk: A systematic review. Obesity Reviews. 2003;**4**(3):157-173

[24] Lipscombe LL et al. The impact of diabetes on survival following breast cancer. Breast Cancer Research and Treatment. 2008;**109**(2):389-395

[25] Peairs AD, Rankin JW, Lee YW. Effects of acute ingestion of different fats on oxidative stress and inflammation in overweight and obese adults. Nutrition Journal. 2011;**10**:122

[26] Wahdan-Alaswad R et al. Glucose promotes breast cancer aggression and reduces metformin efficacy. Cell Cycle. 2013;**12**(24):3759-3769

[27] Renehan AG, Frystyk J, Flyvbjerg A. Obesity and cancer risk: The role of the insulin-IGF axis. Trends in Endocrinology and Metabolism. 2006;**17**(8):328-336

[28] Pollak MN, Schernhammer ES, Hankinson SE. Insulin-like growth factors and neoplasia. Nature Reviews. Cancer. 2004;**4**(7):505-518

[29] Goodwin PJ. Insulin in the adjuvant breast cancer setting: A novel therapeutic target for lifestyle and pharmacologic interventions? Journal of Clinical Oncology. 2008;**26**(6):833-834

[30] Sonnenblick A et al. Impact of diabetes, insulin, and metformin use on the outcome of patients with human epidermal growth factor receptor 2-positive primary breast cancer: Analysis from the ALTTO phase III randomized trial. Journal of Clinical Oncology. 2017;**35**(13):1421-1429

[31] Christopoulos PF, Msaouel P, Koutsilieris M. The role of the insulin-like growth factor-1 system in breast cancer. Molecular Cancer. 2015;**14**:43

[32] Dowling RJ et al. Changes in insulin receptor signaling underlie neoadjuvant metformin administration in breast cancer: A prospective window of opportunity neoadjuvant study. Breast Cancer Research. 2015;**17**:32

[33] Goodwin PJ et al. Effect of metformin vs placebo on and metabolic factors in NCIC CTG MA.32. Journal of the National Cancer Institute. 2015;**107**(3):djv006

[34] Jiralerspong S, Goodwin PJ. Obesity and breast cancer prognosis: Evidence, challenges, and opportunities. Journal of Clinical Oncology. 2016;**34**(35):4203-4216

[35] Alokail MS et al. Combined effects of obesity and type 2 diabetes contribute to increased breast cancer risk in premenopausal women. Cardiovascular Diabetology. 2009;**8**:33

[36] Li YR, Ro V, Tchou JC. Obesity, metabolic syndrome, and breast cancer: From prevention to intervention. Current Surgery Reports. 2018;**6**(3):7

[37] Wang YW et al. Metformin: A review of its potential indications. Drug Design, Development and Therapy. 2017;**11**:2421-2429

[38] Michels KB et al. Type 2 diabetes and subsequent incidence of breast cancer in the Nurses' health study. Diabetes Care. 2003;**26**(6):1752-1758

[39] Chlebowski RT et al. Diabetes, metformin, and breast cancer in postmenopausal women. Journal of Clinical Oncology. 2012;**30**(23):2844-2852

[40] Xu H et al. Metformin use is associated with better survival of breast cancer patients with diabetes: A meta-analysis. The Oncologist. 2015;**20**(11):1236-1244

[41] Hede K. Doctors seek to prevent breast cancer recurrence by lowering insulin levels. Journal of the National Cancer Institute. 2008;**100**(8):530-532

[42] Barzilai N et al. Metformin as a tool to target aging. Cell Metabolism. 2016;**23**(6):1060-1065

[43] Roshan MH, Shing YK, Pace NP. Metformin as an adjuvant in breast cancer treatment. SAGE Open Medicine. 2019;7:2050312119865114

[44] Hadad S et al. Evidence for biological effects of metformin in operable breast cancer: A pre-operative, window-of-opportunity, randomized trial. Breast Cancer Research and Treatment. 2011;**128**(3):783-794

[45] Kalinsky K et al. Presurgical trial of metformin in overweight and obese patients with newly diagnosed breast cancer. Cancer Investigation. 2014;**32**(4):150-157

[46] Bonanni B et al. Dual effect of metformin on breast cancer proliferation in a randomized presurgical trial. Journal of Clinical Oncology. 2012;**30**(21):2593-2600

[47] Liu B et al. Metformin induces unique biological and molecular responses in triple negative breast cancer cells. Cell Cycle. 2009;**8**(13):2031-2040

[48] Varghese S et al. High glucose represses the anti-proliferative and pro-apoptotic effect of metformin in triple negative breast cancer cells. Biomolecules. 2019;**9**(1):16

[49] Wahdan-Alaswad RS et al. Metformin targets glucose metabolism in triple negative breast cancer. Journal of Oncology Translational Research. 2018;**4**(1):E16

[50] Martin-Castillo B et al. A phase 2 trial of neoadjuvant metformin in combination with trastuzumab and chemotherapy in women with early HER2-positive breast cancer: The METTEN study. Oncotarget. 2018;**9**(86):35687-35704

[51] Kim J et al. Anticancer effect of metformin on estrogen receptor-positive and tamoxifen-resistant breast cancer cell lines. Oncology Reports. 2016;**35**(5):2553-2560

[52] Checkley LA et al. Metformin accumulation correlates with organic Cation transporter 2 protein expression and predicts mammary tumor regression In vivo. Cancer Prevention Research. 2017;**10**(3):198-207

[53] Jin HE et al. Reduced antidiabetic effect of metformin and down-regulation of hepatic Oct1 in rats with ethynylestradiol-induced cholestasis. Pharmaceutical Research. 2009;**26**(3):549-559

[54] Shu Y et al. Effect of genetic variation in the organic cation transporter 1 (OCT1) on metformin action. The Journal of Clinical Investigation. 2007;**117**(5):1422-1431

[55] Tzvetkov MV et al. The effects of genetic polymorphisms in the organic cation transporters OCT1, OCT2, and OCT3 on the renal clearance of metformin. Clinical Pharmacology and Therapeutics. 2009;**86**(3):299-306

[56] Jones RG et al. AMP-activated protein kinase induces a p53-dependent

metabolic checkpoint. Molecular Cell. 2005;**18**(3):283-293

[57] Alimova IN et al. Metformin inhibits breast cancer cell growth, colony formation and induces cell cycle arrest in vitro. Cell Cycle. 2009;**8**(6):909-915

[58] Hsieh Li SM et al. Metformin causes cancer cell death through downregulation of p53-dependent differentiated embryo chondrocyte 1. Journal of Biomedical Science. 2018;**25**(1):81

[59] Tanaka R et al. Metformin causes G1-phase arrest via Down-regulation of MiR-221 and enhances TRAIL sensitivity through DR5 up-regulation in pancreatic cancer cells. PLoS One. 2015;**10**(5):e0125779

[60] Ben Sahra I et al. The antidiabetic drug metformin exerts an antitumoral effect in vitro and in vivo through a decrease of cyclin D1 level. Oncogene. 2008;**27**(25):3576-3586

[61] Zhuang Y, Miskimins WK. Cell cycle arrest in metformin treated breast cancer cells involves activation of AMPK, downregulation of cyclin D1, and requires p27Kip1 or p21Cip1. Journal of Molecular Signaling. 2008;**3**:18

[62] Bachman KE et al. The PIK3CA gene is mutated with high frequency in human breast cancers. Cancer Biology & Therapy. 2004;**3**(8):772-775

[63] McAuliffe PF et al. Deciphering the role of PI3K/Akt/mTOR pathway in breast cancer biology and pathogenesis. Clinical Breast Cancer. 2010;**10**(Suppl 3): S59-S65

[64] Sansal I, Sellers WR. The biology and clinical relevance of the PTEN tumor suppressor pathway. Journal of Clinical Oncology. 2004;**22**(14):2954-2963

[65] Kechagioglou P et al. Tumor suppressor PTEN in breast cancer: Heterozygosity, mutations and protein expression. Anticancer Research. 2014;**34**(3):1387-1400

[66] Kalender A et al. Metformin, independent of AMPK, inhibits mTORC1 in a rag GTPase-dependent manner. Cell Metabolism. 2010;**11**(5):390-401

[67] Gwinn DM et al. AMPK phosphorylation of raptor mediates a metabolic checkpoint. Molecular Cell. 2008;**30**(2):214-226

[68] Zhu P et al. Metformin selectively targets tumor-initiating cells in ErbB2-overexpressing breast cancer models. Cancer Prevention Research. 2014;7(2):199-210

[69] Ben Sahra I et al. Metformin in cancer therapy: A new perspective for an old antidiabetic drug? Molecular Cancer Therapeutics. 2010;**9**(5):1092-1099

[70] Cha JH et al. Metformin promotes antitumor immunity via endoplasmic-reticulum-associated degradation of PD-L1. Molecular Cell. 2018;**71**(4): 606-620 e7

[71] Eikawa S et al. Immune-mediated antitumor effect by type 2 diabetes drug, metformin. Proceedings of the National Academy of Sciences of the United States of America. 2015;**112**(6):1809-1814

[72] Ba W et al. Metformin inhibits pro-inflammatory responses via targeting nuclear factor-kappaB in HaCaT cells. Cell Biochemistry and Function. 2019;**37**(1):4-10

[73] Kurelac I et al. The multifaceted effects of metformin on tumor microenvironment. Seminars in Cell & Developmental Biology. 2019;**98**:90-97

[74] Jiralerspong S et al. Obesity, diabetes, and survival outcomes in a large cohort of early-stage breast

cancer patients. Annals of Oncology. 2013;**24**(10):2506-2514

[75] Oliveras-Ferraros C, Vazquez-Martin A, Menendez JA. Genome-wide inhibitory impact of the AMPK activator metformin on [kinesins, tubulins, histones, auroras and polo-like kinases] M-phase cell cycle genes in human breast cancer cells. Cell Cycle. 2009;**8**(10):1633-1636

[76] Rocha GZ et al. Metformin amplifies chemotherapy-induced AMPK activation and antitumoral growth. Clinical Cancer Research. 2011;**17**(12):3993-4005

[77] Bellet M et al. Palbociclib and ribociclib in breast cancer: Consensus workshop on the management of concomitant medication. Therapeutic Advances in Medical Oncology. 2019;**11**:1758835919833867

[78] Vazquez-Martin A et al. The anti-diabetic drug metformin suppresses self-renewal and proliferation of trastuzumab-resistant tumor-initiating breast cancer stem cells. Breast Cancer Research and Treatment. 2011;**126**(2):355-364

[79] Zhao H et al. AMP-activated protein kinase and energy balance in breast cancer. American Journal of Translational Research. 2017;**9**(2):197-213

[80] Huang Z et al. Dual effects of weight and weight gain on breast cancer risk. JAMA. 1997;**278**(17):1407-1411

[81] Nelson HD et al. Risk factors for breast cancer for women aged 40 to 49 years: A systematic review and meta-analysis. Annals of Internal Medicine. 2012;**156**(9):635-648

[82] Marbaniang C, Kma L. Dysregulation of glucose metabolism by oncogenes and tumor suppressors in cancer cells. Asian Pacific Journal of Cancer Prevention. 2018;**19**(9):2377-2390

[83] Lien EC, Lyssiotis CA, Cantley LC. Metabolic reprogramming by the PI3K-Akt-mTOR pathway in cancer. Recent Results in Cancer Research. 2016;**207**:39-72

[84] Lin DS et al. Inflexibility of AMPK-mediated metabolic reprogramming in mitochondrial disease. Oncotarget. 2017;**8**(43):73627-73639

[85] Vaupel P, Schmidberger H, Mayer A. The Warburg effect: Essential part of metabolic reprogramming and central contributor to cancer progression. International Journal of Radiation Biology. 2019;**95**(7):912-919

[86] Chen C et al. Metabolic reprogramming by HIF-1 activation enhances survivability of human adipose-derived stem cells in ischaemic microenvironments. Cell Proliferation. 2017;**50**(5):e12363

[87] Shen L et al. Metabolic reprogramming in triple-negative breast cancer through Myc suppression of TXNIP. Proceedings of the National Academy of Sciences of the United States of America. 2015;**112**(17):5425-5430

[88] Deng XS et al. Metformin targets Stat3 to inhibit cell growth and induce apoptosis in triple-negative breast cancers. Cell Cycle. 2012;**11**(2):367-376

[89] Liu B et al. Potent anti-proliferative effects of metformin on trastuzumab-resistant breast cancer cells via inhibition of erbB2/IGF-1 receptor interactions. Cell Cycle. 2011;**10**(17):2959-2966

[90] Wahdan-Alaswad R et al. Metformin attenuates transforming growth factor beta (TGF-beta) mediated oncogenesis in mesenchymal

stem-like/claudin-low triple negative breast cancer. Cell Cycle. 2016;**15**(8):1046-1059

[91] Wahdan-Alaswad RS, Edgerton SM, Salem HS, Thor AD. Metformin targets cholesterol biosynthesis pathway, GM1 lipid raft stabilization, EGFR signaling and proliferation in triple negative breast cancers. Cancer Therapy and Oncology International Journal. 2018;**9**(3):555765

[92] Wahdan-Alaswad RS et al. Metformin-induced killing of triple-negative breast cancer cells is mediated by reduction in fatty acid synthase via miRNA-193b. Hormones and Cancer. 2014;**5**(6):374-389

[93] Giles ED et al. Obesity and overfeeding affecting both tumor and systemic metabolism activates the progesterone receptor to contribute to postmenopausal breast cancer. Cancer Research. 2012;**72**(24):6490-6501

[94] Lanning NJ et al. Metabolic profiling of triple-negative breast cancer cells reveals metabolic vulnerabilities. Cancer & Metabolism. 2017;**5**:6

[95] Wellberg EA et al. The glucose transporter GLUT1 is required for ErbB2-induced mammary tumorigenesis. Breast Cancer Research. 2016;**18**(1):131

[96] Karlic H et al. Inhibition of the mevalonate pathway affects epigenetic regulation in cancer cells. Cancer Genetics. 2015;**208**(5):241-252

[97] Nilsson S, Huelsenbeck J, Fritz G. Mevalonate pathway inhibitors affect anticancer drug-induced cell death and DNA damage response of human sarcoma cells. Cancer Letters. 2011;**304**(1):60-69

[98] Chimento A et al. Cholesterol and its metabolites in tumor growth: Therapeutic potential of statins in cancer treatment. Frontiers in Endocrinology. 2018;**9**:807

[99] Ding X et al. The role of cholesterol metabolism in cancer. American Journal of Cancer Research. 2019;**9**(2):219-227

[100] Ehmsen S et al. Increased cholesterol biosynthesis is a key characteristic of breast cancer stem cells influencing patient outcome. Cell Reports. 2019;**27**(13):3927-3938 e6

[101] Murtola TJ et al. Statin use and breast cancer survival: A nationwide cohort study from Finland. PLoS One. 2014;**9**(10):e110231

[102] Ahern TP et al. Statin prescriptions and breast cancer recurrence risk: A Danish nationwide prospective cohort study. Journal of the National Cancer Institute. 2011;**103**(19):1461-1468

[103] Borgquist S et al. Statins: A role in breast cancer therapy? Journal of Internal Medicine. 2018;**284**(4):346-357

[104] Sharma A et al. Metformin exhibited anticancer activity by lowering cellular cholesterol content in breast cancer cells. PLoS One. 2019;**14**(1):e0209435

[105] Bajan S, Hutvagner G. Regulation of miRNA processing and miRNA mediated gene repression in cancer. MicroRNA. 2014;**3**(1):10-17

[106] Yerukala Sathipati S, Ho SY. Identifying a miRNA signature for predicting the stage of breast cancer. Scientific Reports. 2018;**8**(1):16138

[107] Cioce M et al. Metformin-induced metabolic reprogramming of chemoresistant ALDHbright breast cancer cells. Oncotarget. 2014;**5**(12):4129-4143

[108] Pulito C et al. microRNAs and cancer metabolism reprogramming:

the paradigm of metformin. Annals of Translational Medicine. 2014;**2**(6):58

[109] Bertoli G, Cava C, Castiglioni I. MicroRNAs: New biomarkers for diagnosis, prognosis, therapy prediction and therapeutic tools for breast cancer. Theranostics. 2015;**5**(10):1122-1143

[110] Rutherford C et al. Phosphorylation of Janus kinase 1 (JAK1) by AMP-activated protein kinase (AMPK) links energy sensing to anti-inflammatory signaling. Science Signaling. 2016;**9**(453):ra109

[111] Hirsch HA, Iliopoulos D, Struhl K. Metformin inhibits the inflammatory response associated with cellular transformation and cancer stem cell growth. Proceedings of the National Academy of Sciences of the United States of America. 2013;**110**(3):972-977

[112] Leonel C et al. Inhibition of epithelial-Mesenchymal transition and metastasis by combined TGFbeta knockdown and metformin treatment in a canine mammary cancer Xenograft model. Journal of Mammary Gland Biology and Neoplasia. 2017;**22**(1):27-41

[113] Vazquez-Martin A et al. Metformin regulates breast cancer stem cell ontogeny by transcriptional regulation of the epithelial-mesenchymal transition (EMT) status. Cell Cycle. 2010;**9**(18):3807-3814

[114] Cufi S et al. Metformin against TGFbeta-induced epithelial-to-mesenchymal transition (EMT): From cancer stem cells to aging-associated fibrosis. Cell Cycle. 2010;**9**(22):4461-4468

[115] Oliveras-Ferraros C et al. Micro(mi)RNA expression profile of breast cancer epithelial cells treated with the anti-diabetic drug metformin: Induction of the tumor suppressor miRNA let-7a and suppression of the TGFbeta-induced oncomiR miRNA-181a. Cell Cycle. 2011;**10**(7):1144-1151

[116] Li C, Kong D. Cancer risks from diabetes therapies: Evaluating the evidence. Pharmacology & Therapeutics. 2014;**144**(1):71-81

[117] Kannarkatt J et al. Metformin and angiogenesis in cancer - revisited. Oncology. 2016;**91**(4):179-184

[118] Orecchioni S et al. The biguanides metformin and phenformin inhibit angiogenesis, local and metastatic growth of breast cancer by targeting both neoplastic and microenvironment cells. International Journal of Cancer. 2015;**136**(6):E534-E544

[119] Wang JC et al. Metformin inhibits metastatic breast cancer progression and improves chemosensitivity by inducing vessel normalization via PDGF-B downregulation. Journal of Experimental & Clinical Cancer Research. 2019;**38**(1):235

[120] Al-Hajj M et al. Prospective identification of tumorigenic breast cancer cells. Proceedings of the National Academy of Sciences of the United States of America. 2003;**100**(7):3983-3988

[121] Bao B et al. Metformin may function as anti-cancer agent via targeting cancer stem cells: The potential biological significance of tumor-associated miRNAs in breast and pancreatic cancers. Annals of Translational Medicine. 2014;**2**(6):59

[122] Saini N, Yang X. Metformin as an anti-cancer agent: Actions and mechanisms targeting cancer stem cells. Acta Biochimica et Biophysica Sinica. 2018;**50**(2):133-143

[123] Iliopoulos D, Hirsch HA, Struhl K. Metformin decreases the dose of chemotherapy for prolonging tumor remission in mouse xenografts involving

multiple cancer cell types. Cancer Research. 2011;**71**(9):3196-3201

[124] Cufi S et al. Metformin-induced preferential killing of breast cancer initiating CD44+CD24−/low cells is sufficient to overcome primary resistance to trastuzumab in HER2+ human breast cancer xenografts. Oncotarget. 2012;**3**(4):395-398

[125] Kheirandish M et al. Anti-cancer effects of metformin: Recent evidences for its role in prevention and treatment of cancer. Current Drug Metabolism. 2018;**19**(9):793-797

[126] Quinn BJ et al. Repositioning metformin for cancer prevention and treatment. Trends in Endocrinology and Metabolism. 2013;**24**(9):469-480

[127] De A, Kuppusamy G. Metformin in breast cancer: Preclinical and clinical evidence. Current Problems in Cancer. 2019:100488. DOI: 10.1016/j.currproblcancer.2019.06.003. [Epub ahead of print]

[128] Hadad SM et al. Evidence for biological effects of metformin in operable breast cancer: Biomarker analysis in a pre-operative window of opportunity randomized trial. Breast Cancer Research and Treatment. 2015;**150**(1):149-155

[129] Jiralerspong S et al. Metformin and pathologic complete responses to neoadjuvant chemotherapy in diabetic patients with breast cancer. Journal of Clinical Oncology. 2009;**27**(20):3297-3302

[130] Dowling RJ et al. Metformin pharmacokinetics in mouse tumors: Implications for human therapy. Cell Metabolism. 2016;**23**(4):567-568

[131] Graham GG et al. Clinical pharmacokinetics of metformin. Clinical Pharmacokinetics. 2011;**50**(2):81-98

[132] Cai H, Everett RS, Thakker DR. Efficacious dose of metformin for breast cancer therapy is determined by cation transporter expression in tumours. British Journal of Pharmacology. 2019;**176**(15):2724-2735

[133] Tang GH et al. Association of Metformin with breast cancer incidence and mortality in patients with type II diabetes: A GRADE-assessed systematic review and meta-analysis. Cancer Epidemiology, Biomarkers & Prevention. 2018;**27**(6):627-635

[134] Cusi K, Consoli A, DeFronzo RA. Metabolic effects of metformin on glucose and lactate metabolism in noninsulin-dependent diabetes mellitus. The Journal of Clinical Endocrinology and Metabolism. 1996;**81**(11):4059-4067

[135] Chae YK et al. Repurposing metformin for cancer treatment: Current clinical studies. Oncotarget. 2016;7(26):40767-40780

[136] Monami M, Dicembrini I, Mannucci E. Thiazolidinediones and cancer: Results of a meta-analysis of randomized clinical trials. Acta Diabetologica. 2014;**51**(1):91-101

[137] Qu C et al. Metformin reverses multidrug resistance and epithelial-mesenchymal transition (EMT) via activating AMP-activated protein kinase (AMPK) in human breast cancer cells. Molecular and Cellular Biochemistry. 2014;**386**(1-2):63-71

Section 4

Metformin and Ageing

Chapter 12

Metformin Modulates the Mechanisms of Ageing

Adriana Florinela Cătoi, Andra Diana Andreicuț, Dan Cristian Vodnar, Katalin Szabo, Andreea Corina, Andreea Arsene, Simona Diana Stefan, Roxana Adriana Stoica and Manfredi Rizzo

Abstract

Living in a time when population is continuously ageing, the challenge and demand for assessing the age-related pathways, potential diseases and longevity have become of major interest. The pharmaceutical industry possesses huge resources in this field, mainly due to the recent discoveries of novel mechanisms of action of old-established, classical drugs. Here we find metformin, a well-established antidiabetic medicine but with new potential benefits, as the most recent reports quote. We present the main pathways of the possible implications of metformin in the modulation of ageing processes, evolution and diseases, focussing on its ageing counteraction, based on the latest scientifically based biochemical reports.

Keywords: metformin, type 2 diabetes, mechanisms of ageing, anti-ageing

1. Introduction

At present, metformin is the preferred first-line drug used for the treatment of type 2 diabetes mellitus (T2DM) [1–4]. However, the journey of metformin (1,1-dimethylbiguanide hydrochloride) has not been a simple one. *Galega officinalis*, also termed as French lilac, Italian fitch, or Spanish sainfoin, the herb metformin derives from, has been known as a traditional medicine since the seventeenth century and was recommended for the treatment of thirst and frequent urination (symptoms of diabetes) by John Hill in 1772. The identification of guanidine and of its related compounds within *Galega officinalis*, which proved to be able to reduce blood glucose in animals, led to the synthesis of metformin (dimethylbiguanide) in 1922. However, it was only in the 1950s that more information on metformin's properties was published and when the name of Glucophage, meaning glucose eater, was suggested by Jean Sterne. Metformin was introduced as a treatment for T2DM in 1958 in the UK and in other European countries, whereas in the USA it was approved only in 1994 and started to be used beginning in 1995 [5]. A milestone multicentre trial, the United Kingdom Prospective Diabetes Study (UKPDS) in 1998, showed that the newly T2DM diagnosed patients receiving metformin for more than a decade displayed significant reduction of the cardiovascular events and of diabetes-related death and highlighted that these effects were independent of the glucose-lowering efficacy. Moreover, the potentially beneficial effects of metformin on the macro- and microvasculature have also been revealed [5–8]. Finally, in a 10-year posttrial analysis, metformin continues to offer cardiovascular benefits [9]. Based on these evidence data, in 2009, the American Diabetes Association (ADA) and the European Association for the Study of Diabetes (EASD) indicated metformin as the first-line therapy for T2DM [10]. Furthermore, metformin holds a significant role in the delay/prevention of T2DM onset, as shown by the randomised trial conducted in the USA, i.e. the Diabetes Prevention Program (DPP). The study highlighted that metformin reduces the incidence of T2DM by 31% compared to placebo in adults at high risk for T2DM (obese and with impaired glucose tolerance) [11–14]. Hence, metformin is also recommended as a pharmacologic tool for the prevention of T2DM in subjects with prediabetes, mainly for those with a BMI ≥ 35 kg/m [2], those aged <60 years, and in women with prior gestational diabetes mellitus [15–17].

Ageing continues to be an intruding topic and an area of great interest, constantly addressed by researchers worldwide. It encompasses a plethora of complex processes that have urged scientists to decipher its underlying mechanisms and to find the possible avenues to postpone its onset and that of its associated diseases [18]. Data from the literature have demonstrated a sustained ageing of the world's population, estimating a total of around 21.8% of subjects over 60 years old in 2050 and 32.2% in 2100 [19]. Installed as a result of the interaction between genetic, epigenetic, environmental and stochastic factors, ageing involves a progressive decline of the body functions as a consequence of the gradual cellular impairment due to a failure of the repair mechanisms [20–23]. Age is a major risk factor for the onset of metabolic, cardiovascular, neurodegenerative, immune and malignant diseases [24]. Ageing has been reported to be conditioned by the genetic factor in a proportion of 25–30%, while the remaining 70–75% is ruled by the environmental factor, making it a possible target for therapeutic tools among which metformin has been found [25, 26].

Beyond its blood glucose-lowering effect, metformin has been described as a drug used for preventing or delaying several conditions associated with ageing [27]. As such, metformin has been proven useful in overweight and obesity [28, 29], hypertension [30], atherosclerosis [31], coronary artery disease [32], dementia [33] and cancer [34]. Moreover, in terms of mortality [35], it has been shown that patients with T2DM under metformin monotherapy had a longer survival than the matched, nondiabetic controls. However, the precise beneficial mechanisms by which metformin performs its non-glycaemic work are yet to be analysed. Hence, given the complex mechanisms of action of metformin, there is a growing interest in approaching and studying the potential anti-ageing effect of this drug. With regard to this interest, some large randomised clinical trials have been recently set up in order to evaluate the potential role of metformin in reducing the burden of age-related diseases. The Investigation of Metformin in Pre-Diabetes on Atherosclerotic Cardiovascular outcomes (VA-IMPACT) trial is a placebo-controlled study started in February 2019 and aimed at shedding light on the potential role of metformin in reducing mortality and cardiovascular morbidity in patients with prediabetes and established atherosclerotic cardiovascular disease. More precisely, the primary outcomes include the time to death from any cause, nonfatal myocardial infarction, stroke, hospitalisation for unstable angina, or symptom-driven coronary revascularisation [27]. The other clinical trial, also a placebo-controlled trial, i.e. Targeting Ageing with Metformin (TAME), investigates subjects who have been diagnosed with one single age-associated disease and will provide insight on the ability of metformin to postpone and/or prevent the installation of a second pathology, such as cancer, CVD and dementia [13, 36]. Finally, more information is needed for a better understanding of the mechanistic targets and therapeutic implications of certain drugs (such as metformin) that might delay/alleviate the development of age-related diseases [37].

Herein, we revisit the mechanisms involved in ageing and the mechanistic target of metformin as a potential anti-ageing drug, and we review the available data on the clinical and experimental results showing the ability of metformin to promote healthspan and longevity.

2. Epidemiological data on the anti-ageing effect of metformin

A large body of evidence has demonstrated that metformin could be considered a geroprotective agent in humans [23]. As explained, the protective role of metformin in survival has been largely demonstrated by the UKPDS multicentre trial in terms of cardiac and all-cause mortality, as compared with usual care [8, 9]. However, given its main role, that is to reduce hyperglycaemia, and knowing that a good control of diabetes correlates with an extended lifespan, the question arises whether metformin could be accounted as a tool to prolong longevity in patients that do not display T2DM. In keeping with this question, a recent systematic review by Campbell et al. [23] summarised the studies in which the effects of metformin on all-cause mortality or diseases of ageing have been compared to the nondiabetic or general population or to diabetics controlling the disease through other means. Overall, the meta-analysis revealed that subjects with T2DM under metformin treatment have a lower rate of all-cause mortality and longer survival than people free of T2DM not using metformin and the general population, suggesting that this drug could be an effective instrument to extend the lifespan of those not affected by T2DM [23, 35, 38–40]. Moreover, the meta-analysis revealed that subjects with T2DM taking metformin had lower rates of all-cause mortality than those following other therapies, such as insulin or sulphonylurea [23]. Given these results, it may be argued that the outcome is attained by the geroprotective role of metformin resulting in delaying or preventing diseases of ageing, such as cancer or cardiovascular disturbances, which are the two most encountered ageing-related diseases [23, 41]. Firstly, in terms of malignancies, Campbell et al. [23] showed that people with T2DM taking metformin had a lower rate of developing any cancer compared with the general population. Moreover, the risk of developing colorectal, breast or lung cancer in individuals with T2DM on metformin treatment, as compared to those using other therapies, was lower. Secondly, subjects with T2DM following metformin therapy displayed a lower rate of any form of cardiovascular disease with respect to those managing their T2DM through any non-metformin therapy. In addition, although the incidence of stroke was also lower with metformin, for myocardial infarction the effect of the drug seems to be non-significant [23].

Finally, apart from the cardiovascular diseases and cancer, there are also other age-related pathologies that could be targeted by metformin, such as cognitive dysfunction. However, the evidence in patients with T2DM is conflicting with some studies showing a protective role of metformin against cognitive decline, whereas others are arguing that metformin treatment could induce neurodegeneration as well as Parkinson's and Alzheimer's disease. Nevertheless, the interpretation of the data is difficult given the possible presence of other concomitant conditions that may contribute to this cognitive decline [42].

3. Mechanisms involved in ageing

Ageing is a complex process that occurs at the molecular, cellular, organ and organismal level that everyone faces in time [43]. It involves the loss of the body's ability to overcome and respond to stress (homeostenosis) by repair and regeneration, thus leading to various disturbances within the human body [24]. Overall, the ageing processes are of a heterogeneous and heterochronic nature. As a heterogeneous process, ageing can evolve at different rates in diverse organisms, while the heterochronic feature implies that cells and tissues within a single organism can age in an asynchronic manner, finally making chronological age different as compared to biological age [24, 43]. Growing body of evidence has shown that ageing involves multiple mechanisms that inter-relate with and modulate each other. In this respect, two elegant reviews have described nine hallmarks of ageing, which have been classified into primary hallmarks (genomic instability, telomere attrition, epigenetic alterations, and loss of proteostasis) as the main culprit of molecular damage, antagonistic hallmarks (deregulated nutrient sensing, mitochondrial dysfunction, and cellular senescence) with beneficial effects when at low levels, by protecting the human organism against damage, but with deleterious effects when at high levels, and finally, the integrative hallmarks (stem cell exhaustion and altered intercellular communication) that arise when the accumulating damage cannot be balanced by homeostatic mechanisms, thus ultimately inducing ageing [22, 36].

Genomic instability has been revealed to be a major stochastic mechanism of ageing [44, 45]. Broadly, deoxyribonucleic acid (DNA) damage can be induced by both exogenous genotoxic factors, such as ionising radiation and ultraviolet irradiation as well as endogenous genotoxic agents, i.e. products of normal metabolism that lead to the formation of reactive oxygen species (ROS) and subsequently to oxidative stress, that may finally result in deleterious effects on the cell. DNA lesions can cause mutations, block transcription and replication but can also trigger DNA damage response (DDR), which implies mechanisms that intervene and arrest cell cycle progression, resulting in the repair of almost all the alterations that occur within the genome. However, when DNA damage is extensive and prevails over repair, DDR effectors trigger cell death (apoptosis) or cell senescence, contributing to ageing and age-related diseases [46, 47]. In fact, in ageing, DNA damage overtakes DNA repair, leading to genomic instability, a fact sustained by studies showing accumulation of DNA alterations in old tissues [48]. On the other hand, genomic instability has been reported to be a driver of accelerated ageing, widely demonstrated by the presence of hypersensitivity to genotoxins and defects in genome maintenance in progeroid syndromes termed as diseases of accelerated ageing. Collectively, DNA damage as a culprit in ageing is highlighted by the accrual of sources of damage, i.e. oxidative stress (the oxidative stress theory of ageing) associated with the mitochondrial theory of ageing, as mitochondria is the primary source of ROS, increased activation of the DDR, mutations and presence of senescent cells along with a decreased capacity for DNA repair [47]. Among these factors oxidative stress is a well-known pathogenic mechanism and seems to be the most important one [49]. The overproduction of ROS along with a reduced antioxidant defence, i.e. oxidative stress, leads to DNA, protein and lipid damage [50, 51]. Also, ROS lead to age-related DNA lesions acting via nuclear factor kappa-light-chain-enhancer of activated B cells (NF-κB) which controls cytokine and chemokine expression and regulates adhesion molecules [45, 52, 53].

Telomeres are chromosomal end structures that play important roles in the protection of DNA from degradation [54]. In each cell division, 20–200 base pairs are lost within the telomeres, and telomerase is in charge of repairing telomeres after cell division. However, when they reach a certain critical length, i.e. shortening or attrition, the cells stop replicating and die [43]. The shortening process, as the telomerase fails to replicate completely the terminal ends of the DNA molecules, has been reported in ageing [55, 56]. Moreover, in humans, damaged telomerase can cause degenerative defects associated with ageing [57, 58].

Epigenetics meaning "above the genes" is termed as the inheritance of changes in gene function with no modifications in the nucleotide sequence of DNA [43, 59]. Epigenetic changes that comprise alterations in DNA itself as DNA methylation and modifications of histones (acetylation and methylation) as well as of other chromatin-associated proteins and chromatin remodelling can also be involved in ageing [22]. Sirtuins, a family of NAD-dependent deacetylases that act on Lys16 of histone H4, are emerging as a link between cellular transformation and lifespan [59]. Of note, epigenetic alterations seem to be reversible, underpinning the anti-ageing interventions [60]. Moreover, Greer et al. [61] showed transgenerational epigenetic inheritance of longevity in *Caenorhabditis elegans* suggesting that manipulation of specific chromatin modifiers in parents can induce an epigenetic memory of longevity in descendants.

Proteostasis or protein stability is an important feature of the cells and involves a complex network that coordinates protein synthesis with polypeptide folding, conservation of protein conformation and protein degradation [62, 63]. When damaged, as a consequence of various external and endogenous stress factors, it leads to the accumulation of protein aggregates holding proteotoxic effects and becomes a contributor to ageing and to age-related diseases [63–65]. In fact, it has been demonstrated that with age, proteostasis becomes compromised, leading to proteotoxicity [43, 62, 66]. More precisely, intracellular damaged protein deposition has been described in age-related diseases such as Alzheimer's and Parkinson's [62, 63, 67]. Finally, evidence data have revealed a double-sense link between DNA damage and proteostasis, which jointly induce an increased cellular lesion [63].

Deregulated nutrient sensing represents another important hallmark of ageing [22, 68]. Nutrient sensing is mediated by specific molecular pathways, such as insulin and insulin-like growth factor 1 (IGF-1 informs the cells about the presence of glucose and has the same intracellular signalling pathway as insulin), termed as "insulin and/IGF1-signalling" pathway (IIS) as well as the mechanistic target of rapamycin (mTOR) that senses nutrients, whereas AMP-activated protein kinase (AMPK) and sirtuins detect the energy levels [22, 43]. All these systems named as "nutrient sensing" pathways regulate metabolism and influence ageing [43]. More precisely, current data show that anabolic signalling induces accelerated ageing, while decreased nutrient signalling (attained through caloric restriction) promotes a healthy span and extends longevity [69, 70].

The "insulin and/IGF1-signalling" pathway (IIS) operates on the forkhead box proteins or FOXO family of transcription factors and on the mTOR complexes and has been reported to be the most conserved ageing-controlling pathway. Indeed, mutations that reduce the functions of insulin and IGF-1 receptor or downregulate the intracellular effectors, i.e. AKT, mTOR and FOXO, result in increased lifespan [22, 69, 71].

The mTOR kinase is part of two complex proteins and is sensitive to high levels of amino acids controlling a wide range of cellular functions, mostly anabolic metabolism [72]. It is noteworthy that mTOR is a target of rapamycin (an mTOR inhibitor), an antibiotic that exerts anti-proliferative effects by acting through this specific pathway. Several studies have shown that mTOR manipulation by inducing downregulation is involved in extending longevity [22, 43].

Finally, the AMPK pathway and sirtuins that sense changes in energy levels, i.e. low levels of ATP, act in the opposite direction as compared to IIS and mTOR, their activation leading to increased energy production and decreased ATP utilisation [22, 43]. In fact, caloric restriction seems to activate the AMPK pathway [73]. Finally, upregulation of both AMPK and sirtuins favours healthy ageing [74].

Mitochondrial dysfunction is a feature of ageing that refers to reduced respiratory chain efficiency, resulting in electron leak and diminished ATP production [75]. The consequence of mitochondrial dysfunction, installed across ageing, is the formation of ROS, and the theory of free radicals as a mechanism inducing ageing has been widely discussed [76]. However, this theory has been re-analysed and reconsidered as emerging data show that oxidative stress up to a specific threshold has, in fact, a beneficial effect in prolonging lifespan [77, 78]. More specifically, it seems that ROS in a certain amount may play a role as a trigger of compensatory homeostatic reactions as a response to the ongoing and increasing stress factors that come along with ageing, resulting in facing damage and maintaining survival [79]. Still, when over the specific threshold, ROS change their purpose and induce deleterious age-related effects [77, 80, 81].

Apart from the ROS theory, accumulating data have revealed that impaired mitochondrial function may contribute to ageing through other mechanisms, such as the increase of permeability in response to stress that triggers inflammatory reactions, the damaged interface between the outer mitochondrial membrane and the endoplasmic reticulum as well as reduced biogenesis of mitochondria [22]. Furthermore, it seems that both endurance training and alternate-day fasting have the ability to improve healthspan through mitochondrial degeneration avoidance [82, 83].

Finally, the mitochondrial dysfunction seems to be related to the hormesis which is deemed as an adaptive response of the organism to low doses of a toxic agent or physical condition, such as ROS, that induces the ability of the organism to tolerate higher doses of the same toxic agent [63]. Hence, although severe mitochondrial dysfunction is deleterious, mild respiratory damage may increase lifespan, possibly subsequently to a hormetic response [84]. In fact, data from the literature have shown that metformin could be considered a mild mitochondrial "toxic agent" as it induces a low energy state and activates AMPK [85]. In this respect, Anisimov et al. [74] showed that when administrated early in life, metformin treatment increases life span in mice.

Senescence is an age hallmark that stands out as a response triggered by genomic instability and telomere attrition resulting in growth arrest, thus limiting the proliferation of aged and damaged cells [22, 46, 47, 86]. A second important feature of senescent cells is the development of a peculiar secretome, termed as the senescence-associated secretory phenotype (SASP), which encompasses cytokines, chemokines and proteases, resulting in a pro-inflammatory state [87, 88]. Under normal conditions the SASP is involved in the recruitment of macrophages, neutrophils and natural killer (NK) cells, thus holding a beneficial effect in eliminating the senescent cells. However, across the ageing process, the senescence cells accumulate resulting in increased cytokine production and recruitment of more immune cells, which jointly contribute to the onset of the inflammageing state, a true driver of ageing [36, 87]. Moreover, a declined activity of the immune system, termed as immunosenescence, is installed in aged people, thus impairing the clearance of senescent cells and, in turn, increasing even more the chronic inflammation state. Collectively, senescence, inflammageing and immunosenescence promote ageing and operate together, rendering aged people more susceptible to age-related diseases [87, 89]. Finally, interestingly, mitochondrial dysfunction can also trigger cellular senescence, a process termed as "mitochondrial dysfunction-associated senescence" (MiDAS). MiDAS support the existence of a strong inter-relation between cellular senescence and metabolic dysfunction, highlighting that targeting metabolism may be a proper way to extend lifespan in humans [36].

Stem cell exhaustion, i.e. the progressive decline in the regenerative potential of the stem cells needed for tissue repair, is another characteristic of ageing. As explained, ageing is accompanied by immunosenescence, a condition that results from reduced haematopoiesis and that has several deleterious consequences [22].

Finally, apart from cellular damage, ageing also implies *altered intercellular communication*. Inflammation is an ageing-associated damage in intercellular communication termed as "inflammageing," as previously described. Inflammageing may result from multiple causes, such as the accumulation of tissue damage, the reduced ability of the immune system to remove pathogens, the increase of senescent cells that produce pro-inflammatory cytokines, immunosenescence that fails to remove the senescent cells, the activation of the NFkB transcription factor, as well as the onset of a dysfunctional autophagic response [22]. Noteworthy, that inflammation is involved in the pathogenesis of obesity and T2DM, diseases that contribute to the onset of ageing [71]. Apart from inflammation, the intercellular communication has been revealed by the bystander effect referring to senescent cells inducing senescence in neighbouring cells via gap-junction-mediated cell–cell cross talk [90].

Given the aforementioned complex hallmarks of ageing, researchers worldwide have searched for proper tools to obtain the delay of ageing and the avoidance of age-related diseases. Here we find metformin, a drug that has been reported to be useful in modulating some of the age-related features. In fact, in cellular and animal models, metformin has been shown to influence and to hold beneficial effects on the following age related hallmarks [91]: (1) genomic instability [92, 93], (2) telomere attrition [94], (3) epigenetic changes [95], (4) proteostasis [96, 97], (5) nutrient-sensing pathways [98, 99], (6) mitochondrial function [100], (7) cellular senescence [101, 102], (8) stem cell function [103], and (9) low-grade inflammation [104].

4. Experimental evidence on the anti-ageing effect of metformin

Evidence-based data have revealed that metformin holds an important role in extending survival and delaying the onset of age-related diseases in nematode *Caenorhabditis elegans* [105, 106] and mice [107], but not in *Drosophila melanogaster* [108, 109]. In this respect, metformin supplementation was shown to increase mean lifespan and to prolong the healthspan of nematode *Caenorhabditis elegans* (an experimental model often used to study ageing and anti-ageing therapies) via AMPK [106]. Moreover, other authors have shown that metformin has the ability to retard ageing in *Caenorhabditis elegans* by metabolic alteration of its trophic microbial partner, *E. coli*. In brief, metformin disrupts the bacterial folate cycle, which reduces the levels of methionine in the worm. Finally, this results in postponing ageing by triggering a metabolic dietary restriction phenomenon and AMPK activation [105, 110]. Based on these results, we might argue another important role of metformin, that of modulating human microbiota, i.e. an increased abundance of *E. coli*, resulting in an increased production of short-chain fatty acids, such as butyrate and propionate, by which metformin might induce significant positive results in T2DM and might interfere with longevity [36, 111, 112].

In a very recent study, Song et al. [113] used the silkworm, a popular experimental model, to investigate the impact of metformin on lifespan and the underlying molecular pathways. They found that metformin prolonged lifespan without reducing body weight, which suggests that it can increase lifespan by remodelling the animal's energy distribution strategy. Also, metformin increased fasting tolerance and levels of the antioxidant glutathione and activated APMK. Finally, these results suggest that activity in this pathway may contribute to metformin-induced lifespan extension in silkworm by increasing stress resistance and anti-oxidative capacity, while reducing energy output for silk product [113].

Studies on ageing and lifespan have also been performed on mice, highlighting the potential anti-ageing effect of metformin, resulting in an extended lifespan [114–116]. Anisimov et al. [116] demonstrated that chronic treatment of female mice with metformin significantly increased mean and maximum lifespan, even without cancer prevention in that model. In a further study, the authors showed that in female mice, metformin increased lifespan and postponed tumours when started at young and middle, but not at the old age [74]. Besides the increase of lifespan in mice, Martin-Montalvo et al. [107] pointed out that metformin seems to mimic some of the benefits of calorie restriction and leads to improved glucose-tolerance test, increased insulin sensitivity and reduced low-density lipoprotein and cholesterol levels without a decrease in the caloric intake. With respect to the mechanisms of action, metformin seems to increase the antioxidant activity, resulting in reductions in both oxidative stress and chronic inflammation [107].

Finally, as previously mentioned, not all experimental models confirm the anti-ageing role of metformin. It is the case of *Drosophila* fruit fly, another animal model where the authors showed that metformin induced a robust activation of AMPK and reduced lipid stores, but did not increase lifespan. Moreover, they found that when administered in high concentrations, metformin is toxic to flies. Finally, it seems that metformin appears to have evolutionarily conserved effects on metabolism but not on fecundity or lifespan [108].

5. Mechanisms of metformin action: A focus on molecular pathways that modulate ageing

The main universally accepted role of metformin is to alleviate hyperglycaemia. This outcome is obtained through the inhibition of hepatic gluconeogenesis [117, 118]. Metformin holds an insulin-sensitising action and insulin-induced suppression of endogenous glucose production [119]. Although other organs have been discussed as a target for metformin, such as the gut [120], liver remains the main ground of action, as reduced hepatic uptake of metformin prevents the lowering blood glucose effect [91]. There are several mechanisms by which metformin downregulates gluconeogenesis. Firstly, metformin induces alterations in cellular energetics [117], i.e. by decreasing cellular respiration through inhibition of the complex I mitochondrial respiratory chain [121, 122]. The result of this inhibition is the increase of the ADP:ATP and AMP:ATP ratios, which subsequently activate the cellular energy state sensor AMP-activated protein kinase (AMPK) [91, 110, 123], the key player of metformin. Once activated, AMPK leads to an increase in ATP production and a decrease in ATP consumption [42]. Noteworthy, AMPK is one of the molecular pathways that can modify the rate of ageing [43]. The importance of the activation of AMPK in obtaining the reduction in hepatic glucose production was investigated by Hawley et al. [85] who showed that an AMPK mutant does not respond to metformin treatment. On the other hand, Foretz et al. [124] showed that in AMPK knockout mice, the inhibition of gluconeogenesis is still present and associated with a reduction in energy state, but this happens in response to higher concentrations of metformin as compared to standard treatment. With regard to therapeutic concentrations of metformin, it seems that AMPK activation is mandatory for the suppression of gluconeogenesis [117, 125]. Finally, we have to mention that the activation of AMPK via inhibition of the complex I mitochondrial respiratory chain has been recently debated [126] as physiological/low concentration of metformin, which cannot induce AMP/ATP change, can still activate AMPK [125].

Another effect mediated by AMPK activation by metformin refers to the inhibitory phosphorylation of acetyl-CoA carboxylase (ACC), which leads to increased fatty acid uptake and β-oxidation and hence to improved lipid metabolism and subsequently to improved insulin sensitivity [127]. Furthermore, activated AMPK decreases glucagon-stimulated cyclic AMP (cAMP) accumulation, cAMP-dependent protein kinase (PKA) activity and downstream PKA target phosphorylation and increases cyclic nucleotide phosphodiesterase 4B (PDE4B). The authors provided a new mechanism by which AMPK antagonises hepatic glucagon signalling via phosphorylation-induced PDE4B activation [128]. Moreover, the decreased PKA activity promotes glucose consumption and inhibits glucose output [129]. Finally, metformin inhibits hepatic gluconeogenesis through AMPK-dependent regulation of the orphan nuclear receptor small heterodimer partner (SHP) [130].

Secondly, AMPK-independent mechanisms by which metformin inhibits hepatic gluconeogenesis have been reported [117]. In this respect, Miller et al. [131] point towards the ability of the drug to inhibit adenylate cyclase, reduce levels of cAMP and PKA activity, abrogate phosphorylation of critical protein targets of PKA, and block glucagon-dependent glucose output from hepatocytes through accumulation of AMP and related nucleotides independently of AMPK [131]. In addition, metformin inhibits the mitochondrial glycerophosphate dehydrogenase, resulting in an altered hepatocellular redox state, reduced conversion of lactate and glycerol to glucose and hence decreased hepatic gluconeogenesis [132].

Taken together, given the important role of metformin in inhibiting hepatic gluconeogenesis and therefore in reducing hyperglycaemia and subsequently hyperinsulinemia, jointly, important accelerators of ageing, several studies regard metformin as a potential anti-ageing drug [42, 117]. Metformin works through complex mechanisms that have been demonstrated to be similar to those associated with caloric restriction, a well-known model that underpins extended lifespan and healthspan. More precisely, it seems that both metformin and caloric restriction induce the same gene expression profile [107, 117, 133].

Another important target involved in changing the rate of ageing is mTOR [117]. TOR responds to insulin, amino acids and hormones and is involved in controlling a wide range of cellular functions, such as glucose metabolism, lipid and protein synthesis, inflammation and mitochondrial function [72]. Metformin has been demonstrated to downregulate mTOR in both a AMPK-dependent and AMPK-independent manner [98, 134–136]. Through stimulation of AMPK, metformin induces suppression of ATP consumption by inhibiting energy needing processes, such as protein synthesis via mTOR [42, 137]. In addition, through downregulation of mTOR signalling and of insulin-like growth factor 1 (IGF-1), metformin influences cell growth, proliferation and autophagy [42].

NF-kB pathway is another key mediator of ageing. As previously described, it is activated by genotoxic, oxidative and inflammatory stress and regulates the expression of cytokines, inflammation, growth factors and genes that regulate apoptosis [45]. Metformin has been demonstrated to inhibit NF-kB resulting in suppressing the inflammatory response via AMPK-dependent and independent pathways [138]. Also, metformin seems to hold the ability to reduce the endogenous ROS production [93] by acting at a mitochondrial level through blockage of the reverse electron flow at the respiratory chain complex 1 [139].

Finally, a very recent pathway has been described by Chen et al. [140]. The authors showed through genetic manipulation that metformin extends the *Caenorhabditis elegans* lifespan and attenuates age-related fitness decline via a mechanism that requires v-ATPase-Ragulator-AXIN/LKB1 of the lysosomal pathway [140].

In toto, the possible molecular mechanisms by which metformin exerts anti-ageing effects are [13, 91]: (1) inhibition of mitochondrial complex 1 in the electron transport chain and decrease of ROS production [139, 141], (2) activation of AMPK [106, 124, 140, 142–144], (3) inhibition of mTOR [106, 134, 135, 140], (4) NF-κB inhibition [101], and (5) reduced IGF-1 signalling [145].

6. Conclusions

Ageing encompasses a cluster of processes that induce a gradual decline of the human body functions, a condition that everyone faces in time. Also, ageing is a risk factor for a gamut of disturbances such as cancer, T2DM and cardiovascular and neurodegenerative diseases. Therefore, researchers worldwide strive to find the adequate tools in order to delay/avoid the onset of age-related diseases and hence promote healthspan. In keeping with this aim, metformin emerges as a drug that, beyond its main role to reduce hyperglycaemia, has antitumor effects and works as a protector against cardiovascular and neurodegenerative diseases making it a potential anti-ageing medicine. Importantly, metformin seems to possess positive effects even in nondiabetic subjects. However, the exact mechanisms of action and the molecular pathways involved in ageing that are modulated by metformin are not fully explained, and further studies are warranted for a better understanding of the beneficial effects of this drug.

Acknowledgements

Mr. Manfredi Rizzo serves as Director, Clinical Medical & Regulatory Affairs, Novo Nordisk Europe East and South. The publication was supported by funds from the National Research Development Projects to finance excellence (PFE)-37/2018–2020 granted by the Romanian Ministry of Research and Innovation.

Author details

Adriana Florinela Cătoi[1]*, Andra Diana Andreicuţ[1], Dan Cristian Vodnar[2], Katalin Szabo[3], Andreea Corina[4,5], Andreea Arsene[6], Simona Diana Stefan[7], Roxana Adriana Stoica[7] and Manfredi Rizzo[8,9]

1 Department of Pathophysiology, Faculty of Medicine, 'Iuliu Haţieganu', University of Medicine and Pharmacy, Cluj-Napoca, Romania

2 Department of Food Science and Technology, University of Agricultural Sciences and Veterinary Medicine, Cluj-Napoca, Romania

3 Institute of Life Sciences, University of Agricultural Sciences and Veterinary Medicine, Cluj-Napoca, Romania

4 Lipids and Atherosclerosis Research Unit, Maimonides Biomedical Research Institute of Cordoba (IMIBIC), Reina Sofia University Hospital, University of Cordoba, Cordoba, Spain

5 CIBER Fisiopatologia de la Obesidad y Nutricion (CIBEROBN), Instituto de Salud Carlos III, Cordoba, Spain

6 Department of General and Pharmaceutical Microbiology, Faculty of Pharmacy, "Carol Davila" University of Medicine and Pharmacy, Bucharest, Romania

7 Diabetes, Nutrition and Metabolic Diseases Department, Faculty of Medicine, "Carol Davila" University of Medicine and Pharmacy, Bucharest, Romania

8 PROMISE Department, University of Palermo, Italy

9 Clinical Medical and Regulatory Affairs, Novo Nordisk - Europe East and South

*Address all correspondence to: florinela12@yahoo.com

References

[1] International Diabetes Federation Guideline Development Group. Global guideline for type 2 diabetes. Diabetes Research and Clinical Practice. 2014;**104**(1):1-52

[2] Inzucchi SE, Bergenstal RM, Buse JB, et al. Management of hyperglycemia in type 2 diabetes: A patient-centered approach: Position statement of the American Diabetes Association and the European Association for the Study of Diabetes. Diabetologia. 2015;**58**(3):429-442

[3] Garber AJ, Abrahamson MJ, Barzilay JI, et al. Consensus statement by the American Association of Clinical Endocrinologists and American College of Endocrinology on the comprehensive type 2 diabetes management algorithm—2017 executive summary. Endocrine Practice. 2017;**23**(2):207-238

[4] Qaseem A, Barry MJ, Humphrey LL, Forciea MA, Clinical Guidelines Committee of the American College of Physicians. Oral pharmacologic treatment of type 2 diabetes mellitus: A clinical practice guideline update from the American College of Physicians. Annals of Internal Medicine. 2017;**166**(4):279-290

[5] Bailey CJ. Metformin: Historical overview. Diabetologia. 2017;**60**(9):1566-1576

[6] Wiernsperger NF. 50 years later: Is metformin a vascular drug with antidiabetic properties ? The British Journal of Diabetes & Vascular Disease. 2007;**7**:204-210

[7] Bailey CJ. Metformin: Effects on micro and macrovascular complications in type 2 diabetes. Cardiovascular Drugs and Therapy. 2008;**22**(3):215-224

[8] UK Prospective Diabetes Study (UKPDS) Group. Effect of intensive blood-glucose control with metformin on complications in overweight patients with type 2 diabetes. Lancet. 1998;**352**(9131):854-865

[9] Holman RR, Paul SK, Bethel MA, Matthews DR, Neil HA. 10-year follow-up of intensive glucose control in type 2 diabetes. The New England Journal of Medicine. 2008;**359**(15):1577-1589

[10] Nathan DM, Buse JB, Davidson MB, et al. Medical management of hyperglycemia in type 2 diabetes: A consensus algorithm for the initiation and adjustment of therapy: A consensus statement of the American Diabetes Association and the European Association for the Study of Diabetes. Diabetes Care. 2009;**32**(1):193-203

[11] Knowler WC, Barrett-Connor E, Fowler SE, et al. Reduction in the incidence of type 2 diabetes with lifestyle intervention or metformin. The New England Journal of Medicine. 2002;**346**(6):393-403

[12] Diabetes Prevention Program Research Group. HbA 1c as a predictor of diabetes and as an outcome in the diabetes prevention program: A randomized clinical trial. Diabetes Care. 2015;**38**(1):51-58

[13] Barzilai N, Crandall JP, KritchevskySB,EspelandMA.Metformin as a tool to target aging. Cell Metabolism. 2016;**23**(6):1060-1065

[14] Hostalek U, Gwilt M, Hildemann S. Therapeutic use of metformin in prediabetes and diabetes prevention. Drugs. 2015;**75**(10):1071-1094

[15] Diabetes Prevention Program Research Group. Long-term safety, tolerability, and weight loss associated with metformin in the diabetes

prevention program outcomes study. Diabetes Care. 2012;**35**(4):731-737

[16] Moin T, Schmittdiel JA, Flory JH, et al. Review of metformin use for type 2 diabetes prevention. American Journal of Preventive Medicine. 2018;**55**(4):565-574

[17] American Diabetes Association. Prevention or delay of type 2 diabetes: Standards of medical care in diabetes—2019. Diabetes Care. 2019;**42**(Suppl 1):S29-S33

[18] Van Ginneken V. Are there any biomarkers of aging? Biomarkers of the brain. Biomedical Journal of Scientific & Technical Research. 2017;**1**:193-206

[19] Lutz W, Sanderson W, Scherbov S. The coming acceleration of global population ageing. Nature. 2008;**451**(7179):716-719

[20] Weinert BT, Timiras PS. Invited review: Theories of aging. Journal of Applied Physiology (Bethesda, MD: 1985). 2003;**95**(4):1706-1716

[21] Garinis GA, van der Horst GT, Vijg J, Hoeijmakers JH. DNA damage and ageing: New-age ideas for an age-old problem. Nature Cell Biology. 2008;**10**(11):1241-1247

[22] López-Otín C, Blasco MA, Partridge L, Serrano M, Kroemer G. The hallmarks of aging. Cell. 2013;**153**(6):1194-1217

[23] Campbell JM, Bellman SM, Stephenson MD, Lisy K. Metformin reduces all-cause mortality and diseases of ageing independent of its effect on diabetes control: A systematic review and meta-analysis. Ageing Research Reviews. 2017;**40**:31-44

[24] Khan SS, Singer BD, Vaughan DE. Molecular and physiological manifestations and measurement of aging in humans. Aging Cell. 2017;**16**(4):624-633

[25] Finlay BB, Pettersson S, Melby MK, Bosch TCG. The microbiome mediates environmental effects on aging. BioEssays. 2019;**2019**:e1800257

[26] Nagpal R, Mainali R, Ahmadi S, et al. Gut microbiome and aging: Physiological and mechanistic insights. Nutrition and Healthy Aging. 2018;**4**(4):267-285

[27] Valencia WM, Palacio A, Tamariz L, Florez H. Metformin and ageing: Improving ageing outcomes beyond glycaemic control. Diabetologia. 2017;**60**(9):1630-1638

[28] Yerevanian A, Soukas AA. Metformin: Mechanisms in human obesity and weight loss. Current Obesity Reports. 2019;**8**(2):156-164

[29] Seifarth C, Schehler B, Schneider HJ. Effectiveness of metformin on weight loss in non-diabetic individuals with obesity. Experimental and Clinical Endocrinology & Diabetes. 2013;**121**(1):27-31

[30] Zhou L, Liu H, Wen X, Peng Y, Tian Y, Zhao L. Effects of metformin on blood pressure in nondiabetic patients: A meta-analysis of randomized controlled trials. Journal of Hypertension. 2017;**35**(1):18-26

[31] Jenkins AJ, Welsh P, Petrie JR. Metformin, lipids and atherosclerosis prevention. Current Opinion in Lipidology. 2018;**29**(4):346-353

[32] Luo F, Das A, Chen J, Wu P, Li X, Fang Z. Metformin in patients with and without diabetes: A paradigm shift in cardiovascular disease management. Cardiovascular Diabetology. 2019;**18**(1):54

[33] Campbell JM, Stephenson MD, De Courten B, Chapman I, Bellman SM, Aromataris E. Metformin use associated with reduced risk of dementia in

patients with diabetes: A systematic review and meta-analysis. Journal of Alzheimer's Disease. 2018;**65**(4):1225-1236

[34] Kobiela J, Dobrzycka M, Jędrusik P, et al. Metformin and colorectal cancer—A systematic review. Experimental and Clinical Endocrinology & Diabetes. 2019;**127**(7):445-454

[35] Bannister CA, Holden SE, Jenkins-Jones S, et al. Can people with type 2 diabetes live longer than those without? A comparison of mortality in people initiated with metformin or sulphonylurea monotherapy and matched, non-diabetic controls. Diabetes, Obesity & Metabolism. 2014;**16**(11):1165-1173

[36] López-Otín C, Galluzzi L, Freije JMP, Madeo F, Kroemer G. Metabolic control of longevity. Cell. 2016;**166**(4):802-821

[37] Piskovatska V, Strilbytska O, Koliada A, Vaiserman A, Lushchak O. Health benefits of anti-aging drugs. Sub-Cellular Biochemistry. 2019;**91**:339-392

[38] Bérard E, Bongard V, Dallongeville J, et al. 14-year risk of all-cause mortality according to hypoglycaemic drug exposure in a general population. PLoS One. 2014;**9**(4):e95671

[39] Bo S, Ciccone G, Rosato R, et al. Cancer mortality reduction and metformin: A retrospective cohort study in type 2 diabetic patients. Diabetes, Obesity & Metabolism. 2012;**14**(1):23-29

[40] Claesen M, Gillard P, De Smet F, Callens M, De Moor B, Mathieu C. Mortality in individuals treated with glucose- lowering agents: A large, controlled cohort study. The Journal of Clinical Endocrinology and Metabolism. 2016;**101**(2):461-469

[41] Mathers CD, Loncar D. Projections of global mortality and burden of disease from 2002 to 2030. PLoS Medicine. 2006;**3**(11):e442

[42] Piskovatska V, Stefanyshyn N, Storey KB, Vaiserman AM, Lushchak O. Metformin as geroprotector: Experimental and clinical evidence. Biogerontology. 2019;**20**(1):33-48

[43] Carmona JJ, Michan S. Biology of healthy aging and longevity. Revista de Investigación Clínica. 2016;**68**(1):7-16

[44] Vijg J, Busuttil RA, Bahar R, Dollé ME. Aging and genome maintenance. Annals of the New York Academy of Sciences. 2005;**1055**:35-47

[45] Kanigur Sultuybek G, Soydas T, Yenmis G. NF - κ B as the mediator of metformin's effect on ageing and ageing-related diseases. Clinical and Experimental Pharmacology & Physiology. 2019;**46**(5):413-422

[46] Hoeijmakers JH. DNA damage, aging, and cancer. The New England Journal of Medicine. 2009;**361**:1475-1485

[47] Niedernhofer LJ, Gurkar AU, Wang Y, Vijg J, Hoeijmakers JHJ, Robbins PD. Nuclear genomic instability and aging. Annual Review of Biochemistry. 2018;**87**:295-322

[48] Lu T, Pan Y, Kao S, et al. Gene regulation and DNA damage in the ageing human brain. Nature. 2004;**429**(6994):883-891

[49] Harman D. Aging: A theory based on free radical and radiation chemistry. Journal of Gerontology. 1956;**11**:298-300

[50] Liochev SI. Reactive oxygen species and the free radical theory of aging. Free Radical Biology & Medicine. 2013;**60**:1-4

[51] Birch-Machin MA, Bowman A. Oxidative stress and ageing. The British Journal of Dermatology. 2016;**175**:26-29

[52] Janssens S, Tschopp J. Signals from within: The DNA-damage-induced NF- κB response. Cell Death and Differentiation. 2006;**13**:773-784

[53] Wu Z, Miyamoto S. Many faces of NF-κB signaling induced by genotoxic stress. Journal of Molecular Medicine. 2007;**85**:1187-1202

[54] Ishikawa N, Nakamura KI, Izumiyama-Shimomura N, et al. Changes of telomere status with aging: An update. Geriatrics & Gerontology International. 2016;**16**(Suppl. 1):30-42

[55] Blackburn EH, Greider CW, Szostak JW. Telomeres and telomerase: The path from maize, Tetrahymena and yeast to human cancer and aging. Nature Medicine. 2006;**12**(10):1133-1138

[56] Blasco MA. Telomere length, stem cells and aging. Nature Chemical Biology. 2007;**3**(10):640-649

[57] Armanois M, Blackburn EH. The telomerase syndromes. Nature Reviews. Genetics. 2012;**13**(10):693-704

[58] Armanios M, Alder JK, Parry EM, Karim B, Strong MA, Greider CW. Short telomeres are sufficient to cause the degenerative defects associated with aging. American Journal of Human Genetics. 2009;**85**(6):823-832

[59] Fraga MF, Esteller M. Epigenetics and aging: The targets and the marks. Trends in Genetics. 2007;**23**(8):413-418

[60] Freije JM, López-Otín C. Reprogramming aging and progeria. Current Opinion in Cell Biology. 2012;**24**(6):757-764

[61] Greer EL, Maures TJ, Ucar D, et al. Transgenerational epigenetic inheritance of longevity in *Caenorhabditis elegans*. Nature. 2011;**479**(7373):365-371

[62] Kaushik S, Cuervo AM. Proteostasis and aging. Nature Medicine. 2015;**21**(12):1406-1415

[63] Hipp MS, Kasturi P, Hartl FU. The proteostasis network and its decline in ageing. Nature Reviews. Molecular Cell Biology. 2019;**20**(7):421-435

[64] Klaips CL, Jayaraj GG, Hartl FU. Pathways of cellular proteostasis in aging and disease. The Journal of Cell Biology. 2018;**217**(1):51-63

[65] Taylor RC, Dillin A. Aging as an event of proteostasis collapse. Cold Spring Harbor Perspectives in Biology. 2011;**3**(5):pii: a004440

[66] Koga H, Kaushik S, Cuervo AM. Protein homeostasis and aging: The importance of exquisite quality control. Ageing Research Reviews. 2011;**10**(2):205-215

[67] Vilchez D, Saez I, Dillin A. The role of protein clearance mechanisms in organismal ageing and age-related diseases. Nature Communications. 2014;**5**:5659

[68] Efeyan A, Comb WC, Sabatini DM. Nutrient sensing mechanisms and pathways. Nature. 2015;**517**(7534):302-310

[69] Fontana L, Patridge L, Longo VD. Extending healthy life span—From yeast to humans. Science. 2010;**328**(5976):321-326

[70] Vermeij WP, Dollé ME, Reiling E, et al. Restricted diet delays accelerated ageing and genomic stress in DNA-repair-deficient mice. Nature. 2016;**537**(7620):427-431

[71] Barzilai N, Huffman DM, Muzumdar RH, Bartke A. The critical

role of metabolic pathways in aging. Diabetes. 2012;**61**:1315-1322

[72] Laplante M, Sabatini DM. mTOR signaling in growth control and disease. Cell. 2012;**149**(2):274-293

[73] Cantó C, Auwerx J. Calorie restriction: Is AMPK as a key sensor and effector? Physiology (Bethesda, Md.). 2011;**26**(4):214-224

[74] Anisimov VN, Berstein LM, Popovich IG, et al. If started early in life, metformin treatment increases life span and postpones tumors in female SHR mice. Aging (Albany NY). 2011;**3**(2):148-157

[75] Green DR, Galluzzi L, Kroemer G. Mitochondria and the autophagy-inflammation-cell death axis in organismal aging. Science. 2011;**333**(6046):1109-1112

[76] Harman D. The free radical theory of aging: Effect of age on serum copper levels. Journal of Gerontology. 1965;**20**:151-153

[77] Hekimi S, Lapointe J, Wen Y. Taking a "good" look at free radicals in the aging process. Trends in Cell Biology. 2011;**21**(10):569-576

[78] Ristow M, Schmeisser S. Extending life span by increasing oxidative stress. Free Radical Biology & Medicine. 2011;**51**(2):327-336

[79] Sena LA, Chandel NS. Physiological roles of mitochondrial reactive oxygen species. Molecular Cell. 2012;**48**(2):158-167

[80] Pantea Stoian A, Mitrofan G, Colceag F, et al. Oxidative stress in diabetes: A model of complex thinking applied in medicine. Revista de Chimie (Bucharest). 2018;**69**(9):2515-2519

[81] Pantea-Stoian A, Ditu G, Diculescu M. Pancreatogenic type 3C diabetes. Journal of Mind and Medical Sciences. 2018;**5**(2):270-277

[82] Safdar A, Bourgeois JM, Daniel I, et al. Endurance exercise rescues progeroid aging and induces systemic mitochondrial rejuvenation in mtDNA mutator mice. Proceedings of the National Academy of Sciences of the United States of America. 2011;**108**(10):4135-4140

[83] Castello L, Maina M, Testa G, et al. Alternate-day fasting reverses the age-associated hypertrophy phenotype in rat heart by influencing the ERK and PI3K signaling pathways. Mechanisms of Ageing and Development. 2011;**132**:305-314

[84] Haigis MC, Yankner BA. The aging stress response. Molecular Cell. 2010;**40**(2):333-344

[85] Hawley SA, Ross FA, Chevtzoff C, et al. Use of cells expressing gamma subunit variants to identify diverse mechanisms of AMPK activation. Cell Metabolism. 2010;**11**(6):554-565

[86] Muñoz-Espín D, Serrano M. Cellular senescence: From physiology to pathology. Nature Reviews. Molecular Cell Biology. 2014;**15**(7):482-496

[87] McHugh D, Gil J. Senescence and aging: Causes, consequences, and therapeutic avenues. The Journal of Cell Biology. 2018;**217**(1):65-77

[88] Kuilman T, Peeper DS. Senescence-messaging secretome: SMS-ing cellular stress. Nature Reviews. Cancer. 2009;**9**(2):81-94

[89] Farr JN, Almeida M. The spectrum of fundamental basic science discoveries contributing to organismal aging. Journal of Bone and Mineral Research. 2018;**33**(9):1568-1584

[90] Nelson G, Wordsworth J, Wang C, et al. A senescent cell bystander effect:

Senescence-induced senescence. Aging Cell. 2012;**11**(2):345-349

[91] Prattichizzo F, Giuliani A, Mensà E, et al. Pleiotropic effects of metformin: Shaping the microbiome to manage type 2 diabetes and postpone ageing. Ageing Research Reviews. 2018;**48**:87-98

[92] Halicka HD, Zhao H, Li J, et al. Genome protective effect of metformin as revealed by reduced level of constitutive DNA damage signaling. Aging (Albany NY). 2011;**3**(10):1028-1038

[93] Algire C, Moiseeva O, Deschênes-Simard X, et al. Metformin reduces endogenous reactive oxygen species and associated DNA damage. Cancer Prevention Research (Philadelphia, PA). 2012;**5**(4):536-543

[94] Garcia-Martin I, Penketh RJA, Janssen AB, et al. Metformin and insulin treatment prevent placental telomere attrition in boys exposed to maternal diabetes. PLoS One. 2018;**13**(12):e0208533

[95] García-Calzón S, Perfilyev A, Männistö V, et al. Diabetes medication associates with DNA methylation of metformin transporter genes in the human liver. Clinical Epigenetics. 2017;**9**:102

[96] Hull RL, Shen Z, Watts MR, et al. Long-term treatment with rosiglitazone and metformin reduces the extent of, but does not prevent, islet amyloid deposition in mice expressing the gene for human islet amyloid polypeptide. Diabetes. 2005;**54**(7):2235-2244

[97] Wolff CA, Reid JJ, Musci RV et al. Differential effects of rapamycin and metformin in combination with rapamycin on mechanisms of proteostasis in cultured skeletal myotubes. The Journals of Gerontology. Series A, Biological Sciences and Medical Sciences. 2019 March. pii: glz058. DOI: 10.1093/gerona/glz058. [Epub ahead of print]

[98] Howell JJ, Hellberg K, Turner M, et al. Metformin inhibits hepatic mTORC1 signaling via dose-dependent mechanisms involving AMPK and the TSC complex. Cell Metabolism. 2017;**25**(2):463-471

[99] Halicka HD, Zhao H, Li J, et al. Potential anti-aging agents suppress the level of constitutive mTOR- and DNA damage-signaling. Aging (Albany NY). 2012;**4**(12):952-965

[100] Andrzejewski S, Gravel S, Pollak M, St-Pierre J. Metformin directly acts on mitochondria to alter cellular bioenergetics. Cancer & Metabolism. 2014;**2**:12

[101] Moiseeva O, Deschênes-Simard X, St-Germain E, et al. Metformin inhibits the senescence-associated secretory phenotype by interfering with IKK/NF-κB activation. Aging Cell. 2013;**12**(3):489-498

[102] Hooten NN, Martin-Montalvo A, Dluzen DF, et al. Metformin-mediated increase in DICER1 regulates microRNA expression and cellular senescence. Aging Cell. 2016;**15**(3):572-581

[103] Xu G, Wu H, Zhang J, et al. Metformin ameliorates ionizing irradiation-induced long-term hematopoietic stem cell injury in mice. Free Radical Biology & Medicine. 2015;**87**:15-25

[104] Tizazu AM, Nyunt MSZ, Cexus O, et al. Metformin monotherapy downregulates diabetes-associated inflammatory status and impacts on mortality. Frontiers in Physiology. 2019;**10**:572

[105] Cabreiro F, Au C, Leung KY, et al. Metformin retards aging in *C. elegans* by altering microbial folate and methionine metabolism. Cell. 2013;**153**(1):228-239

[106] Onken B, Driscoll M. Metformin induces a dietary restriction-like state and the oxidative stress response to extend *C. elegans* healthspan via AMPK, LKB1, and SKN-1. PLoS One. 2010;**5**(1):e8758

[107] Martin-Montalvo A, Mercken EM, Mitchell SJ, et al. Metformin improves healthspan and lifespan in mice. Nature Communications. 2013;**4**:2192

[108] Slack C, Foley A, Partridge L. Activation of AMPK by the putative dietary restriction mimetic metformin is insufficient to extend lifespan in *Drosophila*. PLoS One. 2012;**7**(10):e47699

[109] Anisimov VN. Metformin: Do we finally have an anti-aging drug? Cell Cycle. 2013;**12**(22):3483-3489

[110] Storelli G, Téfit M, Leulier F. Metformin, microbes, and aging. Cell Metabolism. 2013;**17**(6):809-811

[111] Canfora EE, Jocken JW, Blaak EE. Short-chain fatty acids in control of body weight and insulin sensitivity. Nature Reviews. Endocrinology. 2015;**11**(10):577-591

[112] Suceveanu AI, Pantea Stoian A, Parepa I, et al. Gut microbiota patterns in obese and type 2 diabetes (T2D) patients from Romanian Black Sea coast region. Revista de Chimie (Bucharest). 2018;**69**(8):2260-2267

[113] Song J, Jiang G, Zhang J, et al. Metformin prolongs lifespan through remodeling the energy distribution strategy in silkworm, *Bombyx mori*. Aging (Albany NY). 2019;**11**(1):240-248

[114] Anisimov VN, Berstein LM, Egormin PA, et al. Effect of metformin on life span and on the development of spontaneous mammary tumors in HER-2/neu transgenic mice. Experimental Gerontology. 2005;**40**(8-9):685-693

[115] Anisimov VN, Egormin PA, Piskunova TS, et al. Metformin extends life span of HER-2/neu transgenic mice and in combination with melatonin inhibits growth of transplantable tumors in vivo. Cell Cycle. 2010;**9**(1):188-197

[116] Anisimov VN, Berstein LM, Egormin PA, et al. Metformin slows down aging and extends life span of female SHR mice. Cell Cycle. 2008;**7**(17):2769-2773

[117] Novelle MG, Ali A, Diéguez C, Bernier M, de Cabo R. Metformin: A hopeful promise in aging research. Cold Spring Harbor Perspectives in Medicine. 2016;**6**(3):a025932

[118] An H, He L. Current understanding of metformin effect on the control of hyperglycemia in diabetes. The Journal of Endocrinology. 2016;**228**(3):R97-R106

[119] Natali A, Ferrannini E. Effects of metformin and thiazolidinediones on suppression of hepatic glucose production and stimulation of glucose uptake in type 2 diabetes: A systematic review. Diabetologia. 2006;**49**(3):434-441

[120] Buse JB, DeFronzo RA, Rosenstock J, et al. The primary glucose-lowering effect of metformin resides in the gut, not the circulation: Results from short-term pharmacokinetic and 12-week dose-ranging studies. Diabetes Care. 2016;**39**(2):198-205

[121] El-Mir MY, Nogueira V, Fontaine E, Avéret N, Rigoulet M, Leverve X. Dimethylbiguanide inhibits cell respiration via an indirect effect targeted on the respiratory chain complex I. The Journal of Biological Chemistry. 2000;**275**(1):223-228

[122] Owen MR, Doran E, Halestrap AP. Evidence that metformin exerts its anti-diabetic effects through inhibition of complex 1 of the mitochondrial respiratory chain. The Biochemical Journal. 2000;**348**(Pt 3):607-614

[123] Hardie DG. The AMP-activated protein kinase pathway—New players upstream and downstream. Journal of Cell Science. 2004;**117**(Pt 23):5479-5487

[124] Foretz M, Hébrard S, Leclerc J, et al. Metformin inhibits hepatic gluconeogenesis in mice independently of the LKB1/AMPK pathway via a decrease in hepatic energy state. The Journal of Clinical Investigation. 2010;**120**(7):2355-2369

[125] Cao J, Meng S, Chang E, et al. Low concentrations of metformin suppress glucose production in hepatocytes through AMP-activated protein kinase (AMPK). The Journal of Biological Chemistry. 2014;**289**(30):20435-20446

[126] He L, Wondisford FE. Metformin action: Concentrations matter. Cell Metabolism. 2015;**21**(2):159-162

[127] Fullerton MD, Galic S, Marcinko K, et al. Single phosphorylation sites in Acc1 and Acc2 regulate lipid homeostasis and the insulin-sensitizing effects of metformin. Nature Medicine. 2013;**19**(12):1649-1654

[128] Johanns M, Lai Y, Hsu M, et al. AMPK antagonizes hepatic glucagon-stimulated cyclic AMP signalling via phosphorylation-induced activation of cyclic nucleotide phosphodiesterase 4B. Nature Communications. 2016;7:10856

[129] Rena G, Hardie DG, Pearson ER. The mechanisms of action of metformin. Diabetologia. 2017;**60**(9):1577-1585

[130] Kim YD, Park K, Lee Y, et al. Metformin inhibits hepatic gluconeogenesis through AMP-activated protein kinase-dependent regulation of the orphan nuclear receptor SHP. Diabetes. 2008;**57**(2):306-314

[131] Miller RA, Chu Q, Xie J, Foretz M, Viollet B, Birnbaum MJ. Biguanides supress hepatic glucagon signaling by decreasing production of cyclic AMP. Nature. 2013;**494**(7436):256-260

[132] Madiraju AK, Erion DM, Rahimi Y, et al. Metformin suppresses gluconeogenesis by inhibiting mitochondrial glycerophosphate dehydrogenase. Nature. 2014;**510**(7506):542-546

[133] De Cabo R, Carmona-Gutierrez D, Bernier M, Hall MN, Madeo F. The search for antiaging interventions: From elixirs to fasting regimens. Cell. 2014;**157**(7):1515-1526

[134] Nair V, Sreevalsan S, Basha R, et al. Mechanism of metformin-dependent inhibition of mammalian target of rapamycin (mTOR) and Ras activity in pancreatic cancer: Role of specificity protein (Sp) transcription factors. The Journal of Biological Chemistry. 2014;**289**(40):27692-27701

[135] Pérez-Revuelta BI, Hettich MM, Ciociaro A, et al. Metformin lowers Ser-129 phosphorylated α-synuclein levels via mTOR-dependent protein phosphatase 2A activation. Cell Death & Disease. 2014;**5**:e1209

[136] Kalender A, Selvaraj A, Kim SY, et al. Metformin, independent of AMPK, inhibits mTORC1 in a rag GTPase-dependent manner. Cell Metabolism. 2010;**11**(5):390-401

[137] Towler MC, Hardie DG. AMP-activated protein kinase in metabolic control and insulin signaling. Circulation Research. 2007;**100**(3):328-341

[138] Saisho Y. Metformin and inflammation: Its potential beyond glucose-lowering effect. Endocrine, Metabolic & Immune Disorders Drug Targets. 2015;**15**(3):196-205

[139] Batandier C, Guigas B, Detaille D, et al. The ROS production induced by a reverse-electron flux at respiratory-chain complex 1 is hampered by metformin. Journal of Bioenergetics and Biomembranes. 2006;**38**(1):33-42

[140] Chen J, Ou Y, Li Y, Hu S, Shao L, Liu Y. Metformin extends *C. elegans* lifespan through lysosomal pathway. eLife. 2017;**6**:pii: e31268

[141] Bridges HR, Jones AJ, Pollak MN, Hirst J. Effects of metformin and other biguanides on oxidative phosphorylation in mitochondria. The Biochemical Journal. 2014;**462**(3):475-487

[142] Zheng Z, Chen H, Li J, et al. Sirtuin 1-mediated cellular metabolic memory of high glucose via the LKB1/AMPK/ROS pathway and therapeutic effects of metformin. Diabetes. 2012;**61**(1):217-228

[143] Lu J, Shi J, Li M, et al. Activation of AMPK by metformin inhibits TGF-β-induced collagen production in mouse renal fibroblasts. Life Sciences. 2015;**127**:59-65

[144] Cho K, Chung JY, Cho SK, et al. Antihyperglycemic mechanism of metformin occurs via the AMPK/LXRα/POMC pathway. Scientific Reports. 2015;**5**:8145

[145] Liu B, Fan Z, Edgerton SM, Yang X, Lind SE, Thor AD. Potent anti-proliferative effects of metformin on trastuzumab-resistant breast cancer cells via inhibition of erbB2/IGF-1 receptor interactions. Cell Cycle. 2011;**10**(17):2959-2966